Discover How to Eat Out, Eat Well, and Have Fun, Too!

Make the best choices for yourself and your family with this authoritative nutrition guide. With 2.5 million *Counter* books in print, Annette B. Natow and Jo-Ann Heslin bring a wealth of knowledge and experience to the *EATING OUT FOOD COUNTER,* a comprehensive, handy reference that includes nutritional information for more than 80 national restaurant chains. From main dishes to popular snack foods and take-out items, you can take the guesswork out of ordering—and make it easier to pick the best food choices.

Annette B. Natow, Ph.D., R.D., and Jo-Ann Heslin, M.A., R.D., are the authors of twenty-two books on nutrition. Both are former faculty members of Adelphi University and the State University of New York, Downstate Medical Center. They are editors of the *Journal of Nutrition for the Elderly,* serve as editorial board members for the *Environmental Nutrition Newsletter,* and are contributors to magazines and journals.

Books by Annette B. Natow and Jo-Ann Heslin

The Antioxidant Vitamin Counter
Calcium Counts
Count On a Healthy Pregnancy
The Calorie Counter (Second Edition)
The Carbohydrate, Sugar and Fiber Counter
The Cholesterol Counter (Fifth Edition)
The Diabetes Carbohydrate and Calorie Counter
Eating Out Food Counter
The Fat Attack Plan
The Fat Counter (Fifth Edition)
The Food Shopping Counter
Megadoses
The Most Complete Food Counter
No-Nonsense Nutrition for Kids
The Pocket Encyclopedia of Nutrition
The Pocket Fat Counter (Second Edition)
The Pocket Protein Counter
The Pregnancy Nutrition Counter
The Protein Counter
The Sodium Counter

Published by POCKET BOOKS

For information regarding special discounts for bulk purchases, please contact Simon & Schuster Special Sales at 1-800-456-6798 or business@simonandschuster.com

To our families who support us through every project: Harry, Allen, Irene, Sarah, Meryl, Laura, Marty, George, Emily, Steven, Joe, Kristen and Karen.

ACKNOWLEDGMENTS

Without the tireless cooperation of Steven Natow, M.D., and Stephen Llano, the *Eating Out Food Counter* would never have been completed. Our thanks to the companies and restaurant chains for graciously sharing their information. A special thanks to our agent, Nancy Trichter, and our editor, Jane Cavolina.

SOURCES OF DATA

Values in this counter have been obtained from the Composition of Foods, United States Department of Agriculture, Agricultural Handbooks: No. 8–1, Dairy and Egg Products; No. 8–11, Vegetables and Vegetable Products; No. 8–12, Nut and Seed Products; No. 8–14, Beverages; No. 8–18, Baked Products; No. 8–19, Snacks and Sweets; No. 8–21, Fast Foods; Supplements 1989, 1990, 1991, 1992.

"Nutritive Value of Foods," United States Department of Agriculture, Home and Garden Bulletin No. 72.

J. Davies and J. Dickerson, *Nutrient Content of Food Portions.* Cambridge, UK: The Royal Society of Chemistry, 1991.

G. A. Leveille, M. E. Zabik, K. J. Morgan, *Nutrients in Foods.* Cambridge, MA: The Nutrition Guild, 1983.

Information from food labels, manufacturers and processors, and restaurants. The values are based on research conducted through winter 1998. Nutrient values for restaurant menu items and manufacturers' foods may vary from those listed in the book due to reformulation and regional differences. Although restaurant chains use standard recipes, there may be some alteration in foods served in different locations. This can be due to deviation in portion size, the way the food is assembled and normal manufacturing tolerances in product ingredients.

The human being exhibits two psychological tendencies in his diet—one, to stand by the old favorites; the other, to demand variety from day to day.

MARY SWARTZ ROSE, PH.D.
Feeding the Family
The Macmillan Company, 1919

INTRODUCTION

Americans eat out an average of more than four times a week, spending over 44 percent of their food dollars eating away from home. The most popular items ordered are sodas, coffee, milk, lettuce salads, burgers and French fries. On a typical day in 1996, almost half of all adults, 46 percent, ate in a restaurant, with an average check of $4.25 per person. Lunch and brunch are the meals most often eaten out, followed by snack and beverage breaks.

There are all kinds of restaurants, quick service to elegant table service, suiting every lifestyle. Restaurant chains can be fast (or more relaxed), casual (come as you are) or more formal, fun, nutritious, affordable and, most important, they can be found just about everywhere. When you feel like splurging on luscious desserts or if you'd rather have a salad with low calorie dressing, all bases are covered—there is something for everyone.

FAST FACT

Daily specials on restaurant menus are often named for celebrities, but the most popular names for special dishes include "Mom" or "Mother." A survey by Bell Atlantic Corporation found that menu items with "Mother" in their name tend to cost more and contain more fat!

Kids are courted at many restaurant chains. They offer children's menu selections, toys and clubs. They're great when you are looking for a convenient, enjoyable spot for a children's party. Besides having favorite foods, they provide favors like hats and balloons; many even have play areas, sometimes with attendants. Children may be given crayons, paper place mats with creative games to keep them busy and special treats to end the meal. These keep the children happy while the adults enjoy a more relaxed meal. The restaurants benefit, too, as they cultivate a pool of future customers who enjoy returning to the restaurants they loved as children.

FAST FACT

Kids aged 6 to 14 eat in quick-serve restaurants 157 million times a month. Those living in the South eat there twice as often as kids in the West.

Teens, especially boys, seem to be hungry all the time. Three meals a day just doesn't do it for them. Quick-serve and family restaurants are a great place for the "fourth meal" that is often needed to fill them up. Many teens have their first real work experience in these restaurants. It's no wonder that they are favorite spots for meals and snacks.

More and more restaurants are tuned in to environmental, social, humanitarian and health issues. Smoking has been banned in all company owned Arby's restaurants and in all Dunkin' Donuts outlets in the United States and abroad. Other restaurant chains are considering similar moves. Food packaging has been changed to reduce waste and use more recyclable materials, and many franchises actively support local youth activities and athletic teams. Families of critically ill children benefit from the Ronald McDonald houses established by the McDonald Corporation.

Restaurant chains were among the first to voluntarily offer nutrition information for their menu items. Many supply menu advice for people who must monitor their diets because of diabetes or high blood pressure. Some even supply special menus for the hearing and vision impaired. Restaurant chains were also among the first to recognize and accommodate multicultural diversity among their customers. They are ready employers of teens, seniors and others, including those who are developmentally disabled.

Singles, young and old, often find it inconvenient to shop for and prepare food for just one person. It's simpler and takes less time to get a meal to enjoy in a restaurant or to take out and eat at home. For the college set, restaurant chains offer an affordable opportunity to "dine out" and escape from the campus cafeteria. Recognizing this opportunity, some are beginning to open outlets on college campuses.

Only 10 percent of households have traditional homemakers who are not employed outside the home. Working adults, with and without children, account for the vast majority of households. They welcome the convenience of having their evening meal prepared for them. Eating at a restaurant, ordering in, or simply picking up all or part of their dinner, already prepared, simplifies their busy lives.

Seniors are catered to at many restaurant chains, and they respond by eating there over 226,947,000 times a month! There are senior meal selections and senior discounts offered daily and/or on special senior days. Breakfast clubs provide a sociable mealtime that may sometimes be followed by bingo. Many of these restaurants employ seniors, making the environment even more welcoming to older people.

After a morning walk, jog or workout at the gym, a stop at a restaurant is a pleasant opportunity to refuel and be rewarded for your effort. Even President Clinton often included a stop like this in his exercise routine.

FAST FACT

Surveys of mall shoppers by the American Dietetic Association found that over 50 percent visit the mall to eat and to shop. Large malls offer everything from ethnic to exotic foods and drinks.

EATING OUT, EATING WELL

To have a healthy diet, choose a variety of foods, have moderate portions and balance the foods you eat throughout the day. That's easy to do when you eat in restaurants. A wide selection of foods is available, and new and seasonal foods are often added to the menu. Mexican foods are very popular and many chains now serve them. A bean burrito might be a nice change from your usual hamburger and will add variety as well as fiber to your diet.

Eating moderate portions is really easy. All foods served in restaurants are portion controlled. A hamburger eaten on Monday will be the same size as one eaten on Thursday. If portion control is an issue for you, staying with a single instead of a double or triple burger is the best choice. If you want more, you'll have to order seconds, a delaying tactic which can keep you from overeating. It's much easier to "get more" at home.

When you have eaten a high calorie, high fat lunch, balance it with lighter foods at other meals during that day or even the next day. If your meal did not have fruit or vegetables, try to have some later on. It's not hard to eat healthier. Add fruit juice, a steamed vegetable, a baked potato, or salad with low fat dressing or a squeeze of lemon.

How about chicken?

You can usually get grilled or broiled chicken at most restaurants. It's a good idea to remove the skin from the chicken before you eat it. Save fried chicken and chicken nuggets for "once in a blue moon."

If you want a chicken sandwich, hold the creamy dressing and substitute mustard, salsa, ketchup or barbecue sauce. Lettuce and tomato add taste, nutrients and fiber without adding fat.

How about pizza?

Choose vegetable topped pizza with broccoli, tomatoes, onions, peppers and mushrooms most of the time, reserving extra cheese, pepperoni, sausage and other meat toppings for once in a while. A unique, healthy favorite is Hawaiian pizza topped with pineapple and ham. Hungry enough for two slices? Have one of them with a vegetable topping along with one other of your choice. Or try one slice with a large tossed salad.

How about hamburgers?

A plain hamburger topped with lettuce, tomatoes, onions, pickles, ketchup and/or mustard is the best choice. If you love the larger combo burgers or cheeseburgers, why not share one and order a large salad or baked potato as a side.

How about fish?

Choose broiled or grilled fish, saving battered or breaded fried fish for once in a while. This is true for shrimp too.

Choose boiled or steamed shrimp (as in cocktails or salads) or eat it broiled.

How about fries?

Fries are a favorite, so have a small portion topped with ketchup instead of cheese sauce. Other times, try substituting rice or a baked potato, plain or topped with margarine, chives and bacon bits.

How about sandwiches?

Choose multigrain bread and rolls. Go easy on cheese and creamy sauces like mayonnaise. Try spicy mustard or salsa instead. Go heavy on lettuce, onion, sprouts, grated carrots, grilled vegetables and tomatoes. Split it with a friend or save half for later if the sandwich is too big. Wrap sandwiches— burritos, pita or lahvosh filled with meats, cheese, vegetables, eggs and spreads are new additions to the sandwich roster. They're bundled on one end with foil or paper to make them easier to hold. They are portable, different and fun to eat. Wraps bridge the gap between fine dining and quick-serve foods, offering flavorful and sometimes more healthy alternatives to traditional sandwiches.

How about desserts?

Lowfat frozen yogurt with fruit topping is becoming widely available and makes a refreshing and delicious way to end a meal. Some restaurants offer fresh fruit and flavored gelatin at the salad bar. These are great desserts. If you can't resist the double chocolate layer cake, split it or take half home.

How about breakfast?

The most important thing about breakfast is eating it. Breakfast is the meal most likely to be skipped, as often as 23 percent of the time. Adults are more likely to pass on breakfast than children. Breakfast is moving out of the home. According to the American Dietetic Association, 25 percent of consumers eat breakfast away from home, 8 percent in the car!

Breakfast food is the fastest-growing food category. They can range from a full sit-down meal to a cup of convenience-store coffee plus a one-handed food item like a roll or muffin—estimated to be breakfast for as many as 25 percent of commuters.

You can eat out and have a different breakfast every day. A bagel—easy on the cream cheese; pancakes—have syrup, skip the sausage; waffles, ditto; scrambled egg on whole wheat toast. Don't forget yogurt, or cereal with lowfat milk. Add to any of these hot chocolate, lowfat milk, fruit juice or a fresh fruit.

SNACKING

Snacking is the great American pastime. Americans spend over $21 million a day on snacks. It has been estimated that the average American nibbles the equivalent of a fourth meal every day. In fact, because of busy lifestyles, many of us are now snacking on small meals throughout the day, or "grazing," instead of having "three squares." And no matter what you may have heard, eating as many as six to ten good snacks a day may be healthier than you think. Your body functions best when it doesn't go for long periods without food. Having several small meals helps control appetite and weight, lowers cholesterol levels, improves digestion in older adults, and prevents wide swings in blood sugar levels in people with diabetes.

People of all ages benefit from snacking. Small children, because they fill up so quickly, need between-meal snacks to keep them satisfied. Teenage boys, because they are growing so fast, require so much food that they benefit from snacks in addition to their meals. Athletes perform better when they have a high carbohydrate snack before a game or an event. During pregnancy, the increased nutrients needed for the developing baby make snacking smart. Because of body changes, the digestive capacity of older adults may be overwhelmed by large amounts of food. Eating smaller amounts throughout the day is better and may be a way to avoid gaining weight.

In addition to calories, snacks provide lots of nutrients. Yogurt is an excellent source of calcium and other minerals and vitamins; popcorn or nuts add fiber; pretzels and breadsticks have carbohydrates and vitamins; peanut butter has protein; fruits and vegetables—fresh, canned and dried—contain vitamins, minerals and fiber. And all snacks offer a pleasant break and boost energy, alertness and productivity.

The time between eating can be as long as six hours or more, especially in the afternoon. Studies show that not eating for such a long time decreases productivity on the job and increases accidents. According to researchers, a mid-afternoon snack is an excellent mental boost. Students who snacked on either candy or yogurt fifteen minutes before exams had better memory and were more alert than those who did not snack. Another study showed that children in the primary grades who snacked on nuts and raisins had better attitudes toward school.

FAST FACT

Twenty-nine percent of children in the United States spend more than $2.00 a day on snacks; another 27 percent spend $1.00 to $2.00 a day.

ETHNIC EATING

Part of the fun of eating out is having food that is different from what you eat at home. That's why ethnic eating is so popular. Chinese, Italian and Mexican are the most popular ethnic food restaurants. Along with French, Greek and Indian restaurants, they offer a variety of healthy, tasty choices.

Having Chinese Food

Ask for steamed dumplings instead of deep-fried appetizers, and clear soups instead of egg drop. Choose stir-fried, boiled and steamed main dishes with a side of plain, boiled white or brown rice. Try tofu for an interesting main dish. When you have fried noodles or wontons, egg rolls, lobster Cantonese, spareribs, duck or dishes with nuts, split them with others so that you have a smaller portion. If you are watching your salt intake, ask for the food prepared with no salt or MSG. Then season it yourself with light soy sauce, mustard or duck sauce. Sherbet, pineapple chunks and lychees with a fortune cookie are good endings.

Having Italian Food

Start with a mixed salad lightly dressed with vinegar and oil, minestrone soup, eggplant spread (caponata) or a steamed artichoke. Have pasta topped with sautéed or roasted vegetables or with plain tomato sauce (marinara). Other good choices are pasta and beans (pasta e fagioli) and chicken cacciatore. If you sprinkle on grated cheese, use a small amount, just enough for flavor.

When you want a creamy topping, meat or shellfish sauce, order an appetizer or a half portion or split it with others or take half home. Instead of garlic bread, have plain bread, breadsticks or bruschetta (sliced bread topped with chopped tomato). Italian ices, sorbets and fruit poached in wine are good dessert choices.

Having Mexican or Spanish Food

Start with bean soup or gazpacho and go easy on the nachos. Bean burritos with a little cheese, chicken on soft tacos, and rice and beans are good choices. Lean beef or a chicken fajita with steamed tortillas is fine, but limit the refried beans, sour cream and guacamole (avocado) toppings. Use salsa, pico de gallo, red sauce, green sauce and chopped salad to dress the fajitas instead.

Having French Food

Choose steamed mussels or other shellfish, grilled fresh fish and broiled lean meat. Try chicken with a low fat sauce like merengo or diablo. French bread, without butter, is great for mopping up the sauce. Have a Nicoise salad, a tasty tuna dish. Fresh fruit and a small portion of cheese make a good, traditional dessert.

Having Greek Food

Lentil soup or grape leaves stuffed with rice are great for starters. Ask for a Greek salad that is light on the feta cheese and heavy on tomatoes. Or have some cucumbers dressed with yogurt. A lamb roast, marinated, grilled meat or chicken in pita bread (souvlaki), and grilled or roasted chicken are better choices than casseroles of moussaka or pastitsio, which are better shared. Have kebobs of chicken or lamb and vegetables with rice on the side. Try bean salad with lemon dressing (fattoush).

Having Indian Food

Start with mulligatawny (lentil) soup, a chickpea appetizer or a mixed bean salad. Share an order of samosas, fried pastries filled with peas and potatoes. Barbecued chicken or seafood cooked in a tandoori and chicken or seafood curry are good choices, along with rice and stewed vegetables. Try lentil puree (dal) for a tasty change from meat. Condiments like chutney add flavor and are low in fat. Cucumbers with yogurt are a refreshing salad, as is lassi, a yogurt-based drink.

Choose baked and steamed bread (chapati, kulcha) instead of fried flatbread (naan, paratha).

FAST FACT

People living in Washington, DC, Honolulu and Boston spend the most on restaurant food.

EATING IN BY TAKING OUT

In addition to dining out, eating take-out food is a major trend today. Take-out meals have more than doubled in the last ten years. In 1996, more than half of all restaurant purchases were takeout. Delis, supermarkets and most restaurants offer a wide selection of take-out foods. Over 90 percent of all supermarkets feature take-out foods. This is an easy and economical way of eating dishes that you may not have the skill or time to prepare. Only 55 percent of dinners eaten at home include even one homemade dish. When you're short of time, take in a main dish and serve it with a salad or fresh fruit. Because take-out foods often do not have nutritional analyses, in Part Two, "Takeout" (beginning on page 133) you'll find a wide selection of items to help you make good choices.

FAST FACT

Eighty percent of all households in the United States have microwave ovens, making it simple to heat take-out food. By the year 2001, that number will increase to 95 percent. It's predicted that soon new cars will come equipped with microwaves.

IF YOU HAVE HEALTH CONCERNS

Have you been advised to lose weight, lower your fat intake or eat less salt? You can eat healthy foods and follow these diet recommendations when you eat in restaurants.

All the foods we eat are combinations of protein, fat, carbohydrates, vitamins, minerals and fiber. We all need to get enough of these nutrients to stay healthy.

Protein
Don't worry about getting enough protein. Restaurant meals usually have lots of protein in foods like hamburgers, steak, fish, cheese, milk, yogurt and eggs. Most of us get nearly twice as much as we need. And more is not always better. Too much protein does not make you stronger and healthier.

Fat
While many of us may be eating more fat than is good for us, this doesn't mean that some high fat food or even one high fat meal is so bad. It's only part of your overall intake. You can balance it by eating lower fat foods—fruit, vegetables and lowfat milk—at other meals. If, on the other hand, you have been told by your doctor to reduce your fat intake for medical reasons, keep closer tabs on what you are eating and avoid fatty foods whenever you can. This book will help you pick lowfat foods in restaurants and when you take-out so that you stay within the recommended daily guidelines of 30 percent calories from fat. Remember that individual foods need not meet this guideline, but overall fat intake for the day should come close. Balance the extra fat in a cheeseburger by choosing a fat free dressing for your side salad.

Meat, poultry, milk, eggs, cheese and butter all contain cholesterol. In fact, every food that comes from an animal contains cholesterol. To stay within the recommended intake of 300 milligrams of cholesterol per day, balance your cholesterol-containing menu choices with cholesterol-free plant foods—salad, vegetables, margarine, beans, potatoes, pasta and bread.

FAST FACT

Many restaurant chains now include lowfat menu items. They are often noted as "Light," "Lite" or "Guiltless." Heart Smart International, located in Scottsdale, Arizona, performs nutritional analyses of menu items for restaurants. If the items meet the FDA guidelines for healthy eating—which states that "while many factors affect heart disease, diets low in fat and cholesterol may reduce the risk of this disease"—the restaurant is able to designate those menu items as "Heart Smart." To get a list of Heart Smart member restaurants found throughout the country, call 800-762-7819 or visit their web site at www.heartsmart.com.

Carbohydrates

These are the starches and sugars in your food. We know now that starch does not deserve its bad, fattening reputation. Eating more carbohydrates can actually help you lose weight if you don't dress it with lots of fatty add-ons. Pizza, bread, rolls, rice, noodles, beans and pasta are foods that contain carbohydrates and also supply vitamins and minerals.

What about sugar? You really don't have to worry about it unless you have diabetes. If you are diabetic, discuss sugar with your doctor. While it isn't good to overdo sweets, having a sweet dessert at the end of a meal or as an occasional snack is fun and won't hurt.

When you reduce fat, carbohydrates take up the slack. Aim for 50 percent of your daily calories from carbohydrates. Choose two small burgers with more carbohydrates from bread instead of a super burger heavy with meat.

Fiber

Americans eat too little fiber. You can increase your intake by eating more whole grains, fruits, vegetables, beans and seeds. Eating whole fruits and vegetables instead of drinking their juices is one easy way to boost your fiber intake. Another is to choose whole-grain or multigrain rolls instead of plain rolls or top a salad with chickpeas or beans.

Vitamins and Minerals

When you eat a variety of different foods, you increase your chances of getting all the vitamins and minerals you need for good health. Eating more fruits, vegetables and grains helps. Some foods are better sources of certain vitamins and minerals. For example, milk and yogurt are excellent sources of calcium. But many other foods, like vegetables and nuts, contain this mineral too. Even a food additive commonly added to bread and rolls to keep them fresh contains a little calcium. We all know that orange juice is an excellent source of vitamin C, but you may not know that sliced tomato, green peppers and baked potatoes are good sources too.

Sodium is a mineral that we often get too much of—aim for 2,400 to 4,000 milligrams per day. Don't sprinkle on extra salt, ask for fries minus the salt, choose low-sodium dressing when available, and go easy on sauces. Instead, try a sprinkle of pepper, squeeze of lemon, dash of vinegar, salsa or hot sauce.

USING YOUR EATING OUT FOOD COUNTER

This book lists the nutrient content of foods served in over 80 restaurant chains. Included are 4,300 items from ice cream, doughnut and candy shops, cafeterias and restaurants. There are also over 500 take-out foods and over 5,300 snacks. For the first time, information about these nutrient values is at your fingertips. Before the *Eating Out Food Counter* it was impossible to compare so many restaurant and snack foods at one time. For example, when you want to have pizza, you'll find it under the different restaurants that serve it and also among the take-out and snack foods. The choice is up to you.

The *Eating Out Food Counter* is divided into three sections. Part One, "Restaurant Chains," lists the nutrient values in restaurant foods. Part Two lists nutrient values in "Takeout," and Part Three, "Snacks," gives the nutrient values in over 145 different snack categories. Over 10,000 foods are represented in these three lists.

In Part One, restaurant chains are listed alphabetically from Arbys through ZuZu. Within each restaurant list, most menu items are grouped as breakfast menu selections, main menu selections, children's menu selections, salads and salad bars, baked selections, desserts, ice cream and beverages.

In Part Two, takeout items are listed alphabetically in categories from antelope to zucchini. In this list you'll find almost any menu item you might order—from curry, crab cakes, and hamburgers to sandwiches and sushi.

In Part Three, snacks are listed alphabetically in categories from almonds to yogurt, frozen. This list gives you nutrient values for most foods you eat on the run. For each snack category, you will find generic foods listed first in alphabetical order, followed by an alphabetical listing of brand-name foods.

ABBREVIATIONS

avg	=	average
diam	=	diameter
frzn	=	frozen
g	=	gram
in	=	inch
lb	=	pound
lg	=	large
med	=	medium
mg	=	milligram
oz	=	ounce
pkg	=	package
pt	=	pint
prep	=	prepared
qt	=	quart
reg	=	regular
serve	=	serving
sm	=	small
sq	=	square
tbsp	=	tablespoon
tr	=	trace
tsp	=	teaspoon
w/	=	with
w/o	=	without
<	=	less than

EQUIVALENT MEASURES

3 teaspoons	=	1 tablespoon
4 tablespoons	=	1/4 cup
8 tablespoons	=	1/2 cup
12 tablespoons	=	3/4 cup
16 tablespoons	=	1 cup
1000 milligrams	=	1 gram
28 grams	=	1 ounce

Liquid Measurements

2 tablespoons	=	1 ounce
1/4 cup	=	2 ounces
1/2 cup	=	4 ounces
3/4 cup	=	6 ounces
1 cup	=	8 ounces
2 cups	=	1 pint
4 cups	=	1 quart

Dry Measurements

4 ounces	=	1/4 pound
8 ounces	=	1/2 pound
12 ounces	=	3/4 pound
16 ounces	=	1 pound

PART · ONE

RESTAURANT

CHAINS

NOTES

Discrepancies in values are due to rounding. All values for calories, fat, carbohydrate, cholesterol and sodium have been rounded to the nearest whole number.

All **fat** values of foods are given in grams (g).

All **carbohydrate** (CARB) values of foods are given in grams.

All **cholesterol** (CHOL) values of foods are given in milligrams (mg).

All **sodium** (SOD) values of foods are given in milligrams.

tr (trace) is the value used when a food contains less than one calorie, less than one gram of fat or carbohydrate, or less than one milligram of cholesterol or sodium.

A dash (—) indicates data was not available.

FAST FACT

There are more than half a million places to eat out in the U.S.

FOOD	PORTION	CALS	FAT	CARB	CHOL	SOD

ARBY'S
BEVERAGES

FOOD	PORTION	CALS	FAT	CARB	CHOL	SOD
2% Milk	0.5 oz	5	0	1	0	70
Chocolate Shake	1 (12 oz)	451	12	76	36	341
Coca-Cola Classic	1 serv (12 oz)	140	0	39	0	50
Coffee	1 serv (8 oz)	3	0	0	0	3
Diet Coke	1 serv (12 oz)	0	0	0	0	40
Diet Pepsi	1 serv (12 oz)	0	0	0	0	35
Diet 7UP	1 serv (12 oz)	0	0	0	0	35
Dr. Pepper	1 serv (12 oz)	160	0	40	0	55
Hot Chocolate	1 serv (8 oz)	110	1	23	0	120
Iced Tea	1 serv (16 oz)	6	0	1	0	12
Jamocha Shake	1 (12 oz)	384	10	62	36	262
Nehi Orange	1 serv (12 oz)	195	0	52	0	52
Orange Juice	1 serv (6 oz)	82	0	20	0	2
Pepsi Cola	1 serv (12 oz)	150	0	41	0	35
RC Cola	1 serv (12 oz)	165	0	43	0	52
RC Diet Rite	1 serv (12 oz)	1	0	0	0	10
7UP	1 serv (12 oz)	144	0	38	0	34
Upper Ten	1 serv (12 oz)	169	0	42	0	40
Vanilla Shake	1 (12 oz)	360	12	50	36	281

BREAKFAST SELECTIONS

FOOD	PORTION	CALS	FAT	CARB	CHOL	SOD
Bacon	2 strips (0.53 oz)	90	7	0	15	220
Biscuit Plain	1 (2.9 oz)	280	15	34	0	730
Blueberry Muffin	1 (2.3 oz)	230	9	35	25	290
Cinnamon Nut Danish	1 (3.5 oz)	360	11	60	0	105
Croissant Plain	1 (2 oz)	220	12	25	25	230
Egg Portion	1 serv (1.6 oz)	95	8	1	180	54
Ham	1 serv (1.5 oz)	45	1	0	20	405
Sausage	1 (1.3 oz)	163	15	0	25	321
Swiss	1 serv (0.5 oz)	45	3	1	12	175
Table Syrup	1 serv (1 oz)	100	0	25	0	30
Toastix	6 pieces (4.4 oz)	430	21	52	0	550

DESSERTS

FOOD	PORTION	CALS	FAT	CARB	CHOL	SOD
Apple Turnover	1 (3.2 oz)	330	14	48	0	180
Cheesecake Plain	1 serv (3 oz)	320	23	23	95	240
Cherry Turnover	1 (3.2 oz)	320	13	46	0	190
Chocolate Chip Cookie	1 (1 oz)	125	6	16	10	85
Polar Swirl Butterfinger	1 (11.6 oz)	457	18	62	28	318
Polar Swirl Heath	1 (11.6 oz)	543	22	76	39	346
Polar Swirl Oreo	1 (11.6 oz)	329	22	66	35	521

FOOD	PORTION	CALS	FAT	CARB	CHOL	SOD
Polar Swirl Peanut Butter Cup	1 (11.6 oz)	517	24	61	34	385
Polar Swirl Snickers	1 (11.6 oz)	511	19	73	33	351
MAIN MENU SELECTIONS						
Arby's Sauce	1 serv (0.5 oz)	15	tr	4	0	113
Baked Potato Broccoli'n Cheddar	1 (15.7 oz)	571	20	89	12	565
Baked Potato Deluxe	1 (15.3 oz)	736	36	86	59	499
Baked Potato Plain	1 (11.5 oz)	355	tr	82	0	26
Baked Potato w/ Margarine & Sour Cream	1 (14 oz)	578	24	85	25	209
Barbeque Sauce	1 serv (0.5 oz)	30	0	7	0	185
Beef Stock Au Jus	1 serv (2 oz)	10	0	1	0	440
Breaded Chicken Fillet	1 (7.2 oz)	536	28	46	45	1016
Cheddar Cheese Sauce	1 serv (0.75 oz)	35	3	1	4	139
Cheddar Curly Fried	1 serv (4.25 oz)	333	18	40	3	1016
Chicken Cordon Bleu	1 (8.5 oz)	623	33	46	77	1504
Chicken Finger	2 (3.6 oz)	290	16	20	32	677
Curly Fries	1 serv (3.5 oz)	300	15	38	0	853
Fish Fillet Sandwich	1 (7.7 oz)	529	27	50	43	864
French Fries	1 serv (2.5 oz)	246	13	30	0	114
Garden Salad	1 (11.9 oz)	61	1	12	0	40
Grilled Chicken BBQ	1 (7.1 oz)	388	13	47	43	1002
Grilled Chicken Deluxe	1 (8.1 oz)	430	20	41	61	848
Ham 'n Cheese Sandwich	1 (5.9 oz)	359	14	34	53	1283
Ham'n Cheese Melt	1 (4.9 oz)	329	13	34	40	1013
Honey Mayonnaise Reduced Calorie	1 serv (0.5 oz)	70	7	1	20	135
Horsey Sauce	1 serv (0.5 oz)	60	5	2	5	150
Italian Sub	1 (10.1 oz)	675	36	46	836	2089
Italian Sub Sauce	1 serv (0.5 oz)	70	7	1	0	240
Ketchup	1 serv (0.5 oz)	16	0	4	0	143
Light Roast Beef Deluxe	1 (6.4 oz)	296	10	33	42	826
Light Roast Chicken Deluxe	1 (6.8 oz)	276	6	33	33	777
Light Roast Chicken Salad	1 serv (14.4 oz)	149	2	12	29	418
Light Roast Turkey Deluxe	1 (6.8 oz)	260	7	33	33	1262
Mayonnaise	1 serv (0.5 oz)	110	12	0	5	80
Mayonnaise Light Cholesterol Free	1 serv (0.25 oz)	12	1	1	0	64

FOOD	PORTION	CALS	FAT	CARB	CHOL	SOD
Mustard German Style	1 serv (0.16 oz)	5	0	1	0	70
Parmesan Cheese Sauce	1 serv (0.5 oz)	70	7	2	5	130
Potato Cakes	2 (3 oz)	204	12	20	0	397
Roast Beef Arby's Melt w/ Cheddar	1 (5.2 oz)	368	18	36	31	936
Roast Beef Arby-Q	1 (6.4 oz)	431	18	48	37	1321
Roast Beef Bac'n Cheddar Deluxe	1 (8.1 oz)	539	34	38	44	1140
Roast Beef Beef'n Cheddar	1 (6.7 oz)	487	28	40	50	1216
Roast Beef Gaint	1 (8.1 oz)	555	28	43	71	1561
Roast Beef Junior	1 (4.4 oz)	324	14	35	30	779
Roast Beef Regular	1 (5.4 oz)	388	19	33	43	1009
Roast Beef Sub	1 (10.8 oz)	700	42	44	846	2034
Roast Beef Super	1 (8.7 oz)	523	27	50	43	1189
Roast Chicken Club	1 (8.5 oz)	546	31	37	58	1103
Roast Chicken Deluxe	1 (7.6 oz)	433	22	36	34	763
Roast Chicken Santa Fe	1 (6.4 oz)	436	22	35	54	816
Side Salad	1 (5 oz)	23	tr	4	0	15
Sub Roll French Dip	1 (6.8 oz)	475	22	40	55	1411
Sub Roll Hot Ham 'n Swiss	1 (9.3 oz)	500	23	43	68	1664
Sub Roll Pilly Beef'n Swiss	1 (10.4 oz)	755	47	48	91	2025
Sub Roll Triple Cheese Melt	1 (8.4 oz)	720	45	46	91	1797
Tartar Sauce	1 serv (1 oz)	140	15	0	30	220
Turkey Sub	1 (9.8 oz)	550	27	47	65	2084
SALAD DRESSINGS						
Blue Cheese	1 serv (2 oz)	290	31	2	50	580
Buttermilk Ranch Reduced Calorie	1 serv (2 oz)	50	0	12	0	710
Honey French	1 serv (2 oz)	280	23	18	0	400
Italian Reduced Calorie	1 serv (2 oz)	20	1	3	0	1000
Red Ranch	1 serv (0.5 oz)	75	6	5	0	115
Thousand Island	1 serv (2 oz)	260	26	7	30	420
SOUPS						
Boston Clam Chowder	1 serv (8 oz)	190	9	18	25	965
Cream of Broccoli	1 serv (8 oz)	160	8	15	25	1000
Lumberjack Mixed Vegetable	1 serv (8 oz)	90	4	10	5	1150
Old Fashioned Chicken Noodle	1 serv (8 oz)	80	2	11	20	850
Potato w/ Bacon	1 serv (8 oz)	170	7	23	20	905

FOOD	PORTION	CALS	FAT	CARB	CHOL	SOD
Timberline Chili	1 serv (8 oz)	220	10	17	30	1130
Wisconsin Cheese	1 serv (8 oz)	280	18	20	35	1065

AU BON PAIN
BAKED SELECTIONS

FOOD	PORTION	CALS	FAT	CARB	CHOL	SOD
Apple Coffee Cake	1 piece (4.6 oz)	480	24	60	96	285
Bagel Chocolate Chip	1 (5 oz)	380	7	69	5	480
Bagel Dutch Apple w/ Walnut Streussel	1 (5 oz)	360	5	77	0	480
Baguette Loaf	1 slice (1.8 oz)	140	5	29	0	350
Biscotti	1 (1.5 oz)	200	10	24	35	45
Biscotti Chocolate	1 (1.7 oz)	240	13	28	35	50
Braided Roll	1 (1.8 oz)	170	5	26	0	320
Cinnamon Roll	1 (7 oz)	710	26	110	100	740
Cookie Chocolate Chip	1 (2.1 oz)	280	13	40	40	85
Cookie Oatmeal Raisin	1 (2.1 oz)	250	10	40	30	240
Cookie Peanut Butter	1 (2.1 oz)	280	15	32	30	260
Cookie Shortbread	1 (2.4 oz)	390	25	39	65	190
Croissant Almond	1 (4.3 oz)	560	37	50	105	260
Croissant Apple	1 (3.4 oz)	280	10	46	25	180
Croissant Chocolate	1 (3.4 oz)	440	23	53	30	230
Croissant Cinnamon Raisin	1 (3.7 oz)	380	13	61	35	290
Croissant Plain	1 (2.1 oz)	270	15	30	40	240
Croissant Raspberry Cheese	1 (3.5 oz)	380	19	47	60	300
Croissant Sweet Cheese	1 (3.6 oz)	390	22	42	75	330
Danish Cheese Swirl	1 (3.8 oz)	450	28	46	95	410
Danish Lemon Swirl	1 (4 oz)	450	24	53	80	410
Danish Raspberry	1 (3.6 oz)	370	21	42	65	350
Danish Sweet Cheese	1 (3.6 oz)	420	26	42	90	380
Four Grain Loaf	1 slice (1.8 oz)	130	1	25	0	280
French Sandwich Roll	1 (1.8 oz)	120	5	25	0	320
Hazelnut Fudge Brownie	1 (4 oz)	380	18	56	100	150
Holiday Cookie Cranberry Almond Macaroon	1 (1.5 oz)	160	8	22	0	115
Holiday Cookie Cranberry Almond Macaroon w/ Chocolate	1 (1.9 oz)	210	11	27	0	120
Holiday Cookie English Toffee	1 (1.8 oz)	220	12	28	45	110
Holiday Cookie Ginger Pecan	1 (2 oz)	260	15	30	40	115

FOOD	PORTION	CALS	FAT	CARB	CHOL	SOD
Mochaccino Bar	1 (4 oz)	404	24	44	37	294
Muffin Blueberry	1 (4.5 oz)	410	15	64	85	380
Muffin Carrot	1 (5 oz)	480	23	61	55	650
Muffin Chocolate Chip	1 (4.5 oz)	490	20	70	35	560
Muffin Corn	1 (4.6 oz)	470	18	70	65	570
Muffin Low Fat Chocolate Cake	1 (4 oz)	290	3	68	20	630
Muffin Low Fat Triple Berry	1 (4.2 oz)	270	3	60	25	560
Muffin Pumpkin w/ Streusel Topping	1 (5.5 oz)	470	18	74	60	550
Multigrain Loaf	1 slice (1.8 oz)	130	1	26	0	340
Parisienne Loaf	1 slice (1.8 oz)	120	5	25	0	300
Pear Ginger Tea Cake	1 piece (4 oz)	380	20	47	0	202
Pecan Roll	1 (6.8 oz)	900	48	111	50	480
Roll 3 Seed Pecan Raisin	1 (2.7 oz)	250	6	43	0	240
Roll Hearth Sandwich	1 (2.8 oz)	220	2	43	0	410
Rolls Petit Pan	1 (2.5 oz)	200	1	41	0	570
Rye Loaf	1 slice (1.8 oz)	110	2	21	0	310
Scone Cinnamon	1 (4.1 oz)	520	28	60	145	230
Scone Current	1 (3.7 oz)	430	23	47	155	230
Scone Orange	1 (4.1 oz)	440	23	53	155	240
Sourdough Bagel Asiago Cheese	1 (4.2 oz)	380	6	66	15	690
Sourdough Bagel Cinnamon Raisin	1 (4.5 oz)	390	1	83	0	550
Sourdough Bagel Cranberry Walnut	1 (5 oz)	460	4	93	0	590
Sourdough Bagel Everything	1 (4.2 oz)	360	3	72	0	710
Sourdough Bagel Honey 8 Grain	1 (4.2 oz)	360	2	72	0	580
Sourdough Bagel Mocha Chip Swirl	1 (5 oz)	370	4	72	0	480
Sourdough Bagel Plain	1 (4 oz)	350	1	71	0	540
Sourdough Bagel Sesame	1 (4.2 oz)	380	4	71	0	540
Sourdough Bagel Wild Blueberry	1 (4.5 oz)	380	2	80	0	570
Valentine Cookie Chocolate Dipped Shortbread	1 (2.8 oz)	410	27	41	55	160
Valentine Cookie Red Sugar Shortbread Heart	1 (2.4 oz)	350	22	37	60	170

FOOD	PORTION	CALS	FAT	CARB	CHOL	SOD
Valentine Cookie Shortbread	1 (2.4 oz)	340	22	35	60	170
BEVERAGES						
Frozen Java Blast	1 serv (16 oz)	220	2	42	10	120
Frozen Mocha Blast	1 serv (16 oz)	320	3	64	10	150
Hot Apple Cider	1 lg (20 oz)	350	0	87	0	170
Hot Apple Cider	1 med (16 oz)	310	0	77	0	150
Hot Apple Cider	1 sm (10 oz)	190	0	47	0	95
Hot Hazelnut Blast	1 serv (16 oz)	310	6	57	25	180
Hot Mocha Blast	1 lg (17 oz)	310	8	45	30	230
Hot Mocha Blast	1 med (13 oz)	260	6	41	25	180
Hot Mocha Blast	1 sm (9 oz)	160	4	23	15	120
Hot Raspberry Mocha Blast	1 serv (10 oz)	180	4	29	15	115
Hot Raspberry Mocha Blast	1 serv (16 oz)	300	6	52	25	170
Hot Raspberry Mocha Blast	1 serv (20 oz)	350	8	57	30	220
Hot Strawberry Chocolate Blast	1 serv (16 oz)	330	6	57	25	180
Hot Vanilla Chocolate Blast	1 serv (16 oz)	310	6	57	25	180
Iced Caffee Latte	1 lg (20.5 oz)	270	10	26	40	270
Iced Caffee Latte	1 med (12 oz)	150	6	15	25	150
Iced Caffee Latte	1 sm (9 oz)	130	5	12	20	130
Iced Cappuccino	1 lg (20.5 oz)	270	10	26	40	270
Iced Cappuccino	1 med (12 oz)	150	6	15	25	150
Iced Cappuccino	1 sm (9 oz)	110	4	10	15	110
Iced Cocoa	1 lg (20.5 oz)	440	11	66	40	320
Iced Cocoa	1 med (12 oz)	280	6	42	25	190
Iced Cocoa	1 sm (9 oz)	200	6	27	20	160
Iced Hazelnut Blast	1 serv (16 oz)	310	6	54	25	180
Iced Mocha Blast	1 lg (20.5 oz)	360	10	50	40	280
Iced Mocha Blast	1 med (12 oz)	260	6	41	25	180
Iced Mocha Blast	1 sm (9 oz)	180	5	25	20	135
Iced Raspberry Mocha Blast	1 serv (12 oz)	160	4	27	15	100
Iced Raspberry Mocha Blast	1 serv (16 oz)	310	6	54	25	180
Iced Raspberry Mocha Blast	1 serv (24 oz)	330	7	54	25	200
Iced Strawberry Chocolate Blast	1 serv (16 oz)	310	6	54	25	180
Iced Tea Peach	1 lg (16 oz)	170	0	44	0	30

FOOD	PORTION	CALS	FAT	CARB	CHOL	SOD
Iced Tea Peach	1 med (12 oz)	130	0	33	0	20
Iced Tea Peach	1 sm (12 oz)	90	0	22	0	15
Iced Tea Raspberry	1 lg (16 oz)	150	0	38	0	30
Iced Tea Raspberry	1 med (12 oz)	110	0	29	0	20
Iced Tea Raspberry	1 sm (8 oz)	80	0	19	0	15
Iced Vanilla Chocolate Blast	1 serv (16 oz)	310	6	54	25	180
Whipped Cream	1 serv (1.2 oz)	160	11	11	55	0
SALAD DRESSINGS						
Bleu Cheese	1 serv (3 oz)	370	41	8	40	910
Buttermilk Ranch	1 serv (3 oz)	310	32	4	35	270
Caesar	1 serv (3 oz)	380	39	3	25	410
Fat Free Tomato Basil	1 serv (3 oz)	70	0	17	0	650
Greek	1 serv (3 oz)	440	50	2	0	820
Lemon Basil Vinaigrette	1 serv (3 oz)	330	32	15	0	460
Lite Honey Mustard	1 serv (3 oz)	280	17	30	40	560
Lite Italian	1 serv (3 oz)	230	20	15	0	570
Sesame French	1 serv (3 oz)	370	30	26	0	1010
SALADS AND SALAD BARS						
Caesar	1 serv (8.9 oz)	270	10	27	20	800
Chicken Caesar	1 serv (11.4 oz)	360	11	28	65	910
Garden	1 lg (10.6 oz)	160	2	34	0	290
Garden	1 sm (7.5 oz)	100	1	20	0	150
Mozzarella & Roasted Pepper Salad	1 serv (13.7 oz)	340	18	25	60	135
Pesto Chicken Salad	1 serv (10.7 oz)	230	11	11	45	250
Tuna	1 serv (15 oz)	490	27	40	45	750
SANDWICHES AND FILLINGS						
Bagel Spreads Lite Strawberry	1 serv (2 oz)	150	11	6	35	210
Bagel Spreads Lite Vanilla Hazelnut	1 serv (2 oz)	150	11	6	35	210
Cheddar	½ serv (1.5 oz)	170	14	1	45	260
Chicken Tarragon	1 serv (4 oz)	240	17	1	65	170
Club Sandwich Hot Roasted Turkey	1 (14.9 oz)	950	50	80	135	2240
Country Ham	1 serv (3.7 oz)	150	7	1	55	1370
Cracked Pepper Chicken	1 serv (3.9 oz)	140	2	2	72	184
Cream Cheese Lite	1 serv (2 oz)	130	12	2	35	230
Cream Cheese Lite Honey Walnut	1 serv (2 oz)	260	12	8	20	260
Cream Cheese Lite Raspberry	1 serv (2 oz)	200	8	10	20	280
Cream Cheese Lite Sun-Dried Tomato	1 serv (2 oz)	130	11	2	35	230

FOOD	PORTION	CALS	FAT	CARB	CHOL	SOD
Cream Cheese Plain	1 serv (2 oz)	190	18	2	55	210
Grilled Chicken	1 serv (3.9 oz)	140	2	2	72	184
Hot Croissant Ham & Cheese	1 (4.2 oz)	380	20	36	70	690
Hot Croissants Spinach & Cheese	1 (3.6 oz)	270	16	27	40	330
Provolone	½ serv (1.5 oz)	150	11	1	30	370
Roast Beef	1 serv (3.7 oz)	140	5	1	50	550
Sandwich Arizona Chicken	1 (12.7 oz)	720	33	57	125	1190
Sandwich Buffalo Chicken	1 (13.7 oz)	640	19	76	85	1650
Sandwich California Chicken	1 (13.2 oz)	820	44	55	135	1200
Sandwich Fresh Mozzarella Tomato & Pesto	1 (10.5 oz)	650	30	69	55	1090
Sandwich Honey Dijon Chicken	1 (15.3 oz)	730	18	85	135	1990
Sandwich Parmesan Chicken	1 (11.1 oz)	740	24	91	70	1620
Sandwich Steak & Cheese Melt	1 (11.7 oz)	750	32	79	90	1600
Sandwich Thai Chicken	1 (8.3 oz)	420	6	72	20	1320
Swiss	½ serv (1.5 oz)	160	12	1	40	110
Tuna Salad	1 serv (4.5 oz)	360	29	3	50	520
Turkey Breast	1 serv (3.7 oz)	120	1	1	20	1110
Wraps Chicken Caesar	1 (9.9 oz)	630	31	46	80	1140
Wraps Southwestern Tuna	1 (14.4 oz)	950	64	53	110	1230
Wraps Summer Turkey	1 (11.7 oz)	340	9	36	35	1380
SOUPS						
Beef Barley	1 serv (12 oz)	112	3	16	18	980
Beef Barley	1 serv (16 oz)	150	4	22	25	1310
Beef Barley	1 serv (8 oz)	75	2	11	15	660
Beef Stew	1 serv (8 oz)	140	7	14	25	840
Bohemian Cabbage	1 serv (12 oz)	110	5	17	0	960
Bohemian Cabbage	1 serv (16 oz)	140	6	22	0	1280
Bohemian Cabbage	1 serv (8 oz)	70	3	11	0	650
Bread Bowl	1 (9 oz)	640	4	131	0	1950
Broccoli & Cheddar	1 serv (12 oz)	390	33	19	75	1030
Broccoli & Cheddar	1 serv (16 oz)	520	44	25	100	1380
Broccoli & Cheddar	1 serv (8 oz)	260	22	13	50	690
Caribbean Black Bean	1 serv (12 oz)	180	2	32	10	1150

FOOD	PORTION	CALS	FAT	CARB	CHOL	SOD
Caribbean Black Bean	1 serv (16 oz)	250	2	43	10	1540
Caribbean Black Bean	1 serv (8 oz)	120	1	22	5	770
Chicken Chili	1 serv (12 oz)	350	18	31	65	2030
Chicken Chili	1 serv (16 oz)	470	24	41	90	2700
Chicken Chili	1 serv (8 oz)	240	12	21	45	1350
Chicken Noodle	1 serv (12 oz)	120	2	14	25	1000
Chicken Noodle	1 serv (16 oz)	170	3	19	35	1340
Chicken Noodle	1 serv (8 oz)	80	2	10	15	670
Chili	1 serv (12 oz)	340	14	32	50	910
Chili	1 serv (16 oz)	460	19	43	70	1220
Chili	1 serv (8 oz)	230	10	22	35	610
Clam Chowder	1 serv (12 oz)	400	29	24	95	1090
Clam Chowder	1 serv (16 oz)	540	39	32	125	1460
Clam Chowder	1 serv (8 oz)	270	19	16	65	730
Corn Chowder	1 serv (12 oz)	390	24	43	70	1150
Corn Chowder	1 serv (16 oz)	530	33	58	95	1530
Corn Chowder	1 serv (8 oz)	260	16	29	50	760
Cream Of Broccoli	1 serv (12 oz)	330	28	21	60	1160
Cream Of Broccoli	1 serv (16 oz)	440	37	28	80	1550
Cream Of Broccoli	1 serv (8 oz)	220	18	14	40	770
Cream Of Chicken With Wild Rice	1 serv (16 oz)	330	19	33	90	1310
French Onion	1 serv (12 oz)	120	5	17	0	1910
French Onion	1 serv (16 oz)	170	7	23	0	2550
French Onion	1 serv (8 oz)	80	4	12	0	1280
In A Bread Bowl Beef Barley	1 serv (21 oz)	760	7	147	20	2940
In A Bread Bowl Caribbean Black Bean	1 serv (21 oz)	830	5	163	10	3100
In A Bread Bowl Chicken Chili	1 serv (21 oz)	990	22	162	65	3970
In A Bread Bowl Chicken Noodle	1 serv (21 oz)	760	6	146	20	2950
In A Bread Bowl Clam Chowder	1 serv (21 oz)	1050	32	155	100	3040
In A Bread Bowl Cream of Broccoli	1 serv (21 oz)	970	31	152	60	3100
In A Bread Bowl French Onion	1 serv (21 oz)	760	8	148	0	3860
In A Bread Bowl New England Potato & Cheese w/ Ham	1 serv (21 oz)	860	15	152	40	3170
In A Bread Bowl Tomato Florentine	1 serv (21 oz)	760	5	150	10	3490

FOOD	PORTION	CALS	FAT	CARB	CHOL	SOD
In A Bread Bowl Vegetarian Chili	1 serv (21 oz)	870	7	171	0	3550
Louisiana Beans & Rice	1 serv (12 oz)	280	7	37	15	960
Louisiana Beans & Rice	1 serv (16 oz)	360	9	50	20	1320
Louisiana Beans & Rice	1 serv (8 oz)	180	5	25	10	660
New England Potato & Cheese w/ Ham	1 serv (12 oz)	220	12	21	40	1220
New England Potato & Cheese w/ Ham	1 serv (16 oz)	290	15	28	55	1630
New England Potato & Cheese w/ Ham	1 serv (8 oz)	150	8	14	25	820
Potato Leek	1 serv (12 oz)	320	20	28	70	1700
Potato Leek	1 serv (16 oz)	400	25	36	85	2120
Potato Leek	1 serv (8 oz)	200	13	18	45	1060
Santa Fe Chicken Tortilla	1 serv (12 oz)	230	10	32	25	1430
Santa Fe Chicken Tortilla	1 serv (16 oz)	300	13	42	30	1900
Santa Fe Chicken Tortilla	1 serv (8 oz)	150	7	21	15	950
Seafood Gumbo	1 serv (12 oz)	190	9	21	25	870
Seafood Gumbo	1 serv (16 oz)	260	12	28	35	1160
Seafood Gumbo	1 serv (8 oz)	130	6	14	20	580
Tomato Florentine	1 serv (12 oz)	90	2	20	5	1550
Tomato Florentine	1 serv (16 oz)	122	2	27	5	2070
Tomato Florentine	1 serv (8 oz)	61	1	13	5	1030
Tomato Tortellini	1 serv (12 oz)	90	2	15	5	1320
Tomato Tortellini	1 serv (16 oz)	110	2	20	10	1770
Tomato Tortellini	1 serv (8 oz)	60	1	11	5	950
Vegetable Stew	1 serv (12 oz)	100	2	16	5	1460
Vegetable Stew	1 serv (16 oz)	130	2	22	5	1950
Vegetable Stew	1 serv (8 oz)	60	1	11	5	980
Vegetarian Chili	1 serv (12 oz)	210	4	40	0	1610
Vegetarian Chili	1 serv (16 oz)	278	5	53	0	2150
Vegetarian Chili	1 serv (8 oz)	139	3	27	0	1070
Vegetarian Corn & Green Chili Bisque	1 serv (12 oz)	300	16	30	45	1830
Vegetarian Corn & Green Chili Bisque	1 serv (16 oz)	380	20	41	60	2290
Vegetarian Corn & Green Chili Bisque	1 serv (8 oz)	190	10	21	30	1140
Vegetarian Lentil	1 serv (12 oz)	200	1	35	0	1180
Vegetarian Lentil	1 serv (16 oz)	270	1	47	0	1580
Vegetarian Lentil	1 serv (8 oz)	130	0	24	0	790

BASKIN-ROBBINS
FROZEN YOGURT

FOOD	PORTION	CALS	FAT	CARB	CHOL	SOD
Maui Brownie Madness	½ cup	140	3	26	5	80

FOOD	PORTION	CALS	FAT	CARB	CHOL	SOD
Perils Of Pauline	½ cup	140	3	25	5	105
ICE CREAM						
Banana Strawberry	½ cup	130	7	17	25	40
Baseball Nut	½ cup	160	9	18	30	55
Black Walnut	½ cup	160	11	13	30	45
Cherries Jubilee	½ cup	140	7	16	30	40
Chocolate	½ cup	150	9	18	30	60
Chocolate Almond	½ cup	180	11	17	30	55
Chocolate Chip	½ cup	150	10	15	35	45
Chocolate Chip Cookie Dough	½ cup	170	9	20	35	70
Chocolate Fudge	½ cup	160	9	21	30	80
Chocolate Mousse Royale	½ cup	170	10	20	25	60
Chocolate Raspberry Truffle	½ cup	180	9	23	30	60
Chunky Heath Bar	½ cup	170	10	19	30	70
Cookies N Cream	½ cup	170	11	16	30	80
Dirt'N Worms	½ cup	160	8	22	25	80
Egg Nog	½ cup	150	8	16	40	45
Everybody's Favorite Candy Bar	½ cup	170	9	20	30	30
French Vanilla	½ cup	160	10	14	70	45
French Vanilla	½ cup	170	11	15	55	50
Fudge Brownie	½ cup	170	11	19	25	75
Fudge Brownie	½ cup	180	10	20	20	—
German Chocolate Cake	½ cup	180	10	20	25	75
Gold Medal Ribbon	½ cup	150	8	20	30	95
Gold Medal Ribbon	½ cup	150	7	20	20	—
Jamoca	½ cup	140	9	14	35	45
Jamoca Almond Fudge	½ cup	150	8	17	20	65
Jomoca Almond Fudge	½ cup	140	9	17	25	40
Lemon Custard	½ cup	150	8	16	45	55
Lowfat Carmel Apple AlaMod	½ cup	100	2	20	5	75
Lowfat Espresso'N Cream	½ cup	100	3	18	5	60
Mint Chocolate Chip	½ cup	150	10	15	35	35
No Sugar Added Call Me Nuts	½ cup	110	2	21	5	55
No Sugar Added Cherry Cordial	½ cup	100	2	18	5	55
No Sugar Added Mad About Chocolate	½ cup	100	2	19	5	40

FOOD	PORTION	CALS	FAT	CARB	CHOL	SOD
No Sugar Added Pineapple Coconut	½ cup	90	2	16	5	60
No Sugar Added Thin Mint	½ cup	100	3	16	5	65
Nonfat Berry Innocent Cheese	½ cup	110	0	24	0	100
Nonfat Check-It-Out Cherry	½ cup	100	0	22	0	90
Nonfat Jamoca Swirl	½ cup	110	0	23	5	105
Ocean Commotion	½ cup	150	7	20	25	40
Old Fashion Butter Pecan	½ cup	160	11	13	35	35
Oregon Blueberry	½ cup	140	8	16	30	50
Peanut Butter N Chocolate	½ cup	180	12	16	30	95
Pink Bubblegum	½ cup	150	8	19	30	40
Pistachio Almond	½ cup	170	12	13	30	45
Pralines N Cream	½ cup	160	9	19	30	85
Pumpkin Pie	½ cup	130	7	16	30	50
Quarterback Crunch	½ cup	160	10	18	30	75
Reeses Peanut Butter	½ cup	180	11	17	30	70
Rocky Road	½ cup	170	10	19	30	60
Rum Raisin	½ cup	140	7	18	30	40
Strawberry Cheesecake	½ cup	150	9	17	35	65
Triple Chocolate Passion	½ cup	180	11	21	35	70
Vanilla	½ cup	140	8	14	40	40
Very Berry Strawberry	½ cup	130	7	16	25	40
Winter White Chocolate	½ cup	150	9	18	25	50
World Class Chocolate	½ cup	160	9	18	30	55
ICES AND ICE POPS						
Daiquiri Ice	½ cup	110	0	28	0	10
Sherbet Blue Raspberry	½ cup	120	2	25	5	30
Sherbet Orange	½ cup	120	2	26	5	25
Sherbet Rainbow	½ cup	120	2	26	5	25
Sorbet Pink Raspberry Lemon	½ cup	120	0	29	0	10
The Mask Ice	½ cup	120	0	29	0	10
Watermelon Ice	½ cup	110	0	28	0	10
Watermelon Ice	½ cup	110	0	28	0	10
BEN & JERRY'S						
Sugar Cone	1	48	tr	10	0	42
FROZEN YOGURT						
Cherry Garcia	½ cup (3.3 oz)	150	3	29	15	60
Chocolate Chip Cookie Dough	½ cup (3.3 oz)	190	4	34	25	110

FOOD	PORTION	CALS	FAT	CARB	CHOL	SOD
Chocolate Fudge Brownie	½ cup (3.3 oz)	180	3	32	15	100
No Fat Black Raspberry	½ cup (3.4 oz)	140	0	30	5	60
No Fat Vanilla	½ cup (3.4 oz)	140	0	28	5	75
No Fat Vanilla Swirl	½ cup (3.4 oz)	130	0	29	0	70
Peach Raspberry Trifle	½ cup (3.3 oz)	150	2	30	20	65
Vanilla w/ Heath Toffee Crunch	½ cup (3.3 oz)	190	6	30	20	115
ICE CREAM						
Butter Pecan	½ cup (3.1 oz)	270	21	17	60	105
Cherry Garcia	½ cup (3.1 oz)	210	12	20	55	45
Chocolate Chip Cookie Dough	½ cup (3.1 oz)	180	11	17	55	45
Chocolate Fudge Brownie	½ cup (3.1 oz)	230	11	28	35	80
Chubby Hubby	½ cup (3.1 oz)	280	17	26	50	135
Chunky Monkey	½ cup (3.1 oz)	220	13	25	50	45
Coffee Coffee Buzz Buzz	½ cup (3.1 oz)	240	16	23	55	60
Coffee Ole	½ cup (3.1 oz)	200	13	18	65	50
Coffee w/ Heath Toffee Crunch	½ cup (3.1 oz)	250	16	25	55	105
Cool Britannia	½ cup (3.1 oz)	210	12	23	55	55
Deep Deep Chocolate	½ cup (3.1 oz)	210	12	22	40	40
Holy Cannoli	½ cup (3.1 oz)	240	16	20	55	55
Low Fat Blond Brownie Sundae	½ cup (3.1 oz)	160	3	32	25	80
Low Fat Coffee & Biscotti	½ cup (3.1 oz)	160	3	30	30	85
Low Fat Sweet Cream & Cookies	½ cup (3.1 oz)	160	3	30	25	100
Low Fat Vanilla & Chocolate Mint Patty	½ cup (3.1 oz)	170	3	32	20	65
Maple Walnut	½ cup (3.1 oz)	240	13	19	55	40
Mint Chocolate Chunk	½ cup (3.1 oz)	240	16	24	60	55
Mint Chocolate Cookie	½ cup (3.1 oz)	230	14	24	60	110
New York Super Fudge Chunk	½ cup (3.1 oz)	250	16	25	35	45
Peanut Butter Cup	½ cup (3.1 oz)	270	18	21	55	95
Peanut Butter & Jelly	½ cup (3.1 oz)	230	14	23	50	85
Phish Food	½ cup (3.1 oz)	230	12	30	30	70
Pistachio Pistachio	½ cup (3.1 oz)	230	16	18	60	45
Rainforest Crunch	½ cup (3.1 oz)	250	16	21	60	105
Southern Peach	½ cup (3.1 oz)	180	10	20	50	40
Strawberry	½ cup (3.1 oz)	180	10	20	50	40
Sweet Cream Cookie	½ cup (3.1 oz)	230	14	23	60	110

FOOD	PORTION	CALS	FAT	CARB	CHOL	SOD
Vanilla Caramel Fudge	½ cup (3.1 oz)	230	13	25	60	85
Vanilla Chocolate Chunk	½ cup (3.1 oz)	240	16	23	60	55
Vanilla Fudge Brownie	½ cup (3.1 oz)	210	12	23	60	80
Vanilla World's Best	½ cup (3.1 oz)	200	13	17	65	50
Vanilla w/ Heath Toffee Crunch	½ cup (3.1 oz)	250	16	25	60	110
Wavy Gravy	½ cup (3.1 oz)	260	17	24	50	75
White Russian	½ cup (3.1 oz)	200	13	18	65	45
SORBETS						
Cranberry Orange	½ cup (3.2 oz)	110	0	26	0	10
Doonesberry	½ cup (3.2 oz)	100	0	27	0	10
Mango Lime	½ cup (3.2 oz)	110	0	27	0	10
Pina Colada	½ cup (3.2 oz)	110	0	26	0	10
Purple Passion Fruit	½ cup (3.2 oz)	100	0	27	0	10
Strawberry Kiwi	½ cup (3.2 oz)	110	0	27	0	10

BIG BOY
DESSERTS

FOOD	PORTION	CALS	FAT	CARB	CHOL	SOD
Frozen Yogurt Fat Free	1 serv	118	0	27	0	60
Frozen Yogurt Shake	1	156	1	33	2	120
MAIN MENU SELECTIONS						
Baked Cod w/ Salad Baked Potato Roll & Margarine	1 meal	744	21	82	76	655
Baked Potato	1	163	2	37	0	7
Breast of Chicken Pita w/ Mozzarella & Ranch Dressing	1	361	11	23	84	369
Breast of Chicken w/ Mozzarella Salad Baked Potato Roll & Margarine	1 meal	697	20	80	76	613
Cabbage Soup	1 bowl	40	5	7	0	347
Cabbage Soup	1 cup	34	4	6	0	295
Cajun Cod w/ Salad Baked Potato Roll & Margarine	1 meal	736	21	80	76	745
Chicken & Pasta Primavera w/ Salad Roll & Margarine	1 meal	676	14	83	65	875
Chicken 'n Vegetable Stir Fry w/ Salad Baked Potato Roll & Margarine	1 meal	795	18	109	65	845

FOOD	PORTION	CALS	FAT	CARB	CHOL	SOD
Dinner Roll	1	210	5	36	0	340
Plain Egg Beaters Omelette w/ Whole Wheat Bread & Margarine	1 meal	305	10	36	0	603
Promise Margarine	1 pat	25	3	0	0	35
Rice Pilaf	1 serv	153	4	25	10	688
Scrambled Egg Beaters w/ Whole Wheat Bread & Margarine	1 meal	305	10	36	0	603
Southwest Chicken w/ Salad Baked Potato Roll & Margarine	1 meal	702	18	85	76	948
Spaghetti Marinara w/ Salad Roll & Margarine	1 meal	754	11	105	8	754
Turkey Pita w/ Ranch Dressing	1	245	6	23	83	938
Vegetarian Egg Beaters Omelette w/ Whole Wheat Bread & Margarine	1 meal	330	10	40	0	618
Vegetable Stir Fry w/ Salad Baked Potato Roll & Margarine	1 meal	616	14	109	0	774
SALAD DRESSINGS						
Italian Fat Free	1 oz	11	0	3	0	191
Lo Cal Oriental	1 oz	20	2	4	0	189
Lo Cal Ranch	1 oz	41	3	3	8	151
SALADS AND SALAD BARS						
Chicken Breast Salad w/ Roll & Margarine	1 serv	523	16	50	73	654
Oriental Chicken Breast Salad w/ Dinner Roll & Margarine	1 serv	660	20	73	65	855
Tossed Salad	1	35	2	7	0	71

BLIMPIE
6 INCH SUB

FOOD	PORTION	CALS	FAT	CARB	CHOL	SOD
5 Meatball	1 (7.8 oz)	500	22	52	25	970
Blimpie Best	1 (8.5 oz)	410	13	47	50	1480
Cheese Trio	1 (8.2 oz)	510	23	51	60	1060
Club	1 (9.8 oz)	450	13	53	40	1350
Grilled Chicken	1 (9.1 oz)	400	9	52	30	950

FOOD	PORTION	CALS	FAT	CARB	CHOL	SOD
Ham & Swiss	1 (8.2 oz)	400	13	47	35	970
Ham Salami Provolone	1 (9.8 oz)	590	28	52	70	1880
Roast Beef	1 (8.5 oz)	340	5	47	20	870
Steak & Cheese	1 (7.1 oz)	550	26	51	70	1080
Tuna	1 (10.2 oz)	570	32	50	50	790
Turkey	1 (8.2 oz)	320	5	51	10	890
SALADS AND SALAD BARS						
Grilled Chicken Salad	1 serv (16.2 oz)	350	12	13	150	1190

BOJANGLES
BAKED SELECTIONS

FOOD	PORTION	CALS	FAT	CARB	CHOL	SOD
Biscuit	1	243	12	29	2	663
Multi-Grain Roll	1	150	3	26	0	210
Sweet Biscuit Apple Cinnamon	1	330	13	48	tr	540
Sweet Biscuit Bo*Berry	1	220	10	29	tr	410
Sweet Biscuit Cinnamon	1	320	18	37	tr	560
MAIN MENU SELECTIONS						
Biscuit Sandwich Bacon	1	290	17	26	10	810
Biscuit Sandwich Bacon Egg & Cheese	1	550	42	27	160	1250
Biscuit Sandwich Cajun Filet	1	454	21	46	41	949
Biscuit Sandwich Country Ham	1	270	15	26	20	1010
Biscuit Sandwich Egg	1	400	30	26	120	630
Biscuit Sandwich Sausage	1	350	23	26	20	810
Biscuit Sandwich Smoked Sausage	1	380	26	27	20	940
Biscuit Sandwich Steak	1	649	49	13	34	1126
Bo Rounds	1 serv	235	11	31	13	328
Buffalo Bites	1 serv	180	5	5	105	720
Cajun Pintos	1 serv	110	0	18	0	480
Cajun Roast Skinfree Breast	1 serv	143	5	tr	84	562
Cajun Roast Skinfree Leg	1 serv	161	8	tr	125	566
Cajun Roast Skinfree Thigh	1 serv	215	15	tr	95	428
Cajun Roast Wing	1 serv	231	15	3	117	617
Cajun Spiced Breast	1 serv	278	17	12	75	565
Cajun Spiced Leg	1 serv	310	23	11	67	465
Cajun Spiced Thigh	1 serv	264	16	11	96	530
Cajun Spiced Wing	1 serv	355	25	11	94	630

FOOD	PORTION	CALS	FAT	CARB	CHOL	SOD
Chicken Supremes	1 serv	337	16	26	58	629
Corn On The Cob	1 serv	140	2	34	0	20
Dirty Rice	1 serv	166	6	24	10	762
Green Beans	1 serv	25	0	25	0	710
Macaroni & Cheese	1 serv	198	14	12	26	418
Marinated Cole Slaw	1 serv	136	3	26	0	454
Potatoes w/o Gravy	1 serv	80	1	16	0	380
Sandwich Cajun Filet w/ Mayonnaise	1	437	22	41	55	506
Sandwich Cajun Filet w/o Mayonnaise	1	337	11	41	45	401
Sandwich Cajun Steak w/ Horseradish Sauce & Pickles	1	434	26	39	55	985
Sandwich Grilled Filet w/ Mayonnaise	1	335	16	25	61	645
Sandwich Grilled Filet w/o Mayonnaise	1 serv (5.2 oz)	329	7	37	59	418
Seasoned Fries	1 serv	344	19	39	13	480
Southern Style Breast	1 serv	261	16	12	76	702
Southern Style Leg	1 serv	254	15	11	94	446
Southern Style Thigh	1 serv	308	21	14	78	630
Southern Style Wing	1 serv	337	21	19	86	684

BOSTON MARKET
BAKED SELECTIONS

FOOD	PORTION	CALS	FAT	CARB	CHOL	SOD
Brownie	1 (3.3 oz)	450	27	47	80	190
Cookie Chocolate Chip	1 (2.8 oz)	340	17	48	25	240
Cookie Oatmeal Raisin	1 (2.8 oz)	320	13	48	25	260
Honey Wheat Roll	½ roll (2 oz)	150	2	29	0	280

MAIN MENU SELECTIONS

FOOD	PORTION	CALS	FAT	CARB	CHOL	SOD
½ Chicken w/ Skin	1 serv (10 oz)	630	37	2	370	960
¼ Dark Meat Chicken No Skin	1 serv (3.6 oz)	210	10	1	150	320
¼ Dark Meat Chicken w/ Skin	1 serv (4.6 oz)	330	22	2	180	460
¼ White Meat Chicken No Skin Or Wing	1 serv (3.6 oz)	160	4	0	95	350
¼ White Meat Chicken w/ Skin	1 serv (5.4 oz)	330	18	2	175	530
BBQ Baked Beans	¾ cup (7.1 oz)	330	9	53	10	630
Butternut Squash Low Fat	¾ cup (6.8 oz)	160	6	25	15	580
Caesar Salad Entree	1 serv (10 oz)	520	43	16	40	1420

FOOD	PORTION	CALS	FAT	CARB	CHOL	SOD
Caesar Salad w/o Dressing	1 serv (8 oz)	240	13	14	25	780
Caesar Side Salad	1 (4 oz)	210	17	6	20	560
Chicken Caesar Salad	1 serv (13 oz)	670	47	16	120	1860
Chicken Gravy	1 serv (1 oz)	15	1	2	0	170
Chicken Salad Sandwich	1 (10.7 oz)	680	30	63	120	1360
Chicken Sandwich w/ Cheese & Sauce	1 (12.4 oz)	750	33	72	135	1860
Chicken Sandwich w/o Cheese & Sauce Low Fat	1 (10 oz)	430	4	62	65	910
Chunky Chicken Salad	3/4 cup (5.5 oz)	370	27	3	120	800
Cole Slaw	3/4 cup (6.5 oz)	280	16	32	25	520
Corn Bread	1 (2.4 oz)	200	6	33	25	390
Cranberry Relish Low Fat	3/4 cup (7.9 oz)	370	5	84	0	5
Creamed Spinach	3/4 cup (6.4 oz)	280	21	12	65	820
Fruit Salad Low Fat	3/4 cup (5.5 oz)	70	1	17	0	10
Green Bean Casserole	3/4 cup (6 oz)	170	5	10	5	580
Ham & Turkey Club w/ Cheese & Sauce	1 (13.3 oz)	890	44	76	150	2350
Ham & Turkey Club w/o Cheese & Sauce	1 (9.3 oz)	430	6	64	55	1330
Ham Sandwich w/ Cheese & Sauce	1 (11.8 oz)	760	35	71	100	1880
Ham Sandwich w/o Cheese & Sauce	1 (9.3 oz)	450	9	66	45	1600
Ham w/ Cinnamon Apples	1 serv (8 oz)	350	13	35	75	1750
Homestyle Mashed Potatoes & Gravy	3/4 cup (6.6 oz)	200	9	27	25	560
Hot Cinnamon Apples	3/4 cup (6.4 oz)	250	5	56	0	45
Macaroni & Cheese	3/4 cup (6.7 oz)	280	10	12	20	760
Mashed Potatoes	2/3 cup (5.6 oz)	180	8	25	25	390
Meat Loaf & Brown Gravy	1 serv (7 oz)	390	22	19	120	1040
Meat Loaf & Chunky Tomato Sauce	1 serv (8 oz)	370	18	22	120	1170
Meat Loaf Sandwich w/ Cheese	1 (13.8 oz)	860	33	95	165	2270
Meat Loaf Sandwich w/o Cheese	1 (12.3 oz)	690	21	86	120	1610
Mediterranean Pasta Salad	3/4 cup (4.5 oz)	170	10	16	10	490
New Potatoes Low Fat	3/4 cup (4.6 oz)	130	3	25	0	150

FOOD	PORTION	CALS	FAT	CARB	CHOL	SOD
Original Chicken Pot Pie	1 serv (14.9 oz)	750	34	78	115	2380
Rice Pilaf	⅔ cup (5.1 oz)	180	5	32	0	600
Rotisserie Turkey Breast Skinless Low Fat	1 serv (5 oz)	170	1	1	100	850
Steamed Vegetables Low Fat	⅔ cup (3.7 oz)	35	1	7	0	35
Stuffing	¾ cup (6.1 oz)	310	12	44	0	1140
Tortellini Salad	¾ cup (5.6 oz)	380	24	29	90	530
Turkey Sandwich w/ Cheese & Sauce	1 (11.8 oz)	710	28	68	110	1390
Turkey Sandwich w/o Cheese & Sauce	1 (9.3 oz)	400	4	61	60	1070
Whole Kernel Corn Low Fat	¾ cup (5.8 oz)	180	4	30	0	170
Zucchini Marinara	¾ cup (6.6 oz)	80	4	10	0	470
SOUPS						
Chicken Low Fat	¾ cup (6.8 oz)	80	3	4	25	470
Chicken Tortilla	1 cup (8.4 oz)	220	11	19	35	1410

BROWN'S CHICKEN

FOOD	PORTION	CALS	FAT	CARB	CHOL	SOD
Breadsticks w/ Garlic Butter	1	199	4	36	tr	2213
Breast	3.5 oz	284	15	12	67	529
Coleslaw	3.5 oz	131	10	9	6	211
Corn Fritters	3.5 oz	415	25	42	4	552
Corn On Cob	1 ear (3 inch)	126	3	22	1	23
Fettucini Alfredo	1 serv (12 oz)	1507	64	173	51	3018
French Fries	3.5 oz	503	22	44	1	235
Gizzard	3.5 oz	387	20	26	88	795
Leg	3.5 oz	287	16	9	52	542
Liver	3.5 oz	341	19	19	147	704
Mostaccioli w/ Meat	1 serv (12 oz)	835	14	44	17	898
Mostaccioli w/o Meat	1 serv (12 oz)	792	10	146	0	842
Mushrooms	3.5 oz	289	16	30	1	671
Potato Salad	3.5 oz	94	4	13	11	639
Ravioli w/ Meat	1 serv (12 oz)	865	20	138	17	934
Ravioli w/o Meat	1 serv (12 oz)	822	16	140	0	878
Shrimp	3.5 oz	277	10	34	31	778
Thigh	3.5 oz	355	24	13	63	574
Wing	3.5 oz	385	25	17	81	654

BRUEGGER'S BAGELS

FOOD	PORTION	CALS	FAT	CARB	CHOL	SOD
Blueberry	1 (3.5 oz)	300	2	60	0	480
Cinnamon Raisin	1 (3.5 oz)	290	2	60	0	400
Egg	1 (3.5 oz)	280	1	67	25	510

FOOD	PORTION	CALS	FAT	CARB	CHOL	SOD
Everything	1 (3.6 oz)	290	2	55	0	700
Garlic	1 (3.6 oz)	280	2	57	0	440
Honey Grain	1 (3.6 oz)	300	3	58	0	390
Onion	1 (3.6 oz)	280	2	57	0	430
Orange Cranberry	1 (3.5 oz)	290	1	61	0	470
Pesto	1 (3.5 oz)	280	2	55	0	480
Plain	1 (3.5 oz)	280	2	56	0	430
Poppy Seed	1 (3.6 oz)	280	2	57	0	440
Pumpernickel	1 (3.5 oz)	280	2	56	0	390
Salt	1 (3.6 oz)	270	2	55	0	1670
Sesame	1 (3.6 oz)	290	3	57	0	440
Spinach	1 (3.5 oz)	280	1	56	0	490
Sun Dried Tomato	1 (3.5 oz)	280	2	58	0	490
Wheat Bran	1 (3.5 oz)	280	2	55	0	410

BURGER KING
BEVERAGES

FOOD	PORTION	CALS	FAT	CARB	CHOL	SOD
Coca-Cola Classic	1 med (22 fl oz)	260	0	70	0	—
Coffee	1 serv (12 oz)	5	0	1	0	5
Diet Coke	1 med (22 fl oz)	1	0	tr	0	—
Milk 2%	1 (8 oz)	130	5	12	20	120
Shake Chocolate	1 med (10 oz)	320	7	54	20	230
Shake Chocolate Syrup Added	1 med (12 oz)	440	7	84	20	430
Shake Strawberry Syrup Added	1 med (12 oz)	420	6	83	20	260
Shake Vanilla	1 med (10 oz)	300	6	53	20	230
Sprite	1 med (22 fl oz)	260	0	66	0	—
Tropicana Orange Juice	1 serv (11 oz)	140	0	33	0	0

BREAKFAST SELECTIONS

FOOD	PORTION	CALS	FAT	CARB	CHOL	SOD
AM Express Dip	1 serv (1 oz)	80	0	21	0	20
AM Express Grape Jam	1 serv (0.4 oz)	30	0	7	0	0
AM Express Strawberry Jam	1 serv (0.4 oz)	30	0	8	0	5
Biscuit	1 (3.3 oz)	330	18	37	2	950
Biscuit w/ Bacon Egg & Cheese	1 (6 oz)	510	31	39	225	1530
Biscuit w/ Egg	1 (5.3 oz)	420	24	38	205	1110
Biscuit w/ Sausage	1 (4.8 oz)	530	36	38	35	1350
Croissan'wich Sausage Egg & Cheese	1 (5.7 oz)	550	42	22	250	1110
Croissan'wich w/ Sausage & Cheese	1 (3.7 oz)	450	35	21	54	940
French Toast Sticks	1 serv (4.9 oz)	500	27	60	0	490

FOOD	PORTION	CALS	FAT	CARB	CHOL	SOD
Hash Browns	1 sm (2.6 oz)	240	15	25	0	440
Land O'Lakes Whipped Classic Blend	1 serv (0.4 oz)	65	7	0	0	75
MAIN MENU SELECTIONS						
American Cheese	2 slices (0.9 oz)	90	8	0	25	420
BK Big Fish Sandwich	1 (8.8 oz)	720	43	59	80	1180
BK Broiler Chicken Sandwich	1 (8.7 oz)	530	16	45	105	1060
Bacon Bits	1 serv (3 g)	15	1	0	3	70
Big King Sandwich	1 (7.9 oz)	660	43	29	135	920
Broiled Chicken Salad w/o Dressing	1 serv (10.6 oz)	190	8	9	75	500
Bull's Eye Barbecue Sauce	1 serv (0.5 oz)	20	0	5	0	140
Cheeseburger	1 (5 oz)	380	19	28	65	770
Chicken Sandwich	1 (8 oz)	710	43	54	60	1400
Chicken Tenders	8 pieces (4.3 oz)	350	22	17	65	940
Coated French Fries Salted	1 med (4.1 oz)	400	21	50	0	820
Croutons	1 serv (0.2 oz)	30	1	5	0	90
Dipping Sauce Barbecue	1 serv (1 oz)	35	0	9	0	400
Dipping Sauce Honey	1 serv (1 oz)	90	0	23	0	10
Dipping Sauce Ranch	1 serv (1 oz)	170	17	2	0	200
Dipping Sauce Sweet & Sour	1 serv (1 oz)	45	0	11	0	50
Double Cheeseburger	1 (7.5 oz)	600	36	28	135	1060
Double Cheeseburger w/ Bacon	1 (7.6 oz)	640	39	28	145	1240
Double Whopper	1 (12.3 oz)	870	56	45	170	940
Double Whopper w/ Cheese	1 (13.2 oz)	960	63	46	195	1420
Dutch Apple Pie	1 serv (4 oz)	300	15	39	0	230
French Fries Salted	1 med (4.1 oz)	370	20	43	0	240
Garden Salad w/o Dressing	1 (7.5 oz)	100	5	7	15	110
Hamburger	1 (4.5 oz)	330	15	28	55	530
Ketchup	1 serv (0.5 oz)	15	0	4	0	180
King Sauce	1 serv (0.5 oz)	70	7	2	4	70
Lettuce	1 leaf (0.7 oz)	0	0	0	0	0
Mayonnaise	1 serv (1 oz)	210	23	tr	20	160
Mustard	1 serv (3 g)	0	0	0	0	40
Onion	1 serv (0.5 oz)	5	0	1	0	0
Onion Rings	1 serv (4.4 oz)	310	14	41	0	810

FOOD	PORTION	CALS	FAT	CARB	CHOL	SOD
Pickles	4 slices (0.5 oz)	0	0	0	0	140
Side Salad w/o Dressing	1 (4.7 oz)	60	3	4	5	55
Tartar Sauce	1 serv (1 oz)	180	19	0	15	220
Tomato	2 slices (1 oz)	5	0	1	0	0
Whopper	1 (9.5 oz)	640	39	45	90	870
Whopper Jr.	1 (5.9 oz)	420	24	29	60	530
Whopper Jr. w/ Cheese	1 (6.3 oz)	460	28	29	75	770
Whopper w/ Cheese	1 (10.3 oz)	730	46	46	115	1350
SALAD DRESSINGS						
Bleu Cheese	1 serv (1 oz)	160	16	1	30	260
French	1 serv (1 oz)	140	10	11	0	190
Ranch	1 serv (1 oz)	180	19	2	10	170
Reduced Calorie Light Italian	1 serv (1 oz)	15	1	3	0	360
Thousand Island	1 serv (1 oz)	140	12	7	15	190

CAPTAIN D'S
DESSERTS

FOOD	PORTION	CALS	FAT	CARB	CHOL	SOD
Carrot Cake	1 piece (4 oz)	434	23	49	32	414
Cheesecake	1 piece (4 oz)	420	31	30	141	480
Chocolate Cake	1 piece (4 oz)	303	10	49	20	259
Lemon Pie	1 piece (4 oz)	351	10	59	45	135
Pecan Pie	1 piece (4 oz)	458	20	64	4	373
MAIN MENU SELECTIONS						
Baked Potato	1	278	0	—	0	—
Breadstick	1	113	4	—	0	—
Broiled Chicken Lunch	1 serv	503	9	—	82	—
Broiled Chicken Platter	1 serv	802	10	—	82	—
Broiled Chicken Sandwich	1 (8.2 oz)	451	19	29	105	858
Broiled Fish & Chicken Lunch	1 serv	478	8	—	66	—
Broiled Fish & Chicken Platter	1 serv	777	10	—	66	—
Broiled Fish Lunch	1 serv	435	7	—	49	—
Broiled Fish Platter	1 serv	734	7	—	49	—
Broiled Shrimp Lunch	1 serv	421	7	—	155	—
Broiled Shrimp Platter	1 serv	720	8	—	155	—
Cheese	1 slice (1 oz)	54	5	tr	14	206
Cob Corn	1 serv (9.5 oz)	251	2	60	0	13
Cocktail Sauce	1 lg serv (1 fl oz)	34	tr	8	0	252
Cocktail Sauce	1 serv (1 fl oz)	137	tr	34	0	1007
Cole Slaw	1 pt (16 oz)	633	47	47	66	454

FOOD	PORTION	CALS	FAT	CARB	CHOL	SOD
Cole Slaw	1 serv (4 oz)	158	12	12	16	246
Crackers	4 (0.5 oz)	50	1	8	3	147
Cracklins	1 serv (1 oz)	218	17	16	0	741
Dinner Salad w/o Dressing	1 (2.5 oz)	27	1	3	1	67
French Fried Potatoes	1 serv (3.5 oz)	302	10	50	0	152
Fried Okra	1 serv (4 oz)	300	16	34	0	445
Green Beans Seasoned	1 serv (4 oz)	46	2	5	4	752
Hushpuppies	6 (6.7 oz)	756	25	119	0	2790
Hushpuppy	1 (1.1 oz)	126	4	20	0	465
Imitation Sour Cream	1 serv	29	3	—	0	—
Margarine	1 serv	102	12	—	0	—
Non-Dairy Creamer	1 serv	14	1	1	0	8
Rice	1 serv (4 oz)	124	0	28	0	9
Stuffed Crab	1 serv	91	7	16	—	250
Sugar	1 pkg	18	0	3	0	0
Sweet & Sour Sauce	1 lg serv (4 fl oz)	206	0	52	0	18
Sweet & Sour Sauce	1 serv (1.8 fl oz)	52	0	13	0	5
Tartar Sauce	1 lg serv (4 fl oz)	298	27	13	41	633
Tartar Sauce	1 serv (1 fl oz)	75	7	3	10	158
Vegetable Medley	1 serv	36	1	—	0	—
White Beans	1 serv (4 oz)	126	1	22	2	99
SALAD DRESSINGS						
Blue Cheese	1 pkg (1 fl oz)	105	12	tr	14	101
French	1 pkg (1 fl oz)	111	11	4	7	187
Light Italian	1 serv	16	1	—	0	—
Ranch	1 pkg (1 fl oz)	92	10	tr	15	230

CARL'S JR.
BAKED SELECTIONS

FOOD	PORTION	CALS	FAT	CARB	CHOL	SOD
Cheese Danish	1 (4.1 oz)	400	22	49	15	390
Cheesecake Strawberry Swirl	1 serv (3.5 oz)	300	17	31	55	220
Chocolate Cake	1 serv (3 oz)	300	10	49	13	260
Chocolate Chip Cookie	1 (2.5 oz)	370	19	49	25	350
Cinnamon Roll	1 (4.2 oz)	420	13	68	15	570
Muffin Blueberry	1 (4.2 oz)	340	14	49	40	340
Muffin Bran	1 (4.7 oz)	370	13	61	45	410
BEVERAGES						
Coca-Cola Classic	1 reg (16 fl oz)	190	0	51	0	50
Coffee	1 reg (12 oz)	10	0	1	0	25

FOOD	PORTION	CALS	FAT	CARB	CHOL	SOD
Diet 7UP	1 reg (16 oz)	0	0	0	0	90
Diet Coke	1 reg (16 oz)	0	0	0	0	40
Dr. Pepper	1 reg (16 oz)	200	0	52	0	30
Hot Chocolate	1 reg (12 oz)	110	1	24	<5	125
Iced Tea	1 reg (14 fl oz)	5	0	0	0	55
Milk 1%	1 (10 fl oz)	150	3	18	15	180
Minute Maid Orange Soda	1 reg (16 oz)	230	0	59	0	30
Orange Juice	1 (6 fl oz)	90	0	20	0	0
Ramblin' Root Beer	1 reg (16 oz)	230	0	61	0	75
Shake Chocolate	1 sm (13.5 oz)	390	7	74	30	280
Shake Strawberry	1 sm (13.5 oz)	400	7	77	30	240
Shake Vanilla	1 sm (13.5 fl oz)	330	8	54	35	250
Sprite	1 reg (16 fl oz)	190	0	48	0	90
BREAKFAST SELECTIONS						
Bacon	2 strips (0.3 oz)	40	4	0	10	125
Breakfast Burrito	1 (5.3 oz)	430	26	29	460	810
Breakfast Quesadilla Cheese	1 (5.2 oz)	300	14	27	225	750
English Muffin w/ Margarine	1 (2.6 oz)	230	10	30	0	330
French Toast Dips w/o Syrup	1 serv (3.7 oz)	410	25	40	0	380
Grape Jelly	1 serv (0.5 oz)	35	0	9	0	0
Hash Brown Nuggets	1 serv (3.3 oz)	270	17	27	0	410
Sausage	1 patty (1.8 oz)	200	18	0	35	530
Scrambed Eggs	1 serv (3.5 oz)	160	11	1	425	125
Strawberry Jam	1 serv (0.5 oz)	35	0	9	0	0
Sunrise Sandwich	1 (4.6 oz)	370	21	31	225	710
Table Syrup	1 serv (1 oz)	90	0	22	0	22
MAIN MENU SELECTIONS						
American Cheese	1 slice (0.5 oz)	60	5	0	15	270
BBQ Chicken Sandwich	1 (6.7 oz)	310	6	34	55	830
BBQ Sauce	1 serv (1.1 oz)	50	0	11	0	270
Big Burger	1 (6.8 oz)	470	20	46	55	810
Breadstick	1 (0.3 oz)	35	1	7	0	60
Carl's Catch Fish Sandwich	1 (7.5 oz)	560	30	54	60	1220
Chicken Club Sandwich	1 (8.8 oz)	550	29	37	85	1160
Chicken Stars	6 pieces (3 oz)	230	14	11	85	450
CrissCut Fries	1 lg (5.7 oz)	550	34	55	0	1280
Croutons	1 serv (7 g)	35	1	5	0	65
Double Western Bacon Cheeseburger	1 (11.5 oz)	970	57	58	145	1810

FOOD	PORTION	CALS	FAT	CARB	CHOL	SOD
Famous Big Star Hamburger	1 (8.6 oz)	610	38	42	70	890
French Fries	1 reg (4.4 oz)	370	20	44	0	240
Great Stuff Potato Bacon & Cheese	1 (14.2 oz)	630	29	76	40	1720
Great Stuff Potato Broccoli & Cheese	1 (14.2 oz)	530	22	76	15	930
Great Stuff Potato Plain	1 (9.4 oz)	290	0	68	0	40
Great Stuff Potato Sour Cream & Chive	1 (10.9 oz)	430	14	70	10	160
Hamburger	1 (3.1 oz)	200	8	23	25	500
Honey Sauce	1 serv (1 oz)	90	0	23	0	5
Hot & Crispy Sandwich	1 (5 oz)	400	22	35	45	980
Mustard Sauce	1 serv (1 oz)	45	1	10	0	150
Onion Rings	1 serv (5.3 oz)	520	26	63	0	840
Salsa	1 serv (0.9 oz)	10	0	2	0	160
Santa Fe Chicken Sandwich	1 (7.9 oz)	530	30	36	85	1230
Super Star Hamburger	1 (11.2 oz)	820	53	41	120	1030
Sweet N'Sour Sauce	1 serv (1 oz)	50	0	11	0	60
Swiss Cheese	1 slice (0.5 oz)	45	4	0	10	220
Western Bacon Cheeseburger	1 (8.1 oz)	870	35	59	90	1490
Zucchini	1 serv (5.9 oz)	380	23	38	0	1040
SALAD DRESSINGS						
1000 Island	2 fl oz	250	24	7	20	540
Blue Cheese	2 fl oz	310	34	1	25	360
French Fat Free	2 fl oz	70	0	18	0	760
House	2 fl oz	220	22	3	20	440
Italian Fat Free	2 fl oz	15	0	4	0	800
SALADS AND SALAD BARS						
Salad-To-Go Charbroiled Chicken	1 serv (12 oz)	260	9	11	70	530
Salad-To-Go Garden	1 (4.8 oz)	50	3	4	5	75

CARVEL
FROZEN YOGURT

FOOD	PORTION	CALS	FAT	CARB	CHOL	SOD
Vanilla Low Fat No Sugar Added	4 fl oz	110	2	22	—	90
ICE CREAM						
Brown Bonnet Cone	1 (4.7 oz)	380	21	43	40	150
Brown Bonnet Cone No Fat Vanilla	1 (4.7 oz)	300	11	47	—	95
Cake	1 pkg (4 oz)	270	14	33	30	160

FOOD	PORTION	CALS	FAT	CARB	CHOL	SOD
Cake	1 pkg (7 oz)	450	23	54	45	230
Cake Cheesecake	1 serv (4 oz)	280	14	34	30	190
Cake Chocolate Vanilla Chocolate Crunchies	1/15 cake (3.4 oz)	230	12	27	35	95
Cake Cookies & Cream	1 serv (4 oz)	270	14	32	35	160
Cake Fudge Drizzle	1/8 cake (4 oz)	310	17	35	30	170
Cake Fudgie The Whale	1/14 cake (3.6 oz)	290	16	33	30	180
Cake Holiday	1/15 cake (3.4 oz)	240	12	30	30	100
Cake S'mores	1 serv (4 oz)	270	14	33	25	150
Cake Sinfully Chocolate	1 serv (4 oz)	280	14	34	25	150
Cake Strawberries & Cream	1/8 cake (3.8 oz)	240	12	31	35	100
Chocolate	4 fl oz	190	10	22	25	100
Chocolate No Fat	4 fl oz	120	0	28	0	40
Flying Saucer Chocolate	1 (4 oz)	230	9	33	30	140
Flying Saucer Chocolate w/ Sprinkles	1 (4 oz)	330	14	49	30	150
Flying Saucer Low Fat Chocolate	1 (4 oz)	190	3	38	0	130
Flying Saucer Low Fat Vanilla	1 (4 oz)	180	3	36	0	140
Flying Saucer Vanilla	1 (4 oz)	240	10	33	40	150
Flying Saucer Vanilla w/ Sprinkles	1 (4 oz)	340	14	49	40	160
Nature's Crunch	1 (4.2 g)	450	25	55	20	240
Olde Fashion Sundae Butterscotch	1 (8 oz)	500	17	80	60	340
Olde Fashion Sundae Chocolate	1 (8 oz)	470	19	71	55	280
Olde Fashion Sundae Strawberry	1 (8 oz)	420	15	64	55	230
Sheet Cake Chocolate Vanilla Chocolate Crunchies	1/26 cake (3.3 oz)	230	12	27	35	100
Sinful Love Bar	1 (4.2 oz)	460	29	48	20	240
Thick Shake Chocolate	1 (16 oz)	719	31	96	116	418
Thick Shake Low Fat Chocolate	1 (16 oz)	490	1	108	15	330
Thick Shake Low Fat Strawberry	1 (16 oz)	460	1	96	15	290
Thick Shake Low Fat Vanilla	1 (16 oz)	460	1	98	15	280

FOOD	PORTION	CALS	FAT	CARB	CHOL	SOD
Thick Shake No Fat Chocolate	1 (16 oz)	524	8	100	36	346
Thick Shake No Fat Strawberry	1 (16 oz)	453	7	82	36	285
Thick Shake No Fat Vanilla	1 (16 oz)	462	7	84	36	278
Thick Shake Strawberry	1 (16 oz)	648	30	77	116	358
Thick Shake Vanilla	1 (16 oz)	657	30	79	116	350
Vanilla	4 fl oz	200	10	21	40	110
Vanilla No Fat	4 fl oz	120	0	25	0	55
SHERBET						
Black Raspberry	½ cup (3.4 oz)	150	1	33	5	35
Blueberry	½ cup (3.4 oz)	150	1	33	5	30
Lemon	½ cup (3.5 oz)	150	1	31	5	30
Lime	½ cup (3.5 oz)	150	1	31	5	30
Mango	½ cup (3.5 oz)	140	1	30	5	25
Orange	½ cup (3.5 oz)	150	1	31	5	30
Peach	½ cup (3.4 oz)	150	1	32	5	35
Pineapple	½ cup (3.5 oz)	150	1	33	5	40
Strawberry	½ cup (3.5 oz)	150	1	32	5	35

CHICK-FIL-A
BEVERAGES

FOOD	PORTION	CALS	FAT	CARB	CHOL	SOD
Coca-Cola Classic	1 serv (9 oz)	110	0	28	0	10
Diet Coke	1 serv (9 oz)	0	0	0	0	10
Diet Lemonade	1 serv (9 oz)	5	0	2	0	4
Iced Tea Sweetened	1 serv (9 oz)	150	0	38	0	50
Iced Tea Unsweetened	1 serv (9 oz)	0	0	0	0	50
Lemonade	1 serv (9 oz)	90	0	23	0	4
DESSERTS						
Cheesecake	1 slice (3.1 oz)	270	21	7	10	510
Cheesecake w/ Blueberry Topping	1 slice (4.1 oz)	290	23	9	10	550
Cheesecake w/ Strawberry Topping	1 slice (4.1 oz)	290	23	3	10	580
Fudge Nut Brownie	1 (2.6 oz)	350	16	41	30	650
Icedream Cone	1 sm (4.5 oz)	140	4	16	40	240
Icedream Cup	1 sm (7.5 oz)	350	10	50	70	390
Lemon Pie	1 slice (4 oz)	320	16	40	135	280
MAIN MENU SELECTIONS						
Carrot & Raisin Salad	1 sm (2.7 oz)	150	2	28	6	650
Chargrilled Chicken Club Sandwich w/o Dressing	1 (8.2 oz)	390	12	38	70	980

FOOD	PORTION	CALS	FAT	CARB	CHOL	SOD
Chargrilled Chicken Deluxe Sandwich	1 (7.4 oz)	290	3	38	40	640
Chargrilled Chicken Garden Salad	1 serv (14 oz)	170	3	10	25	650
Chargrilled Chicken Sandwich	1 (5.3 oz)	280	3	36	40	640
Chargrilled Chicken w/o Bun Or Pickles	1 piece (2.8 oz)	130	3	0	30	630
Chick-n-Strips	4 (4.2 oz)	230	8	10	20	380
Chick-n-Strips Salad	1 serv (15.9 oz)	290	9	21	20	430
Chicken Deluxe Sandwich	1 (8 oz)	300	9	31	50	870
Chicken Salad Plate	1 serv (16.5 oz)	290	21	40	35	570
Chicken Salad Sandwich On Whole Wheat	1 (5.9 oz)	320	5	42	10	810
Chicken Sandwich	1 (5.9 oz)	290	9	29	50	870
Chicken w/o Bun Or Pickles	1 piece (3.7 oz)	160	8	1	45	690
Cole Slaw	1 sm (2.8 oz)	130	6	11	15	430
Hearty Breast of Chicken Soup	1 cup (7.6 oz)	110	1	10	45	760
Nuggets	8 (3.9 oz)	290	14	12	60	770
Tossed Salad	1 serv (4.6 oz)	70	5	13	0	0
Waffle Potato Fries	1 sm (3 oz)	290	10	49	5	960
Waffle Potato Fries w/o Salt	1 sm (3 oz)	290	10	49	5	80

CHILI'S
DESSERTS

FOOD	PORTION	CALS	FAT	CARB	CHOL	SOD
Diet By Chocolate Cake	1 serv	370	2	79	0	670
Diet By Chocolate Cake w/ Yogurt	1 serv	465	2	99	3	622
Diet By Chocolate Cake w/ Yogurt & Fudge Topping	1 serv	534	3	116	3	703

MAIN MENU SELECTIONS

FOOD	PORTION	CALS	FAT	CARB	CHOL	SOD
Guiltless Grill Chicken Fajitas	1 serv	726	13	108	44	4759
Guiltless Grill Chicken Platter	1 serv	563	7	83	58	3284
Guiltless Grill Chicken Salad w/ Dressing	1 serv	254	3	27	47	1475
Guiltless Grill Chicken Sandwich	1	527	7	70	43	2923
Guiltless Grill Veggie Pasta	1 serv	590	11	98	55	964

FOOD	PORTION	CALS	FAT	CARB	CHOL	SOD
Guiltless Grill Veggie Pasta w/ Chicken	1 serv	696	13	102	97	1399

CHURCH'S CHICKEN

FOOD	PORTION	CALS	FAT	CARB	CHOL	SOD
Apple Pie	1 serv (3.1 oz)	280	12	41	<5	340
Biscuit	1 (2.1 oz)	250	16	26	<5	640
Breast	1 serv (2.8 oz)	200	12	4	65	510
Cajun Rice	1 serv (3.1 oz)	130	7	16	5	260
Cole Slaw	1 serv (3 oz)	92	6	8	0	230
Corn On The Cob	1 serv (5.7 oz)	139	3	24	0	15
French Fries	1 serv (2.7 oz)	210	11	29	0	60
Leg	1 serv (2 oz)	140	9	2	45	160
Okra	1 serv (2.8 oz)	210	16	19	0	520
Potatoes & Gravy	1 serv (3.7 oz)	90	3	14	0	520
Tender Strip	1 (1.1 oz)	80	4	5	15	140
Thigh	1 serv (2.8 oz)	230	16	5	80	520
Wing	1 serv (3.1 oz)	250	16	8	60	540

COLOMBO FROZEN YOGURT

FOOD	PORTION	CALS	FAT	CARB	CHOL	SOD
Alpine Strawberry Nonfat	4 fl oz	100	0	22	0	60
Banana Strawberry Nonfat	4 fl oz	50	0	12	0	10
Brazilian Banana Nonfat	4 fl oz	100	0	22	0	60
Butter Pecan Nonfat	4 fl oz	100	0	22	0	60
Cappuccino Nonfat	4 fl oz	100	0	22	0	60
Cherry Amaretto Nonfat	4 fl oz	50	0	12	0	10
Cherry Vanilla Nonfat	4 fl oz	100	0	22	0	60
Chocolate Nonfat	4 fl oz	50	0	12	0	10
Coconut Cooler Nonfat	4 fl oz	100	0	22	0	60
Cool Berry Blue Nonfat	4 fl oz	100	0	22	0	60
Country Pumpkin Nonfat	4 fl oz	100	0	22	0	60
Double Dutch Chocolate Nonfat	4 fl oz	100	0	22	0	60
Egg Nog Nonfat	4 fl oz	100	0	22	0	60
French Vanilla Lowfat	4 fl oz	110	2	22	5	60
French Vanilla Nonfat	4 fl oz	100	0	22	0	60
Georgia Peach Nonfat	4 fl oz	100	0	22	0	60
German Fudge Chocolate Nonfat	4 fl oz	100	0	22	0	60
Hawaiian Pineapple Nonfat	4 fl oz	100	0	22	0	60
Hazelnut Amaretto Nonfat	4 fl oz	100	0	22	0	60
Honey Almond Nonfat	4 fl oz	100	0	22	0	60
Irish Cream Nonfat	4 fl oz	100	0	22	0	60

FOOD	PORTION	CALS	FAT	CARB	CHOL	SOD
New York Cheesecake Nonfat	4 fl oz	100	0	22	0	60
Old World Chocolate Lowfat	4 fl oz	110	2	22	5	60
Orange Bavarian Creme Nonfat	4 fl oz	100	0	22	0	60
Peanut Butter Lowfat	4 fl oz	110	2	22	5	60
Pecan Praline Nonfat	4 fl oz	100	0	22	0	60
Pina Colada Nonfat	4 fl oz	100	0	22	0	60
Raspberry Nonfat	4 fl oz	50	0	12	0	10
Rockin' Raspberry Nonfat	4 fl oz	100	0	22	0	60
Simply Vanilla Lowfat	4 fl oz	110	2	22	5	60
Simply Vanilla Nonfat	4 fl oz	100	0	22	0	60
Strawberry Nonfat	4 fl oz	50	0	12	0	10
Tropical Tango Nonfat	4 fl oz	100	0	22	0	60
Vanilla Nonfat	4 fl oz	50	0	12	0	10
White Chocolate Almond Nonfat	4 fl oz	100	0	22	0	60
Wild Strawberry Lowfat	4 fl oz	110	2	22	5	60

DAIRY QUEEN
FOOD SELECTIONS

FOOD	PORTION	CALS	FAT	CARB	CHOL	SOD
Chicken Breast Fillet Sandwich	1 (6.7 oz)	430	20	37	55	760
Chicken Strip Basket	1 serv (14.5 oz)	1000	50	102	55	2260
Chili 'n' Cheese Dog	1 (5 oz)	330	21	22	45	1090
DQ Homestyle Bacon Double Cheeseburger	1 (8.9 oz)	610	36	31	130	1380
DQ Homestyle Cheeseburger	1 (5.3 oz)	340	17	29	55	850
DQ Homestyle Double Cheeseburger	1 (7.7 oz)	540	31	30	115	1130
DQ Homestyle Hamburger	1 (4.8 oz)	290	12	29	45	630
DQ Ultimate Burger	1 (9.4 oz)	670	43	29	135	1210
French Fries	1 lg (4.9 oz)	440	23	53	0	790
French Fries	1 med (3.9 oz)	350	18	42	0	630
Grilled Chicken Sandwich	1 (6.5 oz)	310	10	30	50	1040
Hot Dog	1 (3.5 oz)	240	14	19	25	730
Onion Rings	1 serv (4 oz)	320	16	39	0	180

ICE CREAM

FOOD	PORTION	CALS	FAT	CARB	CHOL	SOD
Banana Split	1 (12.9 oz)	510	12	96	30	180

FOOD	PORTION	CALS	FAT	CARB	CHOL	SOD
Blizzard Chocolate Chip Cookie Dough	1 med (15.4 oz)	950	36	143	75	660
Blizzard Chocolate Chip Cookie Dough	1 sm (12 oz)	660	24	99	55	440
Blizzard Chocolate Sandwich Cookie	1 med (11.4 oz)	640	23	97	45	500
Blizzard Chocolate Sandwich Cookie	1 sm (12 oz)	520	18	79	40	380
Breeze Heath	1 med (14.2 oz)	710	18	123	20	580
Breeze Heath	1 sm (10.2 oz)	470	10	85	10	380
Breeze Strawberry	1 med (13.4 oz)	460	1	99	10	270
Breeze Strawberry	1 sm (12 oz)	320	1	68	5	190
Buster Bar	1 (5.2 oz)	450	28	41	15	280
Chocolate Malt	1 med (19.9 oz)	880	22	153	70	500
Chocolate Malt	1 sm (14.7 oz)	650	16	111	55	370
Cone Chocolate	1 med (6.9 oz)	340	11	53	30	160
Cone Chocolate	1 sm (5 oz)	240	8	37	20	115
Cone Dipped	1 med (7.7 oz)	490	24	59	30	190
Cone Dipped	1 sm (5.5 oz)	340	17	42	20	130
Cone Vanilla	1 lg (8.9 oz)	410	12	65	40	200
Cone Vanilla	1 med (6.9 oz)	330	9	53	30	160
Cone Vanilla	1 sm (5 oz)	230	7	38	20	115
Cone Yogurt	1 med (6.9 oz)	260	1	56	5	160
Cup Of Yogurt	1 med (6.7 oz)	230	1	48	5	150
DQ 8 Inch Round Cake Undecorated	1/8 of cake (6.2 oz)	340	12	53	25	250
DQ Fudge Bar No Sugar Added	1 (2.3 oz)	50	0	13	0	70
DQ Lemon Freez'r	1/2 cup (3.2 oz)	80	0	20	0	10
DQ Nonfat Frozen Yogurt	1/2 cup (3 oz)	100	0	21	<5	70
DQ Sandwich	1 (2.1 oz)	150	5	24	5	115
DQ Soft Serve Chocolate	1/2 cup (3.3 oz)	150	5	22	15	75
DQ Soft Serve Vanilla	1/2 cup (3.3 oz)	140	5	22	15	70
DQ Treatzza Pizza Heath	1/8 of pie (2.3 oz)	180	7	28	5	160
DQ Treatzza Pizza M&M	1/8 of pie (2.4 oz)	190	7	29	5	160
DQ Vanilla Orange Bar No Sugar Added	1 (2.3 oz)	60	0	17	0	40
Dilly Bar Chocolate	1 (3 oz)	210	13	21	10	75
Fudge Cake Supreme	1 serv (11.2 oz)	890	38	124	65	960
Misty Slush	1 med (20.9 oz)	290	0	74	0	30
Misty Slush	1 sm (15.9 oz)	220	0	56	0	20
Peanut Buster Parfait	1 (10.7 oz)	730	31	99	35	400

FOOD	PORTION	CALS	FAT	CARB	CHOL	SOD
Shake Chocolate	1 med (18.9 oz)	770	20	130	70	420
Shake Chocolate	1 sm (13.9 oz)	560	15	94	50	310
Starkiss	1 (3 oz)	80	0	21	0	10
Strawberry Shortcake	1 (8.5 oz)	430	14	70	60	360
Sundae Chocolate	1 med (8.2 oz)	400	10	71	30	210
Sundae Chocolate	1 sm (5.7 oz)	280	7	49	20	140
Yogurt Sundae Strawberry	1 med (8.2 oz)	280	1	61	5	160

D'ANGELO SANDWICH SHOPS
SALADS AND SALAD BARS

FOOD	PORTION	CALS	FAT	CARB	CHOL	SOD
D'Lite Chicken	1 serv	325	4	34	49	980
D'Lite Roast Beef	1 serv	350	5	33	63	890
D'Lite Tuna	1 serv	305	2	33	32	805
D'Lite Turkey	1 serv	375	4	33	64	660

SANDWICHES

FOOD	PORTION	CALS	FAT	CARB	CHOL	SOD
D'Lite Pokket Classic Vegetable	1	340	10	48	23	960
D'Lite Pokket Crunchy Vegetable	1	350	10	52	23	1000
D'Lite Pokket Ginger Stir Fry Chicken	1	400	5	55	72	1240
D'Lite Pokket Roast Beef	1	330	6	42	48	710
D'Lite Pokket Spicy Steak	1	425	11	59	41	735
D'Lite Pokket Stuffed Turkey	1	510	8	71	82	880
D'Lite Pokket Turkey	1	350	2	40	79	490
D'Lite Small Sub Crunchy Vegetable	1	385	11	56	23	1045
D'Lite Small Sub Roast Beef	1	365	7	45	48	755
D'Lite Small Sub Stuffed Turkey	1	545	9	75	82	920
D'Lite Small Sub Turkey	1	365	4	43	79	535
Pokket Chicken Stir Fry	1	360	5	46	70	1240

DELTACO
BEVERAGES

FOOD	PORTION	CALS	FAT	CARB	CHOL	SOD
Coffee	1 serv	6	tr	1	0	4
Coke Classic	1 lg	287	0	76	0	35
Coke Classic	1 med	198	0	52	0	24
Coke Classic	1 sm	144	0	38	0	17
Coke Classic Best Value	1 serv	395	0	104	0	48
Diet Coke	1 lg	2	0	tr	0	39

FOOD	PORTION	CALS	FAT	CARB	CHOL	SOD
Diet Coke	1 med	1	0	tr	0	27
Diet Coke	1 sm	1	0	tr	0	20
Diet Coke Best Value	1 serv	2	0	tr	0	53
Iced Tea	1 lg	6	tr	2	0	26
Iced Tea	1 med	4	tr	1	0	18
Iced Tea	1 sm	3	tr	tr	0	13
Iced Tea Best Value	1 serv	8	tr	2	0	36
M&M's Toppers	1 serv	256	8	42	19	112
Milk	1 serv	126	3	15	12	152
Mr Pibb	1 lg	283	0	72	0	47
Mr Pibb	1 med	195	0	49	0	32
Mr Pibb	1 sm	142	0	36	0	23
Mr Pibb Best Value	1 serv	390	0	99	0	64
Orange Juice	1 serv	83	tr	2	0	19
Oreos Toppers	1 serv	257	10	42	19	188
Shake Chocolate	1 med	755	22	135	55	415
Shake Chocolate	1 sm	549	16	98	40	302
Shake Orange	1 med	837	22	162	55	322
Shake Orange	1 sm	609	16	118	40	234
Shake Strawberry	1 med	668	22	120	55	305
Shake Strawberry	1 sm	486	16	87	40	222
Shake Vanilla	1 med	707	25	121	63	353
Shake Vanilla	1 sm	514	18	88	46	257
Snickers Toppers	1 serv	254	10	41	18	128
Sprite	1 lg	287	0	72	0	71
Sprite	1 med	198	0	49	0	49
Sprite	1 sm	144	0	36	0	35
Sprite Best Value	1 serv	395	0	99	0	97
BREAKFAST SELECTIONS						
Burrito Beef And Egg	1	529	27	43	328	929
Burrito Breakfast	1	256	11	30	90	409
Burrito Egg And Cheese	1	443	22	40	305	792
Burrito Egg and Bean	1	470	22	45	305	1035
Burrito Steak And Egg	1	500	25	41	337	1068
CHILDREN'S MENU SELECTIONS						
Kid's Meal Hamburger	1 meal	617	20	96	29	799
Kid's Meal Taco	1 meal	532	17	87	16	373
MAIN MENU SELECTIONS						
American Cheese	1 slice	53	4	tr	14	203
Beans And Cheese	1	122	3	17	9	892
Burrito Chicken	1	264	10	32	36	771
Burrito Combination	1	413	17	46	49	1035
Burrito Del Beef	1	440	20	43	63	878
Burrito Deluxe Chicken	1	549	34	40	83	978

FOOD	PORTION	CALS	FAT	CARB	CHOL	SOD
Burrito Deluxe Combo	1	453	20	49	59	1047
Burrito Deluxe Del Beef	1	479	23	45	73	890
Burrito Green	1	229	8	32	15	714
Burrito Green Regular	1	330	11	46	22	1149
Burrito Macho Beef	1	893	41	84	139	1969
Burrito Macho Combo	1	774	31	87	100	2180
Burrito Red	1	235	8	32	17	656
Burrito Red Regular	1	342	12	46	26	1033
Burrito Spicy Chicken	1	392	11	59	35	1243
Burrito The Works	1	448	18	60	27	1248
Cheeseburger	1	284	13	26	42	852
Chicken Salad	1	254	19	8	58	476
Chicken Salad Deluxe	1	716	47	55	98	1419
Del Burger	1	385	20	35	42	1065
Del Cheeseburger	1	439	25	35	55	1268
Double Del Cheeseburger	1	618	39	36	108	1638
French Fries	1 lg	566	26	76	0	318
French Fries	1 reg	404	19	54	0	227
French Fries	1 sm	242	11	32	0	136
Fries Chili Cheese	1 serv	562	30	58	38	846
Fries Deluxe Chili Cheese	1 serv	600	33	61	48	855
Fries Nacho	1 serv	669	34	80	2	926
Guacamole	1 oz	60	6	2	0	130
Hamburger	1	231	8	26	29	649
Hot Sauce	1 pkg	2	tr	tr	0	38
Nacho Cheese Sauce	1 side order	100	8	4	2	401
Nachos	1 serv	390	32	39	2	504
Nachos Macho	1	1089	61	110	46	1740
Quesadilla	1	257	12	26	30	455
Quesadilla Chicken	1	544	31	38	113	1147
Quesadilla Regular	1	483	27	37	75	871
Quesadilla Spicy Jack	1	254	12	26	30	402
Quesadilla Spicy Jack Chicken	1	537	30	38	114	1214
Quesadilla Spicy Jack Regular	1	476	27	37	76	938
Salsa	2 oz	14	tr	3	tr	308
Salsa Dressing	1 oz	33	3	1	10	85
Soft Taco	1	146	6	17	16	223
Soft Taco Chicken	1	197	11	16	35	401
Soft Taco Deluxe Double Beef	1	211	11	20	35	283
Soft Taco Double Beef	1	178	8	18	25	274

FOOD	PORTION	CALS	FAT	CARB	CHOL	SOD
Sour Cream	1 oz	60	6	tr	20	15
Taco	1	140	8	10	16	99
Taco Chicken	1	186	13	10	35	276
Taco Deluxe Double Beef	1	205	13	13	35	159
Taco Double Beef	1	172	10	12	25	150
Taco Salad	1	235	19	9	31	268
Taco Salad Deluxe	1	741	49	57	83	1280
Tostada	1	140	8	12	15	333

DENNY'S
BEVERAGES

FOOD	PORTION	CALS	FAT	CARB	CHOL	SOD
2% Milk	1 serv (10 oz)	151	6	15	22	152
Chocolate Milk	1 serv (10 oz)	235	9	30	37	189
Coffee French Vanilla	1 serv (8 oz)	76	1	16	2	4
Coffee Hazelnut	1 serv (8 oz)	66	1	14	2	4
Coffee Irish Cream	1 serv (8 oz)	73	1	16	2	4
Grapefruit Juice	1 serv (10 oz)	115	0	29	0	0
Hot Chocolate	1 serv (8 oz)	90	2	18	0	153
Lemonade	1 serv (16 oz)	150	0	35	0	38
Orange Juice	1 serv (10 oz)	126	0	31	0	31
Raspberry Ice Tea	1 serv (16 oz)	78	0	21	0	0
Tomato Juice	1 serv (10 oz)	56	0	11	0	921

BREAKFAST SELECTIONS

FOOD	PORTION	CALS	FAT	CARB	CHOL	SOD
All American Slam	1 serv (15 oz)	1028	87	24	724	1942
Applesauce	1 serv (3 oz)	60	0	15	0	13
Bacon	4 strips (1 oz)	162	18	1	36	640
Bagel Dry	1 (3 oz)	235	1	46	0	495
Banana	1 (4 oz)	110	0	29	0	0
Banana Strawberry Medley	1 serv (4 oz)	108	1	27	0	6
Biscuit Plain	1 (3 oz)	375	22	40	0	750
Biscuit w/ Sausage Gravy	1 serv (7 oz)	570	38	45	24	1475
Blueberry Topping	1 serv (3 oz)	106	0	26	0	15
Canadian Bacon	1 serv (3 oz)	110	5	1	43	1039
Cantaloup	1 serv (3 oz)	32	0	8	0	16
Cheddar Cheese Omelette	1 serv (13 oz)	770	62	24	675	1133
Cherry Topping	1 serv (3 oz)	86	0	21	0	5
Chicken Fried Steak & Eggs	1 serv (14 oz)	723	56	31	452	1505
Country Scramble	1 serv (16 oz)	795	50	67	409	1819
Cream Cheese	1 oz	100	10	1	31	6
Egg	1 (2 oz)	134	12	1	205	61

FOOD	PORTION	CALS	FAT	CARB	CHOL	SOD
Egg Beaters	1 serv (2.3 oz)	71	5	1	1	138
Eggs Benedict	1 serv (19 oz)	860	56	55	525	1943
English Muffin Dry	1 (4 oz)	125	1	24	0	198
Farmer's Omelette	1 serv (18 oz)	912	69	38	633	1816
French Slam	1 serv (14 oz)	1029	71	58	777	1428
French Toast	2 pieces (8 oz)	510	25	51	317	413
Fresh Fruit Mix	1 serv (3 oz)	36	0	9	0	16
Grapefruit	½ (5 oz)	60	0	16	0	0
Grapes	1 serv (3 oz)	55	1	15	0	0
Grits	1 serv (4 oz)	80	0	18	0	520
Ham	1 serv (3 oz)	94	3	2	23	761
Ham'n'Cheddar Omelette	1 serv (14 oz)	743	55	24	657	1518
Hashed Browns	1 serv (4 oz)	218	14	20	0	424
Hashed Browns Covered	1 serv (6 oz)	318	23	21	30	604
Hashed Browns Covered & Smothered	1 serv (8 oz)	359	26	26	30	790
Honeydew	1 serv (3 oz)	31	0	8	0	22
Junior Meals Basic Breakfast	1 serv (9 oz)	558	39	38	230	1103
Junior Meals Junior French Slam	1 serv (7 oz)	461	35	18	386	663
Junior Meals Junior Grand Slam	1 serv (5 oz)	397	25	33	230	1118
Junior Meals Junior Waffle Supreme	1 serv (4 oz)	190	11	20	73	102
Meat Lover's Sampler	1 serv (14 oz)	806	62	24	481	2211
Moon Over My Hammy	1 serv (12 oz)	807	48	46	430	2247
Muffin Blueberry	1 (3 oz)	309	14	42	0	190
Oatmeal	1 serv (4 oz)	100	2	18	0	175
Original Grand Slam	1 serv (10 oz)	795	50	65	460	2237
Pancakes	3 (5 oz)	491	7	95	0	1818
Pork Chop & Eggs	1 serv (12 oz)	555	36	21	469	968
Porterhouse Steak & Eggs	1 serv (18 oz)	1223	95	21	570	1369
Ready To Eat Cereal	1 serv (1 oz)	100	0	23	0	276
Sausage	4 links (3 oz)	354	32	0	64	944
Sausage Cheddar Omelette	1 serv (16 oz)	1036	86	24	721	1841
Scram Slam	1 serv (18 oz)	974	80	30	694	1750
Senior Belgian Waffle Slam	1 serv (6 oz)	399	33	12	302	612
Senior Omelette	1 serv (12 oz)	623	47	27	439	1194
Senior Starter	1 serv (7 oz)	336	24	36	205	541
Senior Triple Play	1 serv (8 oz)	537	25	64	409	1445

FOOD	PORTION	CALS	FAT	CARB	CHOL	SOD
Sirloin Steak & Eggs	1 serv (13 oz)	808	64	21	474	952
Slim Slam	1 serv (14 oz)	638	12	98	34	1772
Southern Slam	1 serv (13 oz)	1065	84	47	484	2449
Strawberries w/ Sugar	1 serv (3 oz)	115	1	26	0	12
Strawberry Topping	1 serv (3 oz)	115	1	26	0	12
Sunshine Slam	1 serv (8 oz)	537	25	64	409	1445
Super Play It Again Slam	1 serv (15 oz)	1192	75	98	690	3555
Syrup	3 tbsp (1.5 oz)	143	0	36	0	26
Syrup Reduced Calorie	1 serv (1.5 oz)	25	0	6	0	96
T-Bone Steak & Eggs	1 serv (16 oz)	1045	82	21	530	1191
Toast Dry	1 slice (1 oz)	92	1	17	0	166
Ultimate Omelette	1 serv (17 oz)	780	62	29	639	1360
Veggie Cheese Omelette	1 serv (16 oz)	714	53	29	644	955
Waffle	1 (6 oz)	304	21	23	146	200
Whipped Cream	1 serv (2 oz)	23	2	2	7	3
Whipped Margarine	1 serv (0.5 oz)	87	10	0	0	117
DESSERTS						
Apple Pie	1 serv (7 oz)	430	20	59	<5	390
Apple Pie w/ Equal	1 serv (7 oz)	370	20	43	<5	360
Banana Split	1 serv (19 oz)	894	43	121	78	177
Blueberry Topping	1 serv (3 oz)	106	0	26	0	15
Cheesecake Pie	1 serv (4 oz)	470	27	48	90	280
Cherry Pie	1 serv (7 oz)	540	21	83	<5	430
Cherry Topping	1 serv (3 oz)	86	0	21	0	5
Chocolate Cake	1 serv (4 oz)	370	17	53	29	374
Chocolate Pecan Pie	1 serv (6 oz)	790	37	107	70	460
Chocolate Shake	1 serv (10 oz)	579	27	77	108	278
Chocolate Topping	1 serv (2 oz)	317	25	27	0	83
Coconut Cream Pie	1 serv (7 oz)	480	26	58	15	440
Double Scoop Sundae	1 serv (6 oz)	375	27	29	74	86
Dutch Apple Pie	1 serv (7 oz)	440	19	65	0	290
French Silk Pie	1 serv (6 oz)	650	43	60	165	220
Fudge Topping	1 serv (2 oz)	201	10	30	3	96
German Chocolate Pie	1 serv (7 oz)	580	33	66	15	460
Hot Fudge Cake Sundae	1 serv (8 oz)	687	38	83	62	486
Ice Cream Float	1 serv (12 oz)	280	10	47	39	109
Key Lime Pie	1 serv (6 oz)	600	27	79	35	300
Lemon Meringue Pie	1 serv (7 oz)	460	17	71	95	310
Pecan Pie	1 serv (6 oz)	600	28	81	50	430
Single Scoop Sundae	1 serv (3 oz)	188	14	14	37	43
Strawberry Topping	1 serv (3 oz)	115	1	26	0	12
Vanilla Shake	1 serv (11 oz)	581	27	77	108	236

FOOD	PORTION	CALS	FAT	CARB	CHOL	SOD
MAIN MENU SELECTIONS						
BBQ Sauce	1 serv (1.5 oz)	47	1	11	0	595
Bacon Cheddar Burger	1 (14 oz)	935	63	43	164	1732
Bacon Lettuce & Tomato Sandwich	1 (6 oz)	634	46	37	54	1116
Baked Potato Plain	1 (6 oz)	186	0	43	0	14
Battered Cod Dinner w/ Tartar Sauce	1 serv (9 oz)	732	47	48	105	1335
Broccoli In Butter Sauce	2 serv (4 oz)	50	2	7	5	280
Brown Gravy	1 serv (1 oz)	13	0	2	0	184
Buffalo Chicken Strips	1 serv (10 oz)	734	42	43	96	1673
Buffalo Wings	12 pieces (15 oz)	856	54	1	500	5552
Carrots In Honey Glaze	2 serv (4 oz)	80	3	12	0	220
Charleston Chicken Sandwich	1 (11 oz)	632	32	53	81	1967
Chicken Quesadilla	1 serv (16 oz)	827	55	43	181	1982
Chicken Fried Chicken	1 serv (6 oz)	327	18	16	65	993
Chicken Fried Steak w/ Gravy	1 serv (4 oz)	265	17	14	27	668
Chicken Gravy	1 serv (1 oz)	14	1	2	2	139
Chicken Melt Sandwich	1 (7 oz)	520	29	43	39	1096
Chicken Strip w/ Dressing	1 serv (10 oz)	635	25	55	95	1510
Chicken Strips	5 pieces (10 oz)	720	33	56	95	1666
Classic Burger	1 (11 oz)	673	40	42	106	1142
Classic Burger w/ Cheese	1 (13 oz)	836	53	43	137	1595
Club Sandwich	1	485	35	40	90	1385
Corn In Butter Sauce	2 serv (4 oz)	120	4	19	5	260
Cornbread Stuffing Plain	1 serv (2 oz)	182	9	20	0	405
Cottage Cheese	1 serv (3 oz)	72	3	2	10	281
Country Gravy	1 serv (1 oz)	17	1	2	0	93
Delidinger Sandwich	1 (14 oz)	852	45	62	80	3142
Deluxe Grilled Cheese Sandwich	1 (7 oz)	482	26	44	1	1135
Dinner Roll	1 (1.5 oz)	132	2	26	0	265
French Fries Unsalted	1 serv (4 oz)	323	14	44	0	130
Fried Fish Sandwich	1 (11 oz)	905	56	74	69	1704
Gardenburger Patty	1 patty (3.4 oz)	160	3	22	10	390
Gardenburger Patty w/ Bun & Fat Free Honey Mustard Dressing	1 serv (11.1 oz)	653	32	72	26	1017

FOOD	PORTION	CALS	FAT	CARB	CHOL	SOD
Green Beans w/ Bacon	2 serv (4 oz)	60	4	6	5	390
Green Peas In Butter Sauce	2 serv (4 oz)	100	2	14	5	360
Grilled Alaskan Salmon	1 serv (7 oz)	296	14	1	102	257
Grilled Chicken Breast	1 serv (4 oz)	130	4	0	67	566
Grilled Chicken Dinner	1 serv (4 oz)	130	4	0	67	560
Grilled Chicken Sandwich	1 (11 oz)	509	19	52	83	1809
Grilled Chopped Steak w/ Gravy	1 serv (10 oz)	400	26	12	91	447
Grilled Mushrooms	1 serv (2 oz)	14	0	2	0	0
Ham & Swiss On Rye	1 (9 oz)	533	31	40	36	1638
Hashed Browns	1 serv (4 oz)	218	14	20	0	424
Herb Toast	1 serv (2 oz)	200	11	21	0	372
Horseradish Sauce	1 serv (1.5 oz)	170	20	3	43	227
Junior Meals Junior Burger	1 serv (3 oz)	261	15	16	41	115
Junior Meals Junior Chicken Strips	1 serv (5 oz)	318	12	28	48	755
Junior Meals Junior Fried Fish	1 serv (5 oz)	465	34	25	68	743
Junior Meals Junior Grilled Cheese	1 serv (4 oz)	375	22	35	1	811
Junior Meals Junior Shrimp Basket	1 serv (4 oz)	291	16	27	60	774
Lunch Basket Charleston Chicken Ranch Melt	1 serv (14 oz)	975	59	68	96	2479
Lunch Basket Chicken Strips	1 serv (8 oz)	568	26	45	70	1239
Lunch Basket Classic Burger	1 serv (12 oz)	674	39	42	121	1161
Lunch Basket Delidinger	1 serv (14 oz)	852	45	62	80	3142
Lunch Basket Five Star Philly	1 serv (10 oz)	657	29	55	97	652
Lunch Basket Patty Melt	1 serv (8 oz)	696	42	39	129	1026
Mashed Potatoes Plain	1 serv (6 oz)	105	1	21	0	378
Mayonnaise	2 tbsp (1 oz)	200	22	1	16	159
Mozzarella Sticks w/ Sauce	8 pieces (10 oz)	756	43	56	48	5423
Onion Ring Basket	1 serv (5 oz)	439	27	44	7	1158
Onion Rings	1 serv (3 oz)	264	16	27	4	695
Patty Melt Sandwich	1 (8 oz)	695	44	39	114	1007
Pork Chop Dinner w/ Gravy	1 serv (8 oz)	386	24	0	121	844

FOOD	PORTION	CALS	FAT	CARB	CHOL	SOD
Porterhouse Steak	1 (14 oz)	708	54	0	161	713
Pot Roast Dinner w/ Gravy	1 serv (7 oz)	260	11	5	140	1085
Rice Pilaf	1 serv (3 oz)	112	2	21	0	328
Roast Turkey & Stuffing	1 serv (12 oz)	701	27	63	100	2346
Sampler	1 serv (15 oz)	1120	59	104	69	3430
Seasoned Fries	1 serv (4 oz)	261	12	35	0	556
Senior Battered Cod	1 serv (5 oz)	465	34	25	68	743
Senior Chicken Fried Steak	1 serv (8 oz)	341	18	29	27	943
Senior Grilled Cheese Sandwich	1 serv	360	25	21	50	1190
Senior Grilled Chicken Breast	1 serv (6 oz)	219	6	16	67	880
Senior Liver w/ Bacon & Onions	1 serv (8 oz)	322	19	20	270	643
Senior Pork Chop	1 serv (4 oz)	193	12	0	60	422
Senior Pot Roast	1 serv (5 oz)	149	6	6	71	818
Senior Roast Turkey & Stuffing	1 serv (8 oz)	596	25	61	51	1750
Senior Sandwich Ham & Swiss	1 serv (9 oz)	497	30	34	36	1537
Senior Sandwich Turkey	1	340	27	26	75	1000
Shrimp Dinner	1 serv (8 oz)	558	32	49	135	1114
Sirloin Steak Dinner	1 serv (5.5 oz)	271	21	0	62	273
Sliced Tomatoes	3 slices (2 oz)	13	0	3	0	6
Sour Cream	1 serv (1.5 oz)	91	9	2	19	23
Steak & Shrimp Dinner w/ Gravy	1 serv (9 oz)	645	42	31	150	1143
Super Bird Sandwich	1 (9 oz)	620	32	48	60	1880
T-Bone Steak Dinner	1 serv (10 oz)	530	40	0	121	534
Turkey Breast On Multigrain	1 (9 oz)	476	26	39	57	1107
SALAD DRESSINGS						
Bleu Cheese	1 oz	124	12	4	18	405
Caesar	1 oz	142	15	1	2	340
Creamy Italian	1 oz	106	10	4	0	306
Fat Free Honey Mustard	1 oz	38	0	9	0	121
French	1 oz	106	10	3	7	274
Oriental Peanut Dressing	1 serv (1 oz)	106	8	6	0	399
Ranch	1 oz	101	11	1	8	215
Reduced Calorie French	1 oz	76	5	8	0	265
Reduced Calorie Italian	1 oz	32	1	3	0	515
Thousand Island	1 oz	104	10	2	21	208

FOOD	PORTION	CALS	FAT	CARB	CHOL	SOD
SALADS AND SALAD BARS						
Buffalo Chicken Salad	1 serv (17 oz)	615	37	36	88	1258
Fried Chicken Salad	1 serv (13 oz)	506	31	30	94	1174
Garden Chicken Delight Salad	1 serv (16 oz)	277	5	30	67	785
Grilled Chicken Caesar Salad w/ Dressing	1 serv (13 oz)	655	47	23	86	1728
Oriental Chicken Salad w/ Dressing	1 serv (20 oz)	568	26	49	67	1656
Side Caesar w/ Dressing	1 serv (6 oz)	338	25	20	7	725
Side Garden Salad w/ Dressing	1 serv (7 oz)	113	4	16	0	147
SOUPS						
Cheese	1 serv (8 oz)	293	23	13	19	895
Chicken Noodle	1 serv (8 oz)	60	2	8	10	640
Clam Chowder	1 serv (8 oz)	214	11	22	5	903
Cream Of Broccoli	1 serv (8 oz)	193	12	15	0	818
Cream Of Potato	1 serv (8 oz)	222	12	23	0	761
Split Pea	1 serv (8 oz)	146	6	18	5	819
Vegetable Beef	1 serv (8 oz)	79	1	11	5	820

DOMINO'S PIZZA
12 INCH MEDIUM PIZZAS

FOOD	PORTION	CALS	FAT	CARB	CHOL	SOD
Add A Topping Anchovies	1 topping serv	23	1	0	9	395
Add A Topping Bacon	1 topping serv	81	7	tr	12	226
Add A Topping Banana Peppers	1 topping serv	3	tr	1	—	92
Add A Topping Canned Mushrooms	1 topping serv	4	tr	1	0	75
Add A Topping Cheddar Cheese	1 topping serv	57	5	tr	15	88
Add A Topping Cooked Beef	1 topping serv	56	5	tr	11	154
Add A Topping Extra Cheese	1 topping serv	48	4	1	7	150
Add A Topping Fresh Mushrooms	1 topping serv	4	tr	1	0	1
Add A Topping Green Olives	1 topping serv	12	1	tr	0	255
Add A Topping Green Peppers	1 topping serv	3	tr	1	0	tr
Add A Topping Ham	1 topping serv	18	1	tr	7	162
Add A Topping Italian Sausage	1 topping serv	55	4	2	11	171

FOOD	PORTION	CALS	FAT	CARB	CHOL	SOD
Add A Topping Onion	1 topping serv	4	tr	1	0	tr
Add A Topping Pepperoni	1 topping serv	62	6	tr	13	199
Add A Topping Pineapple Tidbits	1 topping serv	10	0	2	0	1
Add A Topping Ripe Olives	1 topping serv	14	1	1	0	71
Hand-Tossed Cheese	2 slices (5.2 oz)	347	11	49	15	723
Thin Crust Cheese	¼ pie (3.7 oz)	271	12	31	15	809
14 INCH LARGE PIZZAS						
Add A Topping Anchovies	1 topping serv	23	1	0	9	395
Add A Topping Bacon	1 topping serv	75	6	tr	11	207
Add A Topping Banana Peppers	1 topping serv	3	tr	1	—	81
Add A Topping Canned Mushrooms	1 topping serv	3	tr	1	0	50
Add A Topping Cheddar Cheese	1 topping serv	48	4	tr	12	73
Add A Topping Cooked Beef	1 topping serv	44	4	tr	8	123
Add A Topping Extra Cheese	1 topping serv	45	4	1	7	140
Add A Topping Fresh Mushrooms	1 topping serv	3	tr	1	0	tr
Add A Topping Green Peppers	1 topping serv	2	tr	1	0	tr
Add A Topping Ham	1 topping serv	17	1	tr	7	156
Add A Topping Italian Sausage	1 topping serv	44	3	1	9	137
Add A Topping Onion	1 topping serv	3	tr	1	0	tr
Add A Topping Pepperoni	1 topping serv	55	5	tr	12	177
Add A Topping Pineapple Tidbits	1 topping serv	8	0	tr	0	1
Add A Topping Ripe Olives	1 topping serv	12	1	1	0	63
Deep Dish Cheese	2 slices (6.1 oz)	455	20	54	18	1029
Hand-Tossed Cheese	2 slices (4.8 oz)	317	10	45	14	669
Thin Crust Cheese	⅙ pie (3.5 oz)	253	11	29	14	757
6 INCH DEEP DISH PIZZAS						
Add A Topping Anchovies	1 topping serv	45	2	0	18	790

FOOD	PORTION	CALS	FAT	CARB	CHOL	SOD
Add A Topping Bacon	1 topping serv	82	7	tr	12	226
Add A Topping Banana Peppers	1 topping serv	3	tr	tr	—	73
Add A Topping Canned Mushrooms	1 topping serv	2	tr	tr	0	36
Add A Topping Cheddar Cheese	1 topping serv	86	7	tr	22	132
Add A Topping Cooked Beef	1 topping serv	44	4	tr	8	122
Add A Topping Extra Cheese	1 topping serv	57	5	1	9	180
Add A Topping Fresh Mushrooms	1 topping serv	2	tr	tr	0	tr
Add A Topping Green Olives	1 topping serv	10	1	tr	0	204
Add A Topping Green Peppers	1 topping serv	2	tr	tr	0	tr
Add A Topping Ham	1 topping serv	17	1	tr	7	156
Add A Topping Italian Sausage	1 topping serv	44	3	1	9	137
Add A Topping Onion	1 topping serv	3	tr	1	0	tr
Add A Topping Pepperoni	1 topping serv	50	5	tr	10	159
Add A Topping Pineapple Tidbits	1 topping serv	5	0	1	0	tr
Add A Topping Ripe Olives	1 topping serv	11	1	tr	0	57
Cheese	1 pie (7.6 oz)	595	27	68	23	1300
MAIN MENU SELECTIONS						
Breadstick	1 (0.8 oz)	78	3	11	0	158
Buffalo Wings Barbeque	1 piece (0.9 oz)	50	2	2	26	175
Buffalo Wings Hot	1 piece (0.9 oz)	45	2	1	26	354
Cheesy Bread	1 piece (1 oz)	103	5	11	5	187
Garden Salad	1 lg (7.7 oz)	39	tr	8	0	26
Garden Salad	1 sm (4.3 oz)	22	tr	4	0	14
SALAD DRESSINGS						
Marzetti Blue Cheese	1 serv (1.5 oz)	220	24	2	40	440
Marzetti Creamy Caesar	1 serv (1.5 oz)	200	22	2	10	470
Marzetti Fat Free Ranch	1 serv (1.5 oz)	40	0	10	0	560
Marzetti Honey French	1 serv (1.5 oz)	210	18	14	0	300
Marzetti House Italian	1 serv (1.5 oz)	220	24	1	0	440
Marzetti Light Italian	1 serv (1.5 oz)	20	1	2	0	780
Marzetti Ranch	1 serv (1.5 oz)	260	29	1	5	380

FOOD	PORTION	CALS	FAT	CARB	CHOL	SOD
Marzetti Thousand Island	1 serv (1.5 oz)	200	20	5	25	320

DUNKIN' DONUTS
BAGELS AND CREAM CHEESE

FOOD	PORTION	CALS	FAT	CARB	CHOL	SOD
Bagel Blueberry	1 (4.4 oz)	330	1	70	0	640
Bagel Cinnamon Raisin	1 (4.4 oz)	340	1	72	0	470
Bagel Egg	1 (4.4 oz)	340	2	69	40	670
Bagel Everything	1 (4.4 oz)	340	2	68	0	680
Bagel Garlic	1 (4.4 oz)	330	1	69	0	670
Bagel Onion	1 (4.4 oz)	320	1	66	0	650
Bagel Plain	1 (4.4 oz)	330	1	68	0	690
Bagel Poppy	1 (4.4 oz)	340	3	68	0	680
Bagel Pumpernickel	1 (4.4 oz)	340	2	70	0	660
Bagel Salt	1 (4.4 oz)	320	1	65	0	3170
Bagel Sticks Cinnamon Sugar	1 (2.9 oz)	210	1	45	0	410
Bagel Sticks Jalapeno Cheddar	1 (2.9 oz)	210	1	43	0	490
Bagel Sticks Santa Fe Ranch	1 (2.9 oz)	210	1	43	0	690
Bagel Sticks Spinach Romano	1 (2.9 oz)	210	1	43	0	520
Bagel Whole Wheat	1 (4.4 oz)	320	2	13	0	630
Cream Cheese Classic Lite	2 tbsp (1 oz)	60	5	3	15	115
Cream Cheese Classic Plain	2 tbsp (1 oz)	100	10	1	30	110
Cream Cheese Garden Veggie	2 tbsp (1 oz)	90	9	2	25	200
Cream Cheese Honey Walnut	2 tbsp (1 oz)	100	9	4	10	110
Cream Cheese Savory Chive	2 tbsp (1 oz)	100	10	2	30	125
Cream Cheese Smoked Salmon	2 tbsp (1 oz)	100	9	1	30	95
Cream Cheese Strawberry	2 tbsp (1 oz)	100	9	5	25	100
Super Bagel Glazed Apple Cinnamon	1 (4.6 oz)	350	1	74	0	550

BAKED SELECTIONS

FOOD	PORTION	CALS	FAT	CARB	CHOL	SOD
Bismark	1 (2.8 oz)	310	14	42	0	260
Bow Tie	1 (2.5 oz)	250	10	35	0	300
Brownie Blondie w/ Chocolate Chips	1 (2.4 oz)	300	13	41	25	150

FOOD	PORTION	CALS	FAT	CARB	CHOL	SOD
Brownie Fudge	1 (2.4 oz)	290	13	37	35	85
Brownie Peanut Butter Blondie	1 (2.4 oz)	330	18	36	25	300
Cake Donut Blueberry	1 (2.4 oz)	230	10	30	0	240
Cake Donut Blueberry Crumb	1 (2.6 oz)	260	11	36	0	260
Cake Donut Butternut	1 (2.6 oz)	340	20	35	0	360
Cake Donut Chocolate	1 (2.1 oz)	210	14	19	0	270
Cake Donut Chocolate Coconut	1 (2.4 oz)	250	15	25	0	270
Cake Donut Chocolate Glazed	1 (2.5 oz)	250	14	29	0	280
Cake Donut Cinnamon	1 (2.3 oz)	300	19	29	0	350
Cake Donut Coconut	1 (2.5 oz)	320	20	32	0	360
Cake Donut Double Chocolate	1 (2.6 oz)	260	14	30	0	280
Cake Donut Old Fashioned	1 (2.1 oz)	280	19	24	0	350
Cake Donut Peanut	1 (2.6 oz)	340	22	32	0	360
Cake Donut Powdered	1 (2.4 oz)	310	19	30	0	350
Cake Donut Sugared	1 (2.4 oz)	310	20	28	0	380
Cake Donut Toasted Coconut	1 (2.5 oz)	320	19	33	0	360
Cake Donut Whole Wheat Glazed	1 (2.7 oz)	230	11	31	0	340
Coffee Roll	1 (2.6 oz)	280	13	35	0	300
Coffee Roll Chocolate Frosted	1 (2.7 oz)	290	14	38	0	300
Coffee Roll Cinnamon Raisin	1 (3.1 oz)	330	13	48	0	300
Coffee Roll Maple Frosted	1 (2.7 oz)	300	13	40	0	300
Coffee Roll Vanilla Frosted	1 (2.7 oz)	300	13	40	0	300
Cookie Chocolate Chocolate Chunk	1 (1.5 oz)	200	11	26	30	160
Cookie Chocolate Chunk	1 (1.5 oz)	200	10	26	30	150
Cookie Chocolate Chunk w/ Nut	1 (1.5 oz)	200	11	25	30	150
Cookie Chocolate White Chocolate Chunk	1 (1.5 oz)	200	11	25	30	160
Cookie Oatmeal Raisin Pecan	1 (1.5 oz)	190	9	27	25	150

FOOD	PORTION	CALS	FAT	CARB	CHOL	SOD
Cookie Peanut Butter Chocolate Chunk w/ Nuts	1 (1.5 oz)	210	13	23	25	110
Cookie Peanut Butter Chocolate Chunk w/ Peanuts	1 (1.5 oz)	210	12	22	30	140
Croissant Almond	1 (2.7 oz)	360	21	38	10	300
Croissant Cheese	1 (2.5 oz)	240	15	28	5	260
Croissant Chocolate	1 (2.5 oz)	370	23	40	10	260
Croissant Plain	1 (2.1 oz)	270	17	27	5	260
Crullers/Sticks Dunkin' Donut	1 (2.1 oz)	240	14	26	0	370
Crullers/Sticks Glazed	1 (3 oz)	340	14	49	0	320
Crullers/Sticks Glazed Chocolate	1 (3.2 oz)	410	24	46	0	350
Crullers/Sticks Jelly	1 (3.2 oz)	330	14	48	0	350
Crullers/Sticks Plain	1 (2.1 oz)	260	14	29	0	300
Crullers/Sticks Powdered	1 (2.3 oz)	290	14	35	0	300
Crullers/Sticks Sugar	1 (2.2 oz)	270	14	31	0	300
Eclair	1 (3.2 oz)	290	12	42	0	280
English Muffin	1 (2 oz)	130	1	26	0	520
French Roll	1 (2.1 oz)	140	1	27	0	220
Fritter Apple	1 (3.3 oz)	300	13	41	0	320
Fritter Glazed	1 (2.7 oz)	290	13	39	0	300
Muffin Banana Nut	1 (3.3 oz)	340	12	53	35	210
Muffin Blueberry	1 (3.3 oz)	310	10	51	35	190
Muffin Cherry	1 (3.3 oz)	330	11	53	35	210
Muffin Chocolate Chip	1 (3.3 oz)	400	16	63	35	190
Muffin Corn	1 (3.3 oz)	350	14	51	50	310
Muffin Cranberry Orange Nut	1 (3.5 oz)	310	11	51	30	180
Muffin Honey Raisin Bran	1 (3.3 oz)	330	10	57	15	360
Muffin Lemon Poppy Seed	1 (3.3 oz)	360	13	57	40	440
Muffin Lowfat Apple n' Spice	1 (3.3 oz)	220	2	50	0	480
Muffin Lowfat Banana	1 (3.3 oz)	240	2	54	0	380
Muffin Lowfat Blueberry	1 (3.3 oz)	230	2	51	0	370
Muffin Lowfat Bran	1 (3.3 oz)	260	2	59	0	440
Muffin Lowfat Cherry	1 (3.3 oz)	230	2	53	0	380
Muffin Lowfat Corn	1 (3.3 oz)	250	2	55	0	460
Muffin Lowfat Cranberry Orange	1 (3.3 oz)	230	2	53	0	380

FOOD	PORTION	CALS	FAT	CARB	CHOL	SOD
Muffin Oat Bran	1 (3.2 oz)	290	11	44	0	330
Munchkins Butternut	3 (2 oz)	230	11	30	0	210
Munchkins Chocolate Glazed	3 (2 oz)	180	10	22	0	240
Munchkins Cinnamon	4 (2 oz)	240	13	29	0	290
Munchkins Coconut	3 (1.7 oz)	200	11	22	0	220
Munchkins Glazed Cake	3 (2.1 oz)	220	9	32	0	220
Munchkins Glazed Raised	4 (2.1 oz)	210	7	36	0	170
Munchkins Jelly	3 (1.9 oz)	170	5	28	0	170
Munchkins Lemon	3 (2 oz)	160	6	23	0	160
Munchkins Plain	4 (1.8 oz)	200	12	21	0	290
Munchkins Powdered Sugar	4 (2 oz)	240	13	28	0	290
Munchkins Sugar Raised	6 (1.9 oz)	210	10	26	0	250
Munchkins Toasted Coconut	3 (1.8 oz)	210	11	26	0	220
Tart Apple	1 (3.4 oz)	310	10	45	0	330
Tart Blueberry	1 (3.4 oz)	300	10	48	0	320
Tart Lemon	1 (3.4 oz)	280	11	43	0	340
Tart Raspberry	1 (3.4 oz)	310	10	51	0	350
Tart Strawberry	1 (3.4 oz)	310	10	51	0	340
Turnover Apple	1 (3.8 oz)	350	15	49	0	340
Turnover Blueberry	1 (3.8 oz)	370	15	54	0	330
Turnover Lemon	1 (3.8 oz)	350	15	48	0	360
Turnover Raspberry	1 (3.8 oz)	380	15	57	0	370
Turnover Strawberry	1 (3.8 oz)	380	15	57	0	360
Yeast Donut Apple Crumb	1 (2.6 oz)	250	11	34	0	270
Yeast Donut Apple n' Spice	1 (2.5 oz)	230	10	31	0	250
Yeast Donut Bavarian Kreme	1 (2.5 oz)	250	11	33	0	250
Yeast Donut Black Raspberry	1 (2.4 oz)	240	10	32	0	260
Yeast Donut Boston Kreme	1 (2.8 oz)	270	11	38	0	260
Yeast Donut Chocolate Frosted	1 (2.1 oz)	210	8	31	0	230
Yeast Donut Chocolate Kreme Filled	1 (2.6 oz)	320	16	39	0	250
Yeast Donut Glazed	1 (1.6 oz)	160	7	23	0	200
Yeast Donut Jelly Filled	1 (2.4 oz)	240	10	32	0	260
Yeast Donut Lemon	1 (2.5 oz)	240	11	31	0	250

FOOD	PORTION	CALS	FAT	CARB	CHOL	SOD
Yeast Donut Maple Frosted	1 (2.1 oz)	210	8	32	0	230
Yeast Donut Marble Frosted	1 (2.1 oz)	210	8	32	0	230
Yeast Donut Strawberry	1 (2.4 oz)	240	10	32	0	250
Yeast Donut Strawberry Frosted	1 (2.1 oz)	220	8	32	0	230
Yeast Donut Sugar Raised	1 (1.6 oz)	170	7	23	0	220
Yeast Donut Vanilla Frosted	1 (2.1 oz)	220	8	32	0	230
BEVERAGES						
Coffee Coolatta w/ 2% Milk	1 (15.7 oz)	210	2	45	10	85
Coffee Coolatta w/ Cream	1 (15.7 oz)	370	22	44	75	70
Coffee Coolatta w/ Skim Milk	1 (15.7 oz)	190	0	45	2	85
Coffee Coolatta w/ Whole Milk	1 (15.7 oz)	230	4	45	15	80
Cream	1 serv (1 oz)	60	5	1	20	10
Dark Roast	1 serv (10 oz)	5	0	1	0	5
Decaf	1 serv (10 oz)	0	0	0	0	0
French Vanilla	1 serv (10 oz)	5	0	1	0	5
Hazelnut	1 serv (10 oz)	5	0	1	0	10
Hazelnut Coolatta w/ 2% Milk	1 (15.7 oz)	210	2	43	10	85
Hazelnut Coolatta w/ Cream	1 (15.7 oz)	370	22	42	75	70
Hazelnut Coolatta w/ Skim Milk	1 (15.7 oz)	200	0	43	2	85
Hazelnut Coolatta w/ Whole Milk	1 (15.7 oz)	230	4	43	15	80
Mocha Coolatta w/ 2% Milk	1 (15.7 oz)	220	2	43	10	80
Mocha Coolatta w/ Cream	1 (15.7 oz)	380	22	42	75	70
Mocha Coolatta w/ Skim Milk	1 (15.7 oz)	200	0	43	2	85
Mocha Coolatta w/ Whole Milk	1 (15.7 oz)	230	4	43	15	80
Regular	1 serv (10 oz)	5	0	1	0	5
Vanilla Coolatta w/ 2% Milk	1 (15.7 oz)	220	2	43	10	85

FOOD	PORTION	CALS	FAT	CARB	CHOL	SOD
Vanilla Coolatta w/ Cream	1 (15.7 oz)	380	22	42	75	70
Vanilla Coolatta w/ Skim Milk	1 (15.7 oz)	200	0	43	2	85
Vanilla Coolatta w/ Whole Milk	1 (15.7 oz)	230	4	43	15	80
SANDWICHES						
Croissant Sandwich Broccoli & Cheese	1 (6.1 oz)	370	21	36	20	680
Croissant Sandwich Chicken Salad	1 (7.6 oz)	540	31	37	75	710
Croissant Sandwich Egg & Cheese	1 (5 oz)	430	27	30	280	640
Croissant Sandwich Egg, Bacon & Cheese	1 (5.4 oz)	500	34	30	290	930
Croissant Sandwich Egg, Ham & Cheese	1 (6 oz)	530	29	30	295	1080
Croissant Sandwich Egg, Sausage & Cheese	1 (6.9 oz)	630	49	30	320	1180
Croissant Sandwich Ham & Cheese	1 (6.7 oz)	710	32	29	85	1840
Croissant Sandwich Roast Beef & Cheese	1 (6 oz)	490	27	28	30	680
Croissant Sandwich Seafood Salad	1 (7.6 oz)	480	26	45	50	1020
Croissant Sandwich Tuna Salad	1 (7.5 oz)	540	30	39	50	1140
SOUPS						
Beef Barley	1 serv (8 oz)	90	1	15	10	970
Beef Noodle	1 serv (8 oz)	90	1	12	20	980
Chicken Noodle	1 serv (8 oz)	80	2	12	15	890
Chili	1 serv (8 oz)	170	6	20	20	860
Chili Con Carne w/ Beans	1 serv (8 oz)	300	15	25	45	690
Cream Of Broccoli	1 serv (8 oz)	200	11	17	25	1050
Cream Of Potato	1 serv (8 oz)	190	10	19	25	770
Harvest Vegetable	1 serv (8 oz)	80	2	12	0	1120
Manhattan Clam Chowder	1 serv (8 oz)	70	1	11	5	890
Minestrone	1 serv (8 oz)	100	1	16	0	900
New England Clam Chowder	1 serv (8 oz)	200	10	16	30	1050
Split Pea w/ Ham	1 serv (8 oz)	190	9	20	15	830

FOOD	PORTION	CALS	FAT	CARB	CHOL	SOD

EINSTEIN BROS BAGELS
BAGELS

FOOD	PORTION	CALS	FAT	CARB	CHOL	SOD
Bagel Chips Cinnamon Raisin Swirl	1 serv (1 oz)	90	1	19	0	120
Bagel Chips Plain	1 serv (1 oz)	90	0	18	0	14
Bagel Chips Sourdough Dill	1 serv (1 oz)	90	1	18	0	120
Bagel Chips Sun Dried Tomato	1 serv (1 oz)	90	1	17	0	130
Bagel Chips Sunflower	1 serv (1 oz)	100	2	8	0	190
Bagel Chips Wild Blueberry	1 serv (1 oz)	90	1	19	0	105
Chocolate Chip	1 (4 oz)	380	3	78	0	480
Chopped Garlic	1 (4.2 oz)	377	4	81	0	593
Chopped Onion	1 (4 oz)	340	3	72	0	500
Cinnamon Raisin Swirl	1 (4 oz)	360	1	78	0	480
Cinnamon Sugar	1	330	0	72	0	510
Dark Pumpernickel	1 (3.8 oz)	330	1	72	0	710
Everything	1 (4 oz)	342	2	74	0	653
Honey 8 Grain	1 (4 oz)	320	1	71	0	500
Nutty Banana	1 (4 oz)	370	3	77	0	500
Plain	1 (3.7 oz)	330	1	72	0	520
Poppy Dip'd	1 (3.9 oz)	346	2	73	0	520
Salt	1 (3.9 oz)	330	1	72	0	1626
Sesame Dip'd	1 (4.1 oz)	381	5	74	0	523
Spinach Herb	1 (3.8 oz)	320	1	71	0	510
Sun Dried Tomato	1 (3.8 oz)	320	1	70	0	520
Veggie Confetti	1 (3.8 oz)	330	1	71	0	480
Wild Blueberry	1 (4 oz)	360	1	79	0	510

SANDWICHES AND FILLINGS

FOOD	PORTION	CALS	FAT	CARB	CHOL	SOD
Butter & Margarine Blend	1 serv (0.4 oz)	60	7	0	0	75
Capers	1 tbsp	0	0	0	0	320
Cheddar Cheese	1 serv (0.75 oz)	110	9	1	30	180
Classic New York Lox & Bagel	1 (11.4 oz)	560	24	31	75	1120
Cream Cheese Cheddarpeno	1 serv (1 oz)	90	8	2	30	150
Cream Cheese Chive	1 serv (1 oz)	90	9	2	35	125
Cream Cheese Maple Walnut Raisin	1 serv (1 oz)	100	8	7	25	95
Cream Cheese Plain	1 serv (1 oz)	100	9	2	35	130
Cream Cheese Smoked Salmon	1 serv (1 oz)	90	8	2	35	130

FOOD	PORTION	CALS	FAT	CARB	CHOL	SOD
Cream Cheese Strawberry	1 serv (1 oz)	90	8	4	30	105
Cream Cheese Sun Dried Tomato	1 serv (1 oz)	90	8	3	35	160
Cucumbers	1 serv (1 oz)	0	0	1	0	0
Fruit Spreads	1 tbsp	40	0	10	0	10
Ham	1 serv (2.5 oz)	75	2	1	20	560
Ham & Cheese Sandwich	1 (9.9 oz)	520	15	63	70	1280
Honey	1 tbsp	64	0	18	0	1
Hummus	2 tbsp	60	3	4	0	105
Hummus Sandwich	1 (6 oz)	440	7	62	0	590
Lettuce	1 leaf	0	0	0	0	0
Lite Cream Cheese Plain	1 serv (1 oz)	60	5	2	20	150
Lite Cream Cheese Spinach Dill	1 serv (1 oz)	60	5	2	20	150
Lite Cream Cheese Veggie	1 serv (1 oz)	60	5	3	20	170
Lite Cream Cheese Wildberry	1 serv (1 oz)	70	4	7	15	85
Lowfat Chicken Salad Sandwich	1 (11.6 oz)	440	9	63	45	940
Lowfat Tuna Salad Sandwich	1 (11.6 oz)	440	8	62	30	970
Marshall's Loz	1 serv (2 oz)	90	4	2	10	400
Mayonnaise Lite Reduced Calorie	1 serv (0.5 oz)	50	5	1	5	115
Peanut Butter	1 serv (1.1 oz)	190	16	8	0	140
Peanut Butter & Jelly Sandwich	1 (6 oz)	595	17	99	0	663
Scrambled Egg Sandwich	1 (7.7 oz)	480	17	56	385	630
Scrambled Egg Sandwich w/ Meat & Cheese	1 (8.9 oz)	520	31	57	8	1000
Smoked Turkey	1 serv (2.5 oz)	75	1	0	20	550
Smoked Turkey Sandwich	1 (9.9 oz)	480	14	59	45	1180
Sprouts Alfalfa	1 serv (0.5 oz)	0	0	3	0	10
Sweet Onions	1 serv (1 oz)	0	0	2	0	0
Swiss Cheese	1 serv (0.75 oz)	100	8	0	25	60
Tasty Turkey Sandwich	1 (10 oz)	530	22	61	90	1210
Tomato	1 serv (1.5 oz)	0	0	2	0	0
Turkey Pastrami 99% Fat Free	1 serv (2.5 oz)	75	6	2	0	510

FOOD	PORTION	CALS	FAT	CARB	CHOL	SOD
Turkey Pastrami Sandwich	1 (9.7 oz)	460	12	60	20	—
Veg Out Sandwich	1 (8.9 oz)	350	17	62	3	570
Whitefish Salad Sandwich	1 (9.2 oz)	630	23	59	45	1020

EL POLLO LOCO
MAIN MENU SELECTIONS

FOOD	PORTION	CALS	FAT	CARB	CHOL	SOD
Broccoli Slaw	1 serv (5 oz)	203	17	14	0	365
Burrito BRC	1 (9.3 oz)	482	15	72	15	1250
Burrito Classic Chicken	1 (9.3 oz)	556	22	61	117	1499
Burrito Grilled Steak	1 (11.3 oz)	705	32	68	77	1689
Burrito Loco Grande	1 (13.1 oz)	632	26	67	129	1649
Burrito Smokey Black Bean	1 (9.3 oz)	566	22	78	22	1337
Burrito Spicy Hot Chicken	1 (9.8 oz)	559	22	61	117	1503
Burrito Whole Wheat Chicken	1 (10.8 oz)	592	26	60	146	1199
Chicken Breast	1 piece (3 oz)	160	6	0	110	390
Chicken Leg	1 piece (1.75 oz)	90	5	0	75	150
Chicken Soft Taco	1 (4 oz)	224	12	15	66	585
Chicken Tamale	1 (3.5 oz)	190	8	23	10	480
Chicken Thigh	1 piece (2 oz)	180	12	0	130	230
Chicken Wing	1 (1.5 oz)	110	6	0	80	220
Cole Slaw	1 serv (5 oz)	206	16	12	11	358
Corn-On-Cob	1 ear (5.5 oz)	146	2	33	0	18
Cornbread Stuffing	1 serv (6 oz)	281	12	40	0	832
Crispy Green Beans	1 serv (5 oz)	41	2	6	0	667
Cucumber Salad	1 serv (4.2 oz)	34	0	7	0	11
Fiesta Corn	1 serv (5 oz)	152	6	25	0	397
Flame Broiled Chicken Salad	1 serv (14.9 oz)	167	5	11	56	765
French Fries	1 serv (4.4 oz)	323	14	44	0	330
Garden Salad	1 serv (6.4 oz)	29	0	6	0	20
Gravy	1 serv (1 oz)	14	0	2	2	139
Honey Glazed Carrots	1 serv (5 oz)	104	6	14	0	403
Lime Parfait	1 serv (5 oz)	125	3	25	0	107
Macaroni & Cheese	1 serv (6 oz)	238	12	22	31	919
Mashed Potatoes	1 serv (5 oz)	97	1	21	0	369
Pinto Beans	1 serv (6 oz)	185	4	29	0	744
Polo Bowl	1 serv (19 oz)	504	13	69	56	2068
Potato Salad	1 serv (6 oz)	256	14	30	15	527

FOOD	PORTION	CALS	FAT	CARB	CHOL	SOD
Rainbow Pasta Salad	1 serv (5 oz)	157	1	30	0	533
Salad Shell	1 (5.6 oz)	440	27	42	0	610
Smokey Black Beans	1 serv (5 oz)	255	13	29	11	609
Southwest Cole Slaw	1 serv (5 oz)	178	13	15	8	267
Spanish Rice	1 serv (4 oz)	130	3	24	0	397
Spiced Apples	1 serv (5 oz)	146	0	39	0	139
Steak Bowl	1 serv (15.2 oz)	616	26	62	68	1743
Taco Al Carbon Chicken	1 serv (4.4 oz)	265	12	30	28	223
Taco Al Carbon Steak	1 (4.4 oz)	394	22	30	46	473
Taquito	1 serv (5 oz)	370	17	43	25	690
Tortilla Corn	1 (1.1 oz)	70	1	14	0	35
Tortilla Flour	1 (1 oz)	90	3	13	0	224
Tortilla Wrap Chicken Caesar	1 (10.47 oz)	518	19	59	48	1709
Tortilla Wrap Southwest	1 (11.97 oz)	632	27	69	61	1792
Tostada Salad Chicken	1 serv (14.7 oz)	332	14	26	80	1280
Tostado Salad Steak	1 serv (13.2 oz)	525	31	26	100	1206
SALAD DRESSINGS						
Blue Cheese	1 serv (2 oz)	300	32	2	50	590
Light Italian	1 serv (2 oz)	25	1	3	0	990
Ranch	1 serv (2 oz)	350	39	2	5	500
Thousand Island	1 serv (2 oz)	270	27	9	30	460

FRIENDLY'S

FROZEN YOGURT

FOOD	PORTION	CALS	FAT	CARB	CHOL	SOD
Apple Bettie	½ cup (2.6 oz)	140	3	25	10	75
Chocolate Fudge Brownie	½ cup (2.6 oz)	160	5	25	10	80
Fabulous Fudge Swirl	½ cup (2.6 oz)	140	3	23	10	80
Fudge Berry Swirl	½ cup (2.6 oz)	150	4	25	10	75
Lowfat Perfectly Peach	½ cup (2.6 oz)	110	2	21	10	55
Lowfat Purely Chocolate	½ cup (2.6 oz)	120	3	20	10	65
Lowfat Raspberry Delight	½ cup (2.6 oz)	120	3	21	10	60
Lowfat Simply Vanilla	½ cup (2.6 oz)	120	3	19	10	70
Lowfat Strawberry Patch	½ cup (2.6 oz)	110	2	20	10	55
Mint Chocolate Chip	½ cup (2.6 oz)	130	4	21	10	65
Strawberry Cheesecake Blast	½ cup (2.6 oz)	140	4	22	15	75
Toffee Almond Crunch	½ cup (2.6 oz)	160	5	24	15	85
ICE CREAM						
Black Raspberry	½ cup	150	7	17	30	35
Chocolate Almond Chip	½ cup	170	10	18	35	45
Forbidden Chocolate	½ cup	150	9	14	30	40

FOOD	PORTION	CALS	FAT	CARB	CHOL	SOD
Fudge Nut Brownie	½ cup	200	11	23	25	60
Heath English Toffee	½ cup (2.7 oz)	190	10	24	30	240
Purely Pistachio	½ cup	160	10	16	35	50
Vanilla	½ cup	150	8	16	35	40
Vienna Mocha Chunk	½ cup	180	11	19	30	50

FRULLATI CAFE
BAKED SELECTIONS

FOOD	PORTION	CALS	FAT	CARB	CHOL	SOD
Muffin Banana Nut	1 (4 oz)	394	15	—	31	381
Muffin Cranberry Orange	1 (4 oz)	357	12	—	31	369
Muffin Fat Free Apple Streusel	1 (4 oz)	260	0	—	0	460
Muffin Fat Free Chocolate	1 (4 oz)	260	0	—	0	580
Muffin Fat Free Very Berry	1 (4 oz)	260	0	—	0	500
Muffin Sugar Free Blueberry	1 (4 oz)	308	9	—	12	443
Muffin Wild Blueberry	1 (4 oz)	344	11	—	31	369

BEVERAGES

FOOD	PORTION	CALS	FAT	CARB	CHOL	SOD
Apple Juice	1 serv (12 oz)	131	tr	—	0	8
Carrot Juice	1 serv (12 oz)	111	tr	—	0	80
Celery Juice	1 serv (12 oz)	22	tr	—	0	393
Lemonade	1 serv	209	tr	—	0	18
Lemonade Apple	1 serv	245	tr	—	0	18
Lemonade Cherry	1 serv	237	tr	—	0	21
Lemonade Orange	1 serv	270	tr	—	0	18
Lemonade Strawberry	1 serv	234	tr	—	0	19
Orange Banana Juice	1 serv (12 oz)	150	tr	—	0	3
Orange Juice	1 serv (12 oz)	126	tr	—	0	3
Smoothie A La Frullati	1 lg	426	16	—	20	82
Smoothie A La Frullati	1 sm	275	9	—	10	42
Smoothie Affinity	1 lg	378	16	—	20	82
Smoothie Affinity	1 sm	226	8	—	10	42
Smoothie Fiesta	1 lg	257	1	—	0	9
Smoothie Fiesta	1 sm	234	1	—	0	8
Smoothie Peach Banana	1 lg	289	1	—	0	13
Smoothie Peach Banana	1 sm	266	1	—	0	13
Smoothie Pina Colada	1 lg	387	16	—	82	82
Smoothie Pina Colada	1 sm	236	8	—	10	42
Smoothie Strawberry Banana	1 lg	188	1	—	0	3
Smoothie Strawberry Banana	1 sm	165	1	—	0	3

FOOD	PORTION	CALS	FAT	CARB	CHOL	SOD
Smoothie Strawberry Blueberry	1 lg	113	1	—	0	5
Smoothie Strawberry Blueberry	1 sm	90	1	—	0	5
Smoothie Strawberry Fruit	1 lg	101	1	—	0	2
Smoothie Strawberry Fruit	1 sm	79	1	—	0	2
Smoothie Strawberry Watermelon	1 lg	123	1	—	0	4
Smoothie Strawberry Watermelon	1 sm	100	1	—	0	4
DESSERTS						
Frozen Yogurt	1 lg	263	tr	—	3	132
Frozen Yogurt	1 reg	205	tr	—	3	103
Frozen Yogurt	1 sm	146	tr	—	2	73
Yogurt Smoothie Cappuccino	1 serv	472	3	—	17	250
Yogurt Smoothie Chocolate Fudge	1 serv	555	4	—	17	289
Yogurt Smoothie Fiesta	1 serv	432	4	—	17	249
Yogurt Smoothie Oreo Cookie	1 serv	566	8	—	19	398
Yogurt Smoothie Peach	1 serv	486	4	—	17	248
Yogurt Smoothie Peach Banana	1 serv	519	4	—	17	248
Yogurt Smoothie Peanut Butter	1 serv	630	18	—	17	380
Yogurt Smoothie Pina Colada	1 serv	519	1	—	5	225
Yogurt Smoothie Strawberry Banana	1 serv	514	4	—	17	249
Yogurt Smoothie Strawberry Fruit	1 serv	487	4	—	17	249
Yogurt Smoothie Strawberry Vanilla	1 serv	462	4	—	17	248
Yogurt Smoothie Strawberry Watermelon	1 serv	503	4	—	17	250
SALADS AND SALAD BARS						
Fruit Salad	1 lg	148	1	—	0	25
Fruit Salad	1 sm	99	1	—	0	16
Garden Salad	1 sm	56	1	—	0	86
Garden Salad w/ Italian Fat Free Dressing	1 lg	72	2	—	8	815

FOOD	PORTION	CALS	FAT	CARB	CHOL	SOD
Pasta Salad	1 lg	256	2	—	0	1078
Pasta Salad	1 sm	179	2	—	0	741
SANDWICHES						
Chicken On Croissant	1	481	24	—	109	649
Chicken On Honey Wheat	1	297	8	—	34	854
Chicken On Jewish Rye	1	261	7	—	34	820
Chicken On Pita	1	281	6	—	34	797
Chicken On White	1	291	7	—	35	825
Ham & Cheese On Croissant	1	797	50	—	192	1051
Ham & Cheese On Honey Wheat	1	613	34	—	117	1262
Ham & Cheese On Jewish Rye	1	577	32	—	117	1227
Ham & Cheese On Pita	1	597	32	—	117	1205
Ham & Cheese On White	1	607	33	—	118	1232
Roast Beef On Croissant	1	631	36	—	155	814
Roast Beef On Honey Wheat	1	348	8	—	72	947
Roast Beef On Jewish Rye	1	312	7	—	72	912
Roast Beef On Pita	1	332	7	—	72	889
Roast Beef On White	1	342	8	—	72	917
Tuna On Croissant	1	480	23	—	90	881
Tuna On Honey Wheat	1	295	6	—	16	1086
Tuna On Jewish Rye	1	259	6	—	16	1051
Tuna On Pita	1	280	5	—	16	1028
Tuna On White	1	289	6	—	16	1056
Turkey On Croissant	1	566	33	—	122	1578
Turkey On Honey Wheat	1	342	9	—	56	962
Turkey On Jewish Rye	1	306	8	—	56	927
Turkey On Pita	1	326	7	—	56	904
Turkey On White	1	338	9	—	57	932
Veggie On Croissant	1	510	35	—	83	764
Veggie On Honey Wheat	1	227	7	—	0	897
Veggie On Jewish Rye	1	191	6	—	0	862
Veggie On Pita	1	211	5	—	0	839
Veggie On White	1	221	7	—	0	867
GODFATHER'S PIZZA						
Golden Crust Cheese	¹/₁₀ lg (3.5 oz)	242	9	28	14	363
Golden Crust Cheese	⅛ med (3.1 oz)	212	8	26	12	311

FOOD	PORTION	CALS	FAT	CARB	CHOL	SOD
Golden Crust Combo	1/10 lg (4.9 oz)	305	14	31	25	674
Golden Crust Combo	1/8 med (4.4 oz)	271	12	28	22	562
Original Crust Cheese	1/10 jumbo (5.8 oz)	382	9	53	27	580
Original Crust Cheese	1/10 lg (4 oz)	258	6	36	18	396
Original Crust Cheese	1/4 mini (1.9 oz)	131	3	19	8	183
Original Crust Cheese	1/8 med (3.5 oz)	231	5	24	14	338
Original Crust Combo	1/10 jumbo (8.3 oz)	503	18	56	47	1096
Original Crust Combo	1/10 lg (5.6 oz)	338	12	38	31	740
Original Crust Combo	1/4 mini (2.9 oz)	176	7	21	16	382
Original Crust Combo	1/8 med (5.1 oz)	306	11	36	27	660
GODIVA						
Almond Butter Dome	3 pieces (1.5 oz)	240	17	19	5	20
Bouchee Au Chocolat	1 piece (1.5 oz)	210	11	25	5	40
Bouchee Ivory Raspberry	1 pieces (1 oz)	160	9	17	5	25
Gold Ballotin	3 pieces (1.5 oz)	210	10	27	5	15
Truffle Amaretto Di Saronno	2 pieces (1.5 oz)	210	12	24	5	25
Truffle Deluxe Liqueur	2 pieces (1.5 oz)	210	13	23	5	25
HAAGEN-DAZS **FROZEN YOGURT**						
Brownie Nut Blast	1/2 cup (3.5 oz)	215	8	29	41	66
Chocolate	1/2 cup (3.4 oz)	160	3	26	33	59
Coffee	1/2 cup (3.4 oz)	161	3	26	45	56
Orange Tango	1/2 cup (3.5 oz)	132	1	27	20	26
Pina Colada	1/2 cup (3.4 oz)	139	2	27	25	27
Raspberry Rendezvous	1/2 cup (3.5 oz)	132	1	26	20	27
Soft Serve Coffee	1/2 cup (3.3 oz)	145	4	22	38	79
Soft Serve Nonfat Chocolate	1/2 cup (3.3 oz)	116	tr	24	2	68
Soft Serve Nonfat Chocolate Mousse	1/2 cup (3.3 oz)	86	tr	26	2	70
Soft Serve Nonfat Vanilla	1/2 cup (3.3 oz)	114	tr	23	2	76
Soft Serve Nonfat Vanilla Mousse	1/2 cup (3.3 oz)	78	tr	24	2	66
Strawberry Cheesecake Craze	1/2 cup (3.6 oz)	213	7	30	64	64

FOOD	PORTION	CALS	FAT	CARB	CHOL	SOD
Strawberry Duet	½ cup (3.4 oz)	135	2	27	25	24
Vanilla	½ cup (3.4 oz)	162	3	26	44	58
Vanilla Almond Crunch	½ cup (3.4 oz)	198	5	30	41	88
ICE CREAM						
Bar Chocolate	1 (2.7 oz)	247	17	21	108	73
Bar Coffee	1 (2.7 oz)	249	17	20	111	81
Bar Vanilla	1 (2.7 oz)	251	17	20	111	81
Belgian Chocolate Chocolate	½ cup (3.6 oz)	315	21	28	84	59
Brownies A La Mode	½ cup (3.5 oz)	284	18	25	103	134
Butter Pecan	½ cup (3.7 oz)	304	23	19	100	136
Cappuccino Commotion	½ cup (3.6 oz)	305	21	24	98	102
Caramel Cone Explosion	½ cup (3.6 oz)	298	20	26	93	127
Chocolate	½ cup (3.7 oz)	249	17	21	110	71
Chocolate Chocolate Chip	½ cup (3.7 oz)	282	19	25	97	65
Chocolate Chocolate Mint	½ cup (3.6 oz)	285	20	25	94	64
Coffee	½ cup (3.7 oz)	251	17	20	113	80
Coffee Chip	½ cup (3.6 oz)	285	19	24	98	72
Cookie Dough Dynamo	½ cup (3.6 oz)	298	19	28	92	134
Cookies & Cream	½ cup (3.6 oz)	264	17	23	107	112
Deep Chocolate Peanut Butter	½ cup (3.7 oz)	339	23	25	81	95
Macadamia Brittle	½ cup (3.7 oz)	282	19	23	103	112
Macadamia Nut	½ cup (3.6 oz)	309	24	19	109	114
Midnight Cookies & Cream	½ cup (3.6 oz)	285	18	28	89	131
Peanut Butter Burst	½ cup (2.6 oz)	314	21	25	91	144
Pralines & Cream	½ cup (3.6 oz)	278	17	26	94	174
Rum Raisin	½ cup (3.7 oz)	256	16	21	102	70
Strawberry	½ cup (3.7 oz)	242	16	22	91	74
Strawberry Cheesecake Craze	½ cup (3.7 oz)	273	17	27	97	151
Swiss Chocolate Almond	½ cup (3.6 oz)	288	20	23	97	65
Triple Brownie Overload	½ cup (3.5 oz)	298	20	26	91	101
Vanilla	½ cup (3.7 oz)	252	17	20	113	80
Vanilla Chip	½ cup (3.6 oz)	286	19	24	99	73
Vanilla Fudge	½ cup (3.7 oz)	268	17	24	98	101
Vanilla Swiss Almond	½ cup (3.7 oz)	288	20	21	101	73
SORBET						
Mango	½ cup (4 oz)	107	tr	26	0	1

FOOD	PORTION	CALS	FAT	CARB	CHOL	SOD
Raspberry	½ cup (4 oz)	110	tr	27	0	3
Soft Serve Lemonade	½ cup (3.3 oz)	113	0	28	0	5
Soft Serve Mango	½ cup (3.3 oz)	107	tr	26	0	1
Soft Serve Raspberry	½ cup (3.3 oz)	108	tr	26	0	3
Strawberry	½ cup (4 oz)	118	tr	29	0	1
Zesty Lemon	½ cup (4 oz)	111	0	28	0	5

HARDEE'S
BEVERAGES

FOOD	PORTION	CALS	FAT	CARB	CHOL	SOD
Orange Juice	1 serv (11 oz)	140	tr	34	0	5
Shake Chocolate	1 (12.2 oz)	370	5	67	30	270
Shake Peach	1 (12.1 oz)	390	4	77	25	290
Shake Strawberry	1 (12.7 oz)	420	4	83	20	270
Shake Vanilla	1 (12.2 oz)	350	5	65	20	300

BREAKFAST SELECTIONS

FOOD	PORTION	CALS	FAT	CARB	CHOL	SOD
Apple Cinnamon 'N' Raisin Biscuit	1 (2.18 oz)	200	8	30	0	350
Bacon & Egg Biscuit	1 (5.5 oz)	570	33	45	275	1400
Bacon Egg & Cheese Biscuit	1 (5.9 oz)	610	37	45	280	1630
Big Country Breakfast Bacon	1 serv (9.4 oz)	820	49	62	535	1870
Big Country Breakfast Sausage	1 serv (11.4 oz)	1000	66	62	570	3210
Biscuit 'N' Gravy	1 (7.8 oz)	510	28	55	15	1500
Country Ham Biscuit	1 (3.8 oz)	430	22	45	25	1930
Frisco Breakfast Sandwich Ham	1 (7.4 oz)	500	25	46	290	1370
Ham Biscuit	1 (4 oz)	400	20	47	15	1340
Ham Egg & Cheese Biscuit	1 (6.5 oz)	540	30	48	285	1660
Hash Rounds	1 serv (2.8 oz)	230	14	24	0	560
Jelly Biscuit	1 (3.5 oz)	440	21	57	0	1000
Rise 'N' Shine Biscuit	1 (2.9 oz)	390	21	44	0	1000
Sausage Biscuit	1 (4.1 oz)	510	31	44	25	1360
Sausage & Egg Biscuit	1 (6.3 oz)	630	40	45	285	1480
Three Pancakes	1 serv (4.8 oz)	280	2	56	15	890
Ultimate Omelet Biscuit	1 (5.8 oz)	570	33	45	120	1370

DESSERTS

FOOD	PORTION	CALS	FAT	CARB	CHOL	SOD
Cone Chocolate	1 (4.1 oz)	180	2	34	15	110
Cone Vanilla	1 (4.1 oz)	170	2	34	10	130
Cool Twist Cone Vanilla/ Chocolate	1 (4.1 oz)	180	2	34	10	120
Peach Cobbler	1 serv (6 oz)	310	7	60	0	360

FOOD	PORTION	CALS	FAT	CARB	CHOL	SOD
Sundae Hot Fudge	1 (5.5 oz)	290	6	51	20	310
Sundae Strawberry	1 (5.8 oz)	210	2	43	10	140
MAIN MENU SELECTIONS						
Baked Beans	1 serv (5 oz)	170	1	32	0	600
Big Roast Beef Sandwich	1 (6.5 oz)	460	24	35	70	1230
Cheeseburger	1 (4.3 oz)	310	14	30	40	890
Chicken Fillet Sandwich	1 (7.5 oz)	480	18	54	55	1280
Cole Slaw	1 serv (4 oz)	240	20	13	10	340
Cravin' Bacon Cheeseburger	1 (8.1 oz)	690	46	38	95	1150
Fisherman's Fillet	1 (8.3 oz)	560	27	54	65	1330
French Fries	1 lg (6 oz)	430	18	59	0	190
French Fries	1 med (5 oz)	350	15	49	0	150
French Fries	1 sm (3.4 oz)	240	10	33	0	100
Fried Chicken Breast	1 piece (5.2 oz)	370	15	29	75	1190
Fried Chicken Leg	1 piece (2.4 oz)	170	7	15	45	570
Fried Chicken Thigh	1 piece (4.2 oz)	330	15	30	60	1000
Fried Chicken Wing	1 piece (2.3 oz)	200	8	23	30	740
Frisco Burger	1 (8.1 oz)	720	46	43	95	1340
Gravy	1 serv (1.5 oz)	20	tr	3	0	260
Grilled Chicken Sandwich	1 (7.1 oz)	350	11	38	65	950
Hamburger	1 (3.9 oz)	270	11	29	35	670
Hot Ham 'N' Cheese	1 (5.1 oz)	310	12	34	50	1410
Mashed Potatoes	1 serv (4 oz)	70	tr	14	0	330
Mesquite Bacon Cheeseburger	1 (4.5 oz)	370	18	32	45	970
Mushroom 'N' Swiss Burger	1 (6.8 oz)	490	25	39	80	1100
Quarter Pound Double Cheeseburger	1 (6 oz)	470	27	31	80	1290
Regular Roast Beef	1 (4.3 oz)	320	16	26	43	820
The Boss	1 (7 oz)	570	33	42	85	910
The Works Burger	1 (8.1 oz)	530	30	41	80	1030
SALAD DRESSINGS						
Fat Free French	1 serv (2 oz)	70	0	17	0	580
Ranch	1 serv (2 oz)	290	29	6	25	510
Thousand Island	1 serv (2 oz)	250	23	9	35	540
SALADS AND SALAD BARS						
Garden Salad	1 (10.2 oz)	220	13	11	40	350
Grilled Chicken Salad	1 (11.5 oz)	150	3	11	60	610
Side Salad	1 (4.6 oz)	25	tr	4	0	45

H.SALT SEAFOOD

Chicken	3 oz	108	6	—	69	2

FOOD	PORTION	CALS	FAT	CARB	CHOL	SOD
Cod	3 oz	62	2	—	18	57
Hamburger	3 oz	228	18	—	65	40
Pork Loin	3 oz	254	21	—	55	55
Sirloin Steak	3 oz	239	20	—	58	36
IHOP						
Pancake Buckwheat	1 (2.5 oz)	134	5	19	61	372
Pancake Buttermilk	1 (2 oz)	108	3	17	31	459
Pancake Country Griddle	1 (2.25 oz)	134	4	22	38	497
Pancake Egg	1 (2 oz)	102	5	12	66	213
Pancake Harvest Grain 'N Nut	1 (2.25 oz)	160	8	18	38	391
Waffle	1 (4 oz)	305	15	37	70	468
Waffle Belgian	1 (6 oz)	408	20	49	146	882
Waffle Belgian Harvest Grain 'N Nut	1 (6 oz)	445	28	40	147	876

JACK IN THE BOX
BEVERAGES

FOOD	PORTION	CALS	FAT	CARB	CHOL	SOD
2% Milk	1 serv (8 fl oz)	130	5	14	20	85
Barq's Root Beer	1 reg (20 fl oz)	180	0	50	0	50
Classic Ice Cream Shake Cappuccino	1 reg (11 oz)	630	29	80	90	320
Classic Ice Cream Shake Chocolate	1 reg (11 fl oz)	630	27	85	85	330
Classic Ice Cream Shake Oreo Cookie	1 reg (12 oz)	740	36	91	95	490
Classic Ice Cream Shake Strawberry	1 reg (10 fl oz)	640	28	85	85	300
Classic Ice Cream Shake Vanilla	1 reg (11 oz)	610	31	73	95	320
Coca-Cola Classic	1 reg (20 fl oz)	170	0	46	0	40
Coffee	1 reg (12 fl oz)	5	0	1	0	5
Diet Coke	1 reg (20 fl oz)	0	0	0	0	15
Dr Pepper	1 reg (20 fl oz)	190	0	49	0	25
Iced Tea	1 reg (20 fl oz)	0	0	0	0	0
Minute Maid Lemonade	1 reg (20 fl oz)	190	0	48	0	90
Orange Juice	1 serv (10 oz)	150	0	34	0	20
Sprite	1 reg (20 fl oz)	160	0	41	0	40

BREAKFAST SELECTIONS

FOOD	PORTION	CALS	FAT	CARB	CHOL	SOD
Breakfast Jack	1 (4.2 oz)	300	12	30	185	890
Country Crock Spread	1 pat (5 g)	25	3	0	0	40
Grape Jelly	1 serv (0.5 oz)	40	0	9	0	5
Hash Browns	1 serv (2 oz)	160	11	14	—	310

FOOD	PORTION	CALS	FAT	CARB	CHOL	SOD
Pancake Syrup	1 serv (1.5 oz)	120	0	30	0	5
Pancakes w/ Bacon	1 serv (5.6 oz)	400	12	59	30	980
Sausage Croissant	1 (6.4 oz)	670	48	39	250	940
Sourdough Breakfast Sandwich	1 (5.2 oz)	380	21	31	355	1120
Supreme Croissant	1 (6 oz)	570	20	39	235	1240
Ultimate Breakfast Sandwich	1 (8.5 oz)	620	36	39	245	1800
DESSERTS						
Carrot Cake	1 serv (3.5 oz)	370	16	54	35	340
Cheesecake	1 serv (3.5 oz)	310	18	29	65	210
Hot Apple Turnover	1 (3.8 oz)	340	18	41	0	510
MAIN MENU SELECTIONS						
¼ lb Burger	1 (6 oz)	510	27	39	65	1080
American Cheese	1 slice (0.4 oz)	45	4	0	10	200
Bacon & Cheddar Potato Wedges	1 serv (9.3 oz)	800	58	49	55	1470
Bacon Ultimate Cheeseburger	1 (10.4 oz)	1150	89	31	230	1770
Barbeque Dipping Sauce	1 serv (1 fl oz)	45	0	11	0	300
Cheeseburger	1 (4 oz)	330	15	32	60	760
Chicken & Fries	1 serv (9.3 oz)	730	34	79	65	1690
Chicken Caesar Sandwich	1 (8.3 oz)	520	26	44	55	1050
Chicken Fajita Pita	1 (6.6 oz)	280	9	25	75	840
Chicken Sandwich	1 (5.9 oz)	450	26	38	45	1030
Chicken Strips Breaded	5 pieces (5.3 oz)	360	17	24	80	970
Chicken Supreme Sandwich	1 (8.2 oz)	680	45	46	85	1500
Chili Cheese Curly Fries	1 serv (8.1 oz)	650	41	60	25	1640
Double Cheeseburger	1 (5.3 oz)	450	24	35	75	970
Egg Rolls	3 pieces (6 oz)	440	24	40	35	1020
Egg Rolls	5 pieces (10 oz)	730	41	67	60	1700
Fish & Chips	1 serv (9 oz)	720	35	81	35	1580
French Fries	1 reg (4.1 oz)	360	17	48	0	740
Grilled Chicken Fillet Sandwich	1 (8.1 oz)	520	26	42	140	1240
Hamburger	1 (3.6 oz)	280	12	32	45	560
Jumbo Fries	1 serv (5 oz)	430	20	58	0	890
Jumbo Jack	1 (7.8 oz)	560	36	31	80	680
Jumbo Jack w/ Cheese	1 (8.6 oz)	650	43	32	105	1090
Ketchup	1 pkg (0.3 oz)	10	0	3	0	100
Monster Taco	1 (4 oz)	290	18	21	40	550

FOOD	PORTION	CALS	FAT	CARB	CHOL	SOD
Onion Rings	1 serv (4.2 oz)	460	25	50	0	780
Pilly Cheesesteak Sandwich	1 (7.6 oz)	520	25	41	155	1980
Salsa	1 serv (1 oz)	10	0	2	0	200
Seasoned Curly Fries	1 serv (4.5 oz)	420	24	46	0	1030
Sour Cream	1 serv (1 oz)	60	6	1	20	30
Sourdough Jack	1 (7.8 oz)	670	43	39	110	1180
Soy Sauce	1 serv (0.3 oz)	5	0	tr	0	480
Spicy Crispy Chicken Sandwich	1 (7.9 oz)	560	27	55	50	1020
Stuffed Jalapenos	10 pieces (7.6 oz)	680	40	59	75	2220
Stuffed Jalapenos	7 pieces (5.3 oz)	470	28	41	50	1560
Super Scoop French Fries	1 serv (7 oz)	610	28	82	0	1250
Sweet & Sour Dipping Sauce	1 serv (1 oz)	40	0	11	0	160
Swiss-Style Cheese	1 slice (0.4 oz)	40	3	0	10	190
Taco	1 (2.7 oz)	190	11	15	20	410
Tartar Dipping Sauce	1 pkg (1.5 oz)	220	23	2	20	240
Teriyaki Bowl Chicken	1 serv (17.6 oz)	670	4	128	15	1620
Ultimate Cheeseburger	1 (9.8 oz)	1030	79	30	205	1200
SALAD DRESSINGS						
Blue Cheese	1 serv (2 fl oz)	210	18	11	15	750
Buttermilk House	1 serv (2 fl oz)	290	30	6	20	560
Buttermilk House Dipping Sauce	1 serv (0.9 oz)	130	13	3	10	240
Low Calorie Italian	1 serv (2 fl oz)	25	2	2	0	670
Thousand Island	1 serv (2 fl oz)	250	24	10	20	570
SALADS AND SALAD BARS						
Croutons	1 serv (0.4 oz)	50	2	8	0	105
Garden Chicken Salad	1 serv (8.9 oz)	200	9	8	65	420
Side Salad	1 (3 oz)	50	3	3	10	75

KENNY ROGERS ROASTERS
MAIN MENU SELECTIONS

FOOD	PORTION	CALS	FAT	CARB	CHOL	SOD
½ Chicken w/ Skin	1 serv (9.06 oz)	515	28	2	301	1129
½ Chicken w/o Skin & Wing	1 serv (7.03 oz)	313	10	1	221	876
¼ Chicken Dark Meat w/ Skin	1 serv (4.35 oz)	271	17	1	165	524
¼ Chicken Dark Meat w/o Skin & Wing	1 serv (3.29 oz)	169	7	1	130	454

FOOD	PORTION	CALS	FAT	CARB	CHOL	SOD
¼ Chicken White Meat w/ Skin	1 serv (4.71 oz)	244	11	1	136	604
¼ Chicken White Meat w/o Skin & Wing	1 serv (3.74 oz)	144	2	tr	92	422
Baked Sweet Potato	1 (9 oz)	263	tr	62	0	26
Chicken Caesar Salad	1 serv (9.4 oz)	285	9	18	122	704
Cinnamon Apples	1 serv (5.27 oz)	199	5	41	13	3
Cole Slaw	1 serv (5.05 oz)	225	16	18	13	288
Corn Muffin	1 (2 oz)	175	8	24	0	210
Corn On The Cob	1 (2.25 oz)	68	1	14	0	11
Corn Stuffing	1 serv (7.1 oz)	326	19	34	5	765
Creamy Parmesan Spinach	1 serv (5.3 oz)	119	69	10	12	547
Garlic Parsley Potatoes	1 serv (6.5 oz)	259	12	37	16	867
Honey Baked Beans	1 serv (5 oz)	148	1	32	0	787
Italian Green Beans	1 serv (6.1 oz)	116	8	10	0	374
Macaroni & Cheese	1 serv (5.51 oz)	197	6	24	26	661
Pasta Salad	1 serv (5 oz)	236	12	28	40	296
Pita BBQ Chicken	1 (7.33 oz)	401	7	51	112	1307
Pita Chicken Caesar	1 (9.2 oz)	606	35	34	122	829
Pita Roasted Chicken	1 (10.8 oz)	685	35	42	159	1620
Pot Pie Chicken	1 (12 oz)	708	33	78	69	1500
Potato Salad	1 serv (7.01 oz)	390	27	34	0	628
Real Mashed Potatoes	1 serv (8 oz)	295	14	39	2	478
Rice Pilaf	1 serv (5 oz)	173	5	43	0	146
Roasted Chicken Salad	1 serv (16.9 oz)	292	10	19	218	573
Sandwich Turkey	1 (9.2 oz)	385	12	30	88	923
Side Salad	1 serv (4.73 oz)	23	1	5	0	16
Sour Cream & Dill Pasta Salad	1 serv (5 oz)	233	16	20	16	432
Steamed Vegetables	1 serv (4.25 oz)	48	tr	8	0	59
Sweet Corn Niblets	1 serv (5 oz)	112	1	28	0	385
Tomato Cucumber Salad	1 serv (6 oz)	123	2	10	0	794
Turkey Sliced Breast	1 serv (4.5 oz)	158	2	—	78	586
Zucchini & Squash Santa Fe	1 serv (5 oz)	70	5	8	0	209
SALAD DRESSINGS						
Blue Cheese	1 serv (2.47 oz)	370	39	3	65	720
Buttermilk Ranch	1 serv (2.47 oz)	430	48	2	10	620
Caesar	1 serv (2.47 oz)	340	36	3	15	780
Honey French	1 serv (2.47 oz)	350	29	22	0	490
Honey Mustard	1 serv (2.47 oz)	320	28	18	40	410
Italian Fat Free	1 serv (2.47 oz)	35	0	8	0	1040
Thousand Island	1 serv (2.47 oz)	330	33	8	40	550

FOOD	PORTION	CALS	FAT	CARB	CHOL	SOD
SOUPS						
Chicken Noodle	1 bowl (10 oz)	91	2	12	22	931
Chicken Noodle	1 cup (6 oz)	55	1	7	13	559
KFC						
BBQ Baked Beans	1 serv (5.5 oz)	190	3	33	5	760
Biscuit	1 (2 oz)	180	10	20	0	560
Chicken Pot Pie	1 (13 oz)	770	42	69	70	2160
Chicken Twister	1 (8.7 oz)	550	32	40	85	980
Cole Slaw	1 serv (5 oz)	180	9	21	5	280
Corn On The Cob	1 ear (5.7 oz)	150	2	35	0	20
Cornbread	1 (2 oz)	228	13	25	42	194
Crispy Strips Colonel's	3 (3.25 oz)	261	16	10	40	658
Crispy Strips Spicy Buffalo	3 (4.2 oz)	350	19	22	35	1110
Extra Tasty Crispy Breast	1 (5.9 oz)	470	28	25	80	930
Extra Tasty Crispy Drumstick	1 (2.4 oz)	190	11	8	60	260
Extra Tasty Crispy Thigh	1 (4.2 oz)	370	25	18	70	540
Extra Tasty Crispy Whole Wing	1 (1.9 oz)	200	13	10	45	290
Green Beans	1 serv (4.7 oz)	45	2	7	5	730
Hot & Spicy Breast	1 (6.5 oz)	530	35	23	110	1110
Hot & Spicy Drumstick	1 (2.3 oz)	190	11	10	50	300
Hot & Spicy Thigh	1 (3.8 oz)	370	27	13	90	570
Hot & Spicy Whole Wing	1 (1.9 oz)	210	15	9	50	340
Hot Wings	6 (4.8 oz)	471	33	18	150	1230
Macaroni & Cheese	1 serv (5.4 oz)	180	8	21	10	860
Mashed Potatoes With Gravy	1 serv (4.8 oz)	120	6	17	tr	440
Mean Greens	1 serv (5.4 oz)	70	3	11	10	650
Original Recipe Breast	1 (5.4 oz)	400	24	16	135	1116
Original Recipe Chicken Sandwich	1 (7.3 oz)	497	22	46	52	1213
Original Recipe Drumstick	1 (2.2 oz)	140	9	4	75	422
Original Recipe Thigh	1 (3.2 oz)	250	18	6	95	747
Original Recipe Whole Wing	1 (1.6 oz)	140	10	5	55	414
Potato Salad	1 serv (5.6 oz)	230	14	23	15	540
Potato Wedges	1 serv (4.8 oz)	280	13	28	5	750
Tender Roast Breast w/ Skin	1 (4.9 oz)	251	11	1	151	830
Tender Roast Breast w/o Skin	1 (4.2 oz)	169	4	1	112	797

FOOD	PORTION	CALS	FAT	CARB	CHOL	SOD
Tender Roast Drumstick w/ Skin	1 (1.9 oz)	97	4	tr	85	271
Tender Roast Drumstick w/o Skin	1 (1.2 oz)	67	2	tr	63	259
Tender Roast Thigh w/ Skin	1 (3.2 oz)	207	12	<2	120	504
Tender Roast Thigh w/o Skin	1 (2.1 oz)	106	6	tr	84	312
Tender Roast Wing w/ Skin	1 (1.8 oz)	121	8	1	74	331
Value BBQ Chicken Sandwich	1 (5.3 oz)	256	8	28	57	782

KRYSTAL
BEVERAGES

Chocolate Shake	1 (16 fl oz)	275	10	44	32	178

BREAKFAST SELECTIONS

Biscuit	1 (2.5 oz)	244	12	31	2	437
Biscuit Bacon	1 (2.9 oz)	306	17	32	14	726
Biscuit Bacon, Egg & Cheese	1 (4.7 oz)	421	26	33	153	899
Biscuit Country Ham	1 (3.7 oz)	334	17	31	23	1147
Biscuit Egg	1 (4 oz)	327	19	32	134	481
Biscuit Gravy	1 (7.5 oz)	419	26	40	23	980
Biscuit Sausage	1 (4.1 oz)	437	30	31	49	668
Sunriser	1 (3.8 oz)	259	17	17	162	544

DESSERTS

Apple Pie	1 serv (4.5 oz)	300	10	49	0	420
Donut Plain	1 (1.3 oz)	150	9	17	5	135
Donut w/ Chocolate Icing	1 (1.8 oz)	212	11	27	5	165
Donut w/ Vanilla Icing	1 (1.8 oz)	198	9	29	5	135
Lemon Meringue Pie	1 serv (4 oz)	340	9	57	50	190
Pecan Pie	1 serv (4 oz)	450	23	56	55	290

MAIN MENU SELECTIONS

Bacon Cheeseburger	1 (7.4 oz)	521	34	29	89	1083
Big K	1 (8 oz)	540	35	29	93	1283
Burger Plus	1 (6.5 oz)	415	26	28	63	614
Burger Plus w/ Cheese	1 (7.1 oz)	473	31	28	77	867
Cheese Krystal	1 (2.5 oz)	187	10	16	29	453
Chili	1 lg (12 oz)	327	12	41	28	1283
Chili	1 reg (8 oz)	218	8	27	19	855
Chili Cheese Pup	1 (2.7 oz)	211	13	14	31	642
Chili Pup	1 (2.5 oz)	182	10	13	24	597
Corn Pup	1 (2.3 oz)	214	14	17	24	710

FOOD	PORTION	CALS	FAT	CARB	CHOL	SOD
Crispy Crunchy Chicken Sandwich	1 (5.75 oz)	467	24	48	56	949
Double Cheese Krystal	1 (4.5 oz)	337	19	25	57	815
Double Krystal	1 (4 oz)	277	14	24	43	547
Fries	1 lg (5.3 oz)	463	23	59	16	203
Fries	1 reg (4.1 oz)	358	18	45	12	157
Fries	1 sm (3 oz)	262	13	33	9	115
Krys Kross Fries	1 serv (4.3 oz)	486	29	52	31	604
Krys Kross Fries Chili Cheese	1 serv (6.8 oz)	625	39	57	61	1111
Krys Kross Fries w/ Cheese	1 serv (5.3 oz)	515	31	54	31	803
Krystal	1 (2.2 oz)	158	7	16	22	324
Plain Pup	1 (1.9 oz)	160	9	12	20	470

LITTLE CAESARS
MAIN MENU SELECTIONS

FOOD	PORTION	CALS	FAT	CARB	CHOL	SOD
Crazy Bread	1 piece (1.4 oz)	106	3	16	0	114
Crazy Sauce	1 serv (6 oz)	170	tr	14	0	381
Deli-Style Sandwich Ham & Cheese	1 (11.6 oz)	728	35	71	54	1602
Deli-Style Sandwich Italian	1 (11.9 oz)	740	37	71	62	1831
Deli-Style Sandwich Veggie	1 (11.9 oz)	647	29	74	29	1195
Hot Oven-Baked Sandwich Cheeser	1 (12.1 oz)	822	39	75	580	2244
Hot Oven-Baked Sandwich Meatsa	1 (15 oz)	1036	56	75	130	3302
Hot Oven-Baked Sandwich Pepperoni	1 (11.2 oz)	899	47	74	58	2428
Hot Oven-Baked Sandwich Supreme	1 (13.1 oz)	894	46	77	700	2367
Hot Oven-Baked Sandwich Veggie	1 (13.7 oz)	669	23	79	58	1534

PIZZA

FOOD	PORTION	CALS	FAT	CARB	CHOL	SOD
Baby Pan!Pan!	1 serv (8.4 oz)	616	24	67	47	1466
Pan!Pan! Cheese	1 med slice (2.9 oz)	181	6	22	15	379
Pan!Pan! Pepperoni	1 med slice (3 oz)	199	8	22	15	452
Pizza!Pizza! Cheese	1 med slice (3.2 oz)	201	7	24	17	281
Pizza!Pizza! Pepperoni	1 med slice (3.3 oz)	220	9	24	17	358

FOOD	PORTION	CALS	FAT	CARB	CHOL	SOD
SALAD DRESSINGS						
1000 Island	1 serv (1.5 oz)	183	17	6	30	542
Blue Cheese	1 serv (1.5 oz)	160	14	8	17	600
Caesar	1 serv (1.5 oz)	255	27	3	13	404
French	1 serv (1.5 oz)	166	16	5	0	553
Greek	1 serv (1.5 oz)	268	30	tr	9	202
Italian	1 serv (1.5 oz)	200	21	3	12	468
Italian Fat Free	1 serv (1.5 oz)	15	0	3	0	420
Ranch	1 serv (1.5 oz)	221	22	5	18	340
SALADS AND SALAD BARS						
Antipasto Salad	1 serv (8.4 oz)	176	12	7	19	542
Caesar Salad	1 serv (5 oz)	140	5	14	11	372
Greek Salad	1 serv (10.3 oz)	168	10	12	37	653
Tossed Salad	1 serv (8.5 oz)	116	3	19	0	170

LONG JOHN SILVER'S
MAIN MENU SELECTIONS

FOOD	PORTION	CALS	FAT	CARB	CHOL	SOD
Batter-Dipped Chicken	1 piece (2 oz)	120	6	11	15	400
Batter-Dipped Fish	1 piece (3 oz)	170	11	12	30	470
Batter-Dipped Shrimp	1 piece (0.4 oz)	35	3	2	10	95
Breaded Chicken Strips	1 piece (1.15 oz)	100	5	6	10	360
Breaded Clams	1 serv (3 oz)	300	17	31	40	670
Breaded Fish	1 piece (1.6 oz)	110	5	11	20	340
Cheese Sticks	1 serv (1.6 oz)	160	9	12	10	360
Chicken Salsa	1 reg (11 oz)	690	32	81	20	1690
Corn Cobbette w/ Butter	1 piece (3.3 oz)	140	8	19	0	0
Corn Cobbette w/o Butter	1 (3.1 oz)	80	1	19	0	0
Fish Cajun	1 lg (23 oz)	1450	70	85	60	3630
Flavorbaked Chicken	1 piece (2.6 oz)	110	3	tr	55	600
Flavorbaked Fish	1 piece (2.3 oz)	90	3	1	35	320
Fries	1 lg (5 oz)	420	24	46	0	830
Fries	1 reg (3 oz)	250	15	28	0	500
Honey Mustard Sauce	1 serv (0.4 oz)	20	0	5	0	60
Hushpuppy	1 (0.8 oz)	60	3	9	0	25
Ketchup	1 serv (.32 oz)	10	0	2	0	110
Popcorn Chicken Munchers	1 serv (4 oz)	380	23	20	35	1030
Popcorn Fish Munchers	1 serv (4 oz)	300	14	29	50	1220
Popcorn Shrimp Munchers	1 serv (4 oz)	320	15	33	85	1440
Rice	1 serv (3 oz)	140	3	26	0	210
Sandwich Batter Dipped Fish No Sauce	1 (5.4 oz)	320	13	40	30	800

FOOD	PORTION	CALS	FAT	CARB	CHOL	SOD
Sandwich Flavorbaked Chicken	1 (5.8 oz)	290	10	27	60	970
Sandwich Flavorbaked Fish	1 (6 oz)	320	14	28	55	930
Sandwich Ultimate Fish	1 (6.4 oz)	430	21	44	35	1340
Shrimp Sauce	1 serv (0.4 oz)	15	0	3	0	180
Side Salad	1 (4.3 oz)	25	0	4	0	15
Slaw	1 serv (3.4 oz)	140	6	20	0	260
Sweet'N'Sour Sauce	1 serv (0.4 oz)	20	0	5	0	45
Tartar Sauce	1 serv (0.4 oz)	35	2	5	0	35
Wraps Chicken Cajun	1 lg (22 oz)	1440	71	165	50	3730
Wraps Chicken Cajun	1 reg (11 oz)	720	35	83	25	1860
Wraps Chicken Ranch	1 lg (22 oz)	1450	72	165	50	3620
Wraps Chicken Ranch	1 reg (11 oz)	730	36	82	25	1810
Wraps Chicken Salsa	1 lg (22 oz)	1370	64	162	35	3370
Wraps Chicken Tartar	1 lg (22 oz)	1450	72	165	45	3560
Wraps Chicken Tartar	1 reg (11 oz)	730	36	83	25	1780
Wraps Fish Cajun	1 reg (11.5 oz)	730	35	85	30	1820
Wraps Fish Ranch	1 lg (23 oz)	1460	72	170	60	3520
Wraps Fish Ranch	1 reg (11.5 oz)	730	36	85	30	1760
Wraps Fish Salsa	1 lg (23 oz)	1380	64	167	45	3280
Wraps Fish Salsa	1 reg (11.5 oz)	690	32	84	25	1640
Wraps Fish Tartar	1 lg (23 oz)	1470	72	170	55	3460
Wraps Fish Tartar	1 reg (11.5 oz)	730	36	85	25	1730
Wraps Popcorn Shrimp Cajun	1 lg (22 oz)	1450	71	172	95	3660
Wraps Popcorn Shrimp Cajun	1 reg (11 oz)	720	35	86	50	1830
Wraps Popcorn Shrimp Ranch	1 lg (22 oz)	1460	72	171	100	3560
Wraps Popcorn Shrimp Ranch	1 reg (11 oz)	720	35	86	50	1830
Wraps Popcorn Shrimp Salsa	1 lg (22 oz)	1380	64	169	85	3310
Wraps Popcorn Shrimp Salsa	1 reg (11 oz)	690	32	84	40	1660
Wraps Popcorn Shrimp Tartar	1 lg (22 oz)	1460	72	172	95	3500
Wraps Popcorn Shrimp Tartar	1 reg (11 oz)	730	36	86	45	1750
SALAD DRESSINGS						
Fat-Free French	1 serv (1.5 oz)	50	0	14	0	360
Fat-Free Ranch	1 serv (1.5 oz)	50	0	13	0	380
Italian	1 serv (1 oz)	130	14	2	0	280

FOOD	PORTION	CALS	FAT	CARB	CHOL	SOD
Malt Vinegar	1 serv (0.3 oz)	0	0	0	0	15
Ranch Dressing	1 serv (1 oz)	170	18	1	5	260
Thousand Island	1 serv (1 oz)	110	10	5	15	280

LYONS RESTAURANTS
MAIN MENU SELECTIONS

FOOD	PORTION	CALS	FAT	CARB	CHOL	SOD
Light & Healthy Halibut Brochette	1 serv	502	7	—	47	—
Light & Healthy Lime & Cilantro Chicken	1 serv	511	9	—	101	—

MACHEEZMO MOUSE
CHILDREN'S MENU SELECTIONS

FOOD	PORTION	CALS	FAT	CARB	CHOL	SOD
El Bento Kid	1 serv (7 oz)	235	1	35	63	330
Quesadilla Kid Cheese	1 serv (5 oz)	360	13	42	40	535
Quesadilla Kid Chicken	1 serv (7 oz)	430	15	42	100	565
Taco Kid Cheese	1 serv (6 oz)	285	5	47	20	344
Taco Kid Chicken	1 (8 oz)	355	7	47	80	374

MAIN MENU SELECTIONS

FOOD	PORTION	CALS	FAT	CARB	CHOL	SOD
Beans	1 oz	35	0	7	0	30
Bento Stick	1 oz	30	1	0	63	68
Boss Sauce	1 oz	30	0	8	0	140
Broccoli	1 oz	4	0	1	0	5
Burrito Chicken	1 (13 oz)	580	11	85	110	748
Burrito Combo	1 (14 oz)	630	12	87	124	933
Burrito Vegetarian	1 (14 oz)	655	8	123	20	890
Cheese	1 oz	81	5	1	20	180
Chicken	1 oz	35	1	0	30	15
Chili	1 oz	43	1	1	22	100
Chips	1 oz	140	6	19	0	80
Cilantro	1 oz	8	0	1	0	15
Dinner Rice, Beans, Broccoli	1 serv (10 oz)	328	tr	72	0	330
Dinner Rice, Beans, Salad	1 serv (12 oz)	344	tr	76	0	370
El Bento	1 serv (16 oz)	600	2	121	63	776
El Bento Deluxe	1 serv (20 oz)	740	7	136	65	902
Enchilada Chicken	1 (12 oz)	533	13	71	92	825
Enchilada Chili	1 (12 oz)	549	13	73	76	995
Enchilada Sauce	1 oz	6	0	2	0	65
Enchilada Veggie	1 (14 oz)	623	11	106	32	955
Fresh Greens	1 oz	2	0	0	0	5
Green Sauce	1 oz	5	0	1	0	110
Guacamole	1 oz	100	3	19	0	110
Marinated Veggies	1 oz	10	tr	3	0	20

FOOD	PORTION	CALS	FAT	CARB	CHOL	SOD
Mexican Cheese	1 oz	100	8	0	24	280
Mustard Dressing	1 oz	25	tr	3	0	200
Power Salad Chicken	1 serv (16 oz)	275	1	44	63	444
Power Salad Veggie	1 serv (13 oz)	200	tr	44	0	275
Rice	1 oz	45	tr	11	0	50
Salad Chicken	1 serv (15 oz)	430	8	56	110	655
Salad Veggie Taco	1 serv (16 oz)	655	14	110	20	755
Salsa	1 oz	4	0	1	0	45
Snack Famouse #5	1 serv (14 oz)	585	5	114	20	747
Snack Nacho Grande	1 serv (9 oz)	841	41	84	62	960
Snack Quesadilla Cheese	1 serv (6 oz)	377	13	42	42	610
Snack Quesadilla Chicken	1 serv (10 oz)	450	15	42	102	650
Snack Tacos Chicken	1 serv (6 oz)	290	8	34	82	295
Snack Tacos Chili	1 serv (6 oz)	314	8	36	66	465
Snack Tacos Veggie	1 serv (6 oz)	290	6	48	22	325
Sour Cream	1 oz	23	0	4	0	25
Tortilla Corn	3 (1 oz)	60	0	15	0	5
Tortilla Flour	1 oz	80	3	16	0	70
Tortilla Wheat	1 oz	80	3	15	0	65
Veggie Deluxe	1 serv (18 oz)	665	6	136	2	733
Yogurt Nonfat	1 oz	20	tr	2	0	22
MANHATTAN BAGEL						
Blueberry	1 (4 oz)	260	tr	54	0	560
Cheddar Cheese	1 (4 oz)	270	4	48	10	560
Chocolate Chip	1 (4 oz)	290	3	56	0	530
Cinnamon Raisin	1 (4 oz)	280	tr	57	0	560
Egg	1 (4 oz)	270	2	53	0	710
Everything	1 (4 oz)	290	3	54	0	2000
Garlic	1 (4 oz)	270	tr	55	0	560
Jalapeno Cheddar	1 (4 oz)	260	2	53	0	310
Marble	1 (4 oz)	260	tr	52	0	540
Oat Bran	1 (4 oz)	260	1	53	0	470
Oat Bran Raisin Walnut	1 (4 oz)	270	3	54	0	450
Onion	1 (4 oz)	270	tr	55	0	560
Plain	1 (4 oz)	260	tr	52	0	560
Poppy	1 (4 oz)	300	4	54	0	560
Pumpernickel	1 (4 oz)	250	1	52	0	530
Rye	1 (4 oz)	260	1	52	0	560
Salt	1 (4 oz)	260	tr	53	0	7100
Sesame	1 (4 oz)	310	5	55	0	560
Spinach	1 (4 oz)	270	tr	54	0	580
Sun-Dried Tomato	1 (4 oz)	260	1	53	0	340
Whole Wheat	1 (4 oz)	260	tr	52	0	470

FOOD	PORTION	CALS	FAT	CARB	CHOL	SOD
MAX & IRMA'S						
Black Bean Roll Up	1 serv	401	8	—	13	534
Fat Free French	2 tbsp	126	tr	—	0	1034
Fat Free Honey Mustard	2 tbsp	60	0	—	0	280
Fruit Smoothie	1 serv	114	tr	—	0	3
Garden Grill	1 serv	467	7	—	12	911
Garlic Breadstick	1	156	6	—	0	293
Gourmet Garden Grill	1 serv	484	8	—	12	912
Grilled Zucchini & Mushroom Pasta	1 serv	448	10	—	13	—
Grilled Zucchini & Mushroom Pasta w/ Chicken	1 serv	621	18	—	78	—
Hula Bowl w/ Fat Free Honey Mustard Dressing	1 serv	526	8	—	91	1309
Lo-Cal Ranch	2 tbsp	54	6	—	7	141
Tijuana Tortilla Wrap	1	692	15	—	54	1958
MCDONALD'S						

(FAST FACT: The first McDonalds was opened in 1948 in San Bernardino, California. There are now 22,246 worldwide with almost 10,000 outside the United States.)

FOOD	PORTION	CALS	FAT	CARB	CHOL	SOD
BAKED SELECTIONS						
Apple Pie Baked	1 (2.7 oz)	260	13	34	0	200
Chocolate Chip Cookie	1 (1.2 oz)	170	10	22	20	120
Cinnamon Roll	1 (3.3 oz)	400	20	47	75	340
Danish Apple	1 (3.7 oz)	360	16	51	40	290
Danish Cheese	1 (3.7 oz)	410	22	47	70	340
Lowfat Muffin Apple Bran	1 (4 oz)	300	3	61	0	380
BEVERAGES						
Coca-Cola Classic	1 sm (16 oz)	150	0	40	0	15
Coca-Cola Classic	1 child serv (12 oz)	110	0	29	0	10
Coca-Cola Classic	1 lg (32 oz)	310	0	86	0	30
Coca-Cola Classic	1 med (21 oz)	210	0	58	0	20
Diet Coke	1 child serv (12 oz)	0	0	0	0	20
Diet Coke	1 lg (32 oz)	0	0	0	0	60
Diet Coke	1 med (21 oz)	0	0	0	0	30
Diet Coke	1 sm (16 oz)	1	0	0	0	30
Hi-C Orange	1 child serv (12 oz)	120	0	32	0	20

FOOD	PORTION	CALS	FAT	CARB	CHOL	SOD
Hi-C Orange	1 lg (32 oz)	350	0	94	0	60
Hi-C Orange	1 med (21 oz)	240	0	64	0	40
Hi-C Orange	1 sm (16 oz)	160	0	44	0	30
Milk 1%	1 serv (8 oz)	100	3	13	10	115
Orange Juice	1 serv (6 oz)	80	0	20	0	20
Shake Chocolate	1 sm (14.5 oz)	360	9	60	40	250
Shake Strawberry	1 sm (14.5 oz)	360	9	60	40	180
Shake Vanilla	1 sm (14.5 oz)	360	9	59	40	250
Sprite	1 child serv (12 oz)	110	0	28	0	40
Sprite	1 lg (32 oz)	310	0	83	0	115
Sprite	1 med (21 oz)	210	0	56	0	80
Sprite	1 sm (16 fl oz)	150	0	39	0	55
BREAKFAST SELECTIONS						
Bacon Egg & Cheese Biscuit	1 (5.5 oz)	470	25	36	235	1250
Biscuit	1 (2.9 oz)	290	15	34	0	780
Breakfast Burrito	1 (4.1 oz)	320	19	23	195	600
Egg McMuffin	1 (4.8 oz)	290	14	27	235	710
English Muffin	1 (1.9 oz)	140	2	25	0	210
Hash Browns	1 serv (1.9 oz)	130	8	14	0	330
Hotcakes Margarine & Syrup	2 serv (7.8 oz)	570	16	100	15	750
Hotcakes Plain	1 serv (5.3 oz)	310	7	53	15	610
Sausage	1 (1.5 oz)	170	16	0	35	290
Sausage Biscuit	1 (4.5 oz)	470	31	35	35	1080
Sausage Biscuit With Egg	1 (6.2 oz)	550	37	35	245	1160
Sausage McMuffin	1 (3.9 oz)	360	23	26	45	740
Sausage McMuffin With Egg	1 (5.7 oz)	440	28	27	255	810
Scrambled Eggs	2 (3.6 oz)	160	11	1	425	170
DESSERTS						
McDonaldland Cookies	1 pkg (1.5 oz)	180	5	32	0	190
Nuts For Sundaes	1 serv (7 g)	40	4	2	0	0
Reduced Fat Ice Cream Cone Vanilla	1 (3.2 oz)	150	5	23	20	75
Sundae Hot Caramel	1 (6.4 oz)	360	10	61	35	180
Sundae Hot Fudge	1 (6.3 oz)	340	12	52	30	170
Sundae Strawberry	1 (6.2 oz)	290	7	50	30	95
MAIN MENU SELECTIONS						
Arch Deluxe	1 (8.4 oz)	550	31	39	55	1010
Arch Deluxe With Bacon	1 (8.7 oz)	590	34	39	60	1150
Barbeque Sauce	1 pkg (1 oz)	45	0	10	0	250

FOOD	PORTION	CALS	FAT	CARB	CHOL	SOD
Big Mac	1 (7.5 oz)	560	31	45	85	1070
Cheeseburger	1 (4.2 oz)	320	13	35	40	820
Chicken McNuggets	4 pieces (2.5 oz)	190	11	10	40	340
Chicken McNuggets	6 pieces (3.7 oz)	290	17	15	60	510
Chicken McNuggets	9 pieces (5.6 oz)	430	26	23	90	770
Crispy Chicken Deluxe	1 (7.8 oz)	500	25	43	55	1100
Fish Filet Deluxe	1 (8 oz)	560	28	54	30	1060
French Fries	1 lg (5.2 oz)	450	22	57	0	290
French Fries	1 sm (2.4 oz)	210	10	26	0	135
French Fries	1 super (6.2 oz)	540	26	68	0	350
Grilled Chicken Deluxe	1 (7.8 oz)	440	20	38	60	1040
Grilled Chicken Deluxe Plain w/o Mayonnaise	1 (7.2 oz)	300	5	38	50	930
Grilled Chicken Salad Deluxe	1 serv (9 oz)	120	2	7	45	240
Hamburger	1 (3.7 oz)	260	9	34	30	580
Honey	1 pkg (0.5 oz)	45	0	12	0	0
Honey Mustard	1 pkg (0.5 oz)	40	5	3	10	85
Hot Mustard	1 pkg (1 oz)	60	4	7	5	240
Light Mayonnaise	1 pkg (0.4 oz)	40	4	tr	5	85
Quarter Pounder	1 (6 oz)	420	21	37	70	820
Quarter Pounder With Cheese	1 (7 oz)	530	30	38	95	1290
Sweet 'N Sour Sauce	1 pkg (1 oz)	50	0	11	0	140
SALAD DRESSINGS						
Caesar	1 pkg (2.1 oz)	160	14	7	20	450
Fat Free Herb Vinaigrette	1 pkg (2.1 oz)	50	0	11	0	330
Ranch	1 pkg (2.1 oz)	230	21	10	20	550
Reduced Calorie Red French	1 pkg (2.1 oz)	160	8	23	0	490
SALADS AND SALAD BARS						
Croutons	1 pkg (0.4 oz)	50	2	7	0	80
Garden Salad	1 serv (6.2 oz)	35	0	7	0	20

MORRISON'S
DESSERTS

FOOD	PORTION	CALS	FAT	CARB	CHOL	SOD
Boston Cream Cake	1 slice	218	4	—	—	171
MAIN MENU SELECTIONS						
Baked Potato	1	220	tr	—	—	16
Broccoli	1 serv (4 oz)	37	2	—	—	310
Cabbage	1 serv (4 oz)	36	tr	—	—	190

FOOD	PORTION	CALS	FAT	CARB	CHOL	SOD
Cantaloupe Compote	1 serv (4 oz)	130	1	—	—	30
Cauliflower	1 serv (4 oz)	68	5	—	—	178
Chicken Stew & Dumplings	1 serv (7 oz)	362	14	—	—	468
Chicken Teriyaki	1 serv (5.5 oz)	232	10	—	—	1187
French Bread	1 slice	207	2	—	—	413
Grilled Chicken Pecan Salad	1 serv (6 oz)	298	8	—	—	635
Lima Beans	1 serv (4 oz)	170	4	—	—	300
Okra & Tomatoes	1 serv (5 oz)	40	2	—	—	233
Pinto Beans	1 serv (4 oz)	105	4	—	—	332
Plain Jell-O	1 serv (3 oz)	131	tr	—	—	109
Rutabagas	1 serv (4 oz)	33	1	—	—	147
Sliced Tomato	4 slices	40	1	—	—	20
Soft Roll	1 (2 oz)	170	4	—	—	200
Strawberries & Banana Bowl	1 serv (6 oz)	203	1	—	—	4
Strawberries Peaches & Bananas	1 serv (6 oz)	203	1	—	—	4
Turnip Greens	1 serv (4 oz)	30	2	—	—	365
Watermelon	1 serv (6 oz)	102	1	—	—	6
Yellow Squash	1 serv (4 oz)	22	1	—	—	179
SALADS AND SALAD BARS						
Garden Salad	1 serv (2.5 oz)	75	2	—	—	163
Tossed Salad	1 serv (3 oz)	30	tr	—	—	18

MRS. FIELDS

FOOD	PORTION	CALS	FAT	CARB	CHOL	SOD
Brownie Double Fudge	1 (3.1 oz)	420	20	56	35	125
Brownie Fudge Walnut	1 (3.4 oz)	500	29	54	40	135
Brownie Pecan Fudge	1 (2.8 oz)	390	21	48	40	135
Brownie Pecan Pie	1 (3 oz)	400	21	48	55	160
Cookie Chewy Fudge	1 (1.7 oz)	230	12	32	25	100
Cookie Milk Chocolate Chip	1 (1.7 oz)	240	12	32	35	210
Cookie Milk Chocolate w/ Walnuts	1 (1.7 oz)	250	13	30	30	200
Cookie Oatmeal Raisin	1 (1.7 oz)	220	10	31	30	230
Cookie Peanut Butter	1 (1.7 oz)	240	13	27	40	280
Cookie Semi-Sweet Chocolate	1 (1.7 oz)	230	12	32	30	210
Cookie Triple Chocolate	1 (1.7 oz)	230	12	31	30	210
Muffin Banana Walnut	1 (3.9 oz)	460	24	53	45	390
Muffin Blueberry	1 (4 oz)	390	15	58	45	470
Muffin Chocolate Chip	1 (4 oz)	450	19	65	40	470

FOOD	PORTION	CALS	FAT	CARB	CHOL	SOD
Muffin Mandarin Orange	1 (4 oz)	420	17	59	45	490
Peanut Butter Dream Bar	1 (5 oz)	750	40	85	40	270
PRETZELS						
Hot Sam Bavarian	1 lg (5.1 oz)	390	0	83	0	780
Hot Sam Bavarian	1 reg (2.5 oz)	200	0	42	0	390
Hot Sam Bavarian Stix	10 (5 oz)	390	0	83	0	780
Hot Sam Sweet Dough	1 (4.5 oz)	360	3	73	0	780
Hot Sam Sweet Dough Blueberry	1 (4.5 oz)	400	4	81	0	610

MY FAVORITE MUFFIN

FOOD	PORTION	CALS	FAT	CARB	CHOL	SOD
Basic Muffin	⅓ muffin	220	10	30	0	190
Double Chocolate	⅓ muffin	190	8	30	0	230
Fat Free Bavarian	⅓ muffin	100	0	24	0	140
Fat Free Bavarian Chocolate	⅓ muffin	130	0	31	0	200

NATHAN'S
BEVERAGES

FOOD	PORTION	CALS	FAT	CARB	CHOL	SOD
Lemonade	16 fl oz	189	0	46	—	5
Lemonade	22 fl oz	260	0	64	—	7
Lemonade	32 fl oz	378	0	93	—	10
MAIN MENU SELECTIONS						
Breaded Chicken Sandwich	1 (7.2 oz)	510	25	48	56	927
Charbroiled Chicken Sandwich	1 (4.5 oz)	288	5	24	53	861
Cheese Steak Sandwich	1 (6.1 oz)	485	26	37	73	579
Chicken 2 Pieces	1 serv (7.1 oz)	693	44	26	211	958
Chicken 4 Pieces	1 serv (14.2 oz)	1382	88	52	422	1912
Chicken Platter 2 Pieces	1 serv (14.8 oz)	1096	66	72	212	1413
Chicken Platter 4 Pieces	1 serv (21.9 oz)	1788	109	99	425	2369
Chicken Salad	1 serv (12.7 oz)	154	4	9	49	345
Double Burger	1 (7.3 oz)	671	41	32	154	460
Filet of Fish Platter	1 serv (22 oz)	1455	74	137	147	1837
Filet of Fish Sandwich	1 (5.2 oz)	403	15	46	32	714
Frank Nuggets	11 pieces (5.1 oz)	563	38	40	73	1173
Frank Nuggets	15 pieces (6.9 oz)	764	52	54	99	1594
Frank Nuggets	7 pieces (3.2 oz)	357	24	25	46	744
Frankfurter	1 (3.2 oz)	310	19	22	45	820
French Fries	1 serv (8.6 oz)	514	26	62	0	61
Fried Clam Platter	1 serv (13.1 oz)	1024	51	119	49	1826

FOOD	PORTION	CALS	FAT	CARB	CHOL	SOD
Fried Clam Sandwich	1 (5.4 oz)	620	29	72	44	1417
Fried Shrimp	1 serv (4.4 oz)	348	11	47	71	869
Fried Shrimp Platter	1 serv (12.6 oz)	796	34	100	83	1436
Hamburger	1 (4.7 oz)	434	23	32	77	281
Knish	1 (5.9 oz)	318	7	53	2	822
Pastrami Sandwich	1 (4.1 oz)	325	12	34	48	1013
Sauteed Onions	1 serv (3.5 oz)	39	1	6	0	16
Super Burger	1 (7.6 oz)	533	32	34	86	525
Turkey Sandwich	1 (4.9 oz)	270	2	34	27	1458
SALADS AND SALAD BARS						
Garden Salad	1 serv (10.9 oz)	193	13	10	36	261

OLIVE GARDEN

FOOD	PORTION	CALS	FAT	CARB	CHOL	SOD
Garden Fare Apple Carmellina	1 serv (12.2 oz)	560	2	131	5	190
Garden Fare Dinner Capellini Pomodoro	1 serv (21.1 oz)	610	16	98	5	940
Garden Fare Dinner Capellini Primavera	1 serv (20.1 oz)	400	7	68	15	950
Garden Fare Dinner Capellini Primavera w/ Chicken	1 serv (23.8 oz)	560	10	71	95	1030
Garden Fare Dinner Chicken Giardino	1 serv (20.6 oz)	550	11	71	85	1000
Garden Fare Dinner Linguine Alla Marinara	1 serv (16.3 oz)	500	9	89	0	160
Garden Fare Dinner Penne Fra Diavolo	1 serv (14.3 oz)	420	7	77	10	940
Garden Fare Dinner Shrimp Primavera	1 serv (28.4 oz)	740	15	104	290	1630
Garden Fare Lunch Capellini Pomodoro	1 serv (11.7 oz)	360	9	57	5	540
Garden Fare Lunch Capellini Primavera	1 serv (11.2 oz)	260	5	42	15	560
Garden Fare Lunch Capellini Primavera w/ Chicken	1 serv (14.9 oz)	420	8	45	90	640
Garden Fare Lunch Chicken Giardino	1 serv (12.8 oz)	360	9	47	50	900
Garden Fare Lunch Linguine Alla Marinara	1 serv (10.2 oz)	310	6	54	0	105
Garden Fare Lunch Penne Fra Diavolo	1 serv (10.2 oz)	300	5	57	10	640
Garden Fare Lunch Shrimp Primavera	1 serv (15.2 oz)	410	8	60	145	840
Minestrone Soup	1 serv (6 oz)	80	1	15	0	450

FOOD	PORTION	CALS	FAT	CARB	CHOL	SOD
PERKINS						
Low Fat Brownie	1 (5.4 oz)	260	1	—	—	—
Low Fat Muffin Banana	1 (5.8 oz)	330	3	—	—	—
Low Fat Muffin Blueberry	1 (5.8 oz)	270	3	—	—	—
Low Fat Muffin Honey Bran	1 (5.8 oz)	270	3	—	—	—
Low Fat Muffin Plain	1 (5.8 oz)	300	3	—	—	—
PICCADILLY CAFETERIA						
BAKED SELECTIONS						
Corn Sticks	1 (2 oz)	165	10	17	26	385
French Bread	1 slice	132	2	24	6	199
Garlic Bread	1 serv (15.8 oz)	1154	24	195	48	1718
Mexican Corn Bread	1 piece	220	14	21	31	547
Roll	1 (2 oz)	130	2	23	0	195
Roll Whole Wheat	1 (1.7 oz)	117	1	22	19	159
Texas Toast	1 serv (15.5 oz)	1088	17	195	48	1633
BEVERAGES						
Iced Tea	1 serv (6.5 oz)	2	0	tr	0	0
Punch	1 serv (9 oz)	133	0	34	0	1
DESSERTS						
Apple Pie	1 slice (7.2 oz)	439	19	67	0	476
Cantaloupe	1 serv (5.5 oz)	55	tr	13	0	14
Cantaloupe	1 serv (9 oz)	89	1	21	0	23
Chocolate Cream Pie	1 slice (7.5 oz)	512	25	65	66	655
Custard	1 cup (5.4 oz)	183	1	39	25	358
Custard Pie	1 slice (6.2 oz)	412	18	54	18	630
Dole Whip Topping	1 serv (3 oz)	68	1	15	0	14
Fresh Fruit Plate	1 serv (21.1 oz)	389	5	81	11	306
Gelatin	1 serv (4.75 oz)	128	4	22	14	94
Honeydew Melon	1 serv (5.5 oz)	55	tr	14	0	16
Honeydew Melon	1 serv (9 oz)	89	tr	23	0	26
Lemon Chiffon Pie	1 slice (6.3 oz)	481	20	61	32	645
Pound Cake	1 slice (3.8 oz)	371	17	51	76	744
Watermelon	1 serv (11 oz)	100	1	22	0	6
MAIN MENU SELECTIONS						
Au Jus	1 serv (3 oz)	5	tr	1	0	537
Baby Lima Beans	1 serv (4.5 oz)	151	6	19	0	371
Baked Potato	1	218	tr	50	0	16
Baked Potato w/ Topping	1	350	15	51	33	119
Beef Chopped Steak Fried	1 serv (4 oz)	311	23	4	59	457
Beef Leg Roast	1 serv (4 oz)	311	18	1	92	472
Beef Liver Fried	1 serv (4.5 oz)	430	29	15	418	404

FOOD	PORTION	CALS	FAT	CARB	CHOL	SOD
Beef Tips Braised	1 serv (10 oz)	470	26	41	56	828
Black-eyed Peas w/ Pork Jowls	1 serv (4 oz)	108	6	9	7	386
Broccoli Buttered	1 serv (4 oz)	77	6	5	0	273
Broccoli & Rice Au Gratin	½ cup	184	9	20	18	577
Carrots Young Buttered	½ cup	90	6	9	0	512
Cauliflower Buttered	1 serv	80	6	6	0	260
Chicken Baked w/o Skin	¼ chicken	352	11	tr	168	401
Chicken Teriyaki	1 serv (4 oz)	445	22	14	124	1432
Chicken Teriyaki Polynesian	1 serv (4 oz)	537	27	34	104	2051
Corn	1 serv (4.5 oz)	128	7	17	0	423
Cornbread Stuffing	1 serv (4.5 oz)	164	9	12	26	597
Crackers	4 (0.4 oz)	51	1	8	—	172
Cranberry Sauce	1 serv (1.5 oz)	64	tr	17	0	12
Eggplant Escalloped	½ cup	180	10	19	15	928
Fish Baked	1 serv (7 oz)	195	10	3	54	532
Green Beans	1 serv (4.5 oz)	77	6	5	7	552
Ham Baked	1 serv (4 oz)	224	10	6	67	1703
Macaroni & Cheese	½ cup	317	11	38	22	1752
Mashed Potatoes	1 serv (4.8 oz)	120	3	20	0	62
Meatballs Baked & Spaghetti	1 serv (11.5 oz)	108	5	7	23	419
New Potatoes Boiled	½ cup	148	12	12	0	852
Okra Smothered	1 serv (4 oz)	121	10	9	0	633
Onion Sauce	1 serv (4 oz)	152	7	30	0	481
Rice	½ cup	99	tr	22	0	9
Rice Polynesian	1 serv (4 oz)	140	6	20	0	627
Spaghetti Baked	1 serv (9.5 oz)	256	10	33	13	448
Squash Baked Italian	1 serv (4.75 oz)	73	3	8	8	1072
Squash Mixed Yellow & Zucchini	1 serv (4 oz)	72	5	6	0	390
Squash Yellow Baked French Style	⅓ cup	86	5	9	5	405
Turkey Breast	1 serv (3 oz)	99	2	tr	—	612
Vegetables Unseasoned	1 serv (5 oz)	29	tr	6	0	23
SALADS AND SALAD BARS						
Broccoli Salad	1 serv (4 oz)	202	20	6	13	252
Cabbage Combination Salad	1 serv (4.5 oz)	50	tr	15	0	1164
Carrot & Raisin Salad	1 serv (4.5 oz)	321	23	30	10	280
Cole Slaw w/ Cream	1 serv (4 oz)	182	18	5	9	344
Cucumber & Celery Salad	1 serv (4 oz)	82	6	6	0	686

FOOD	PORTION	CALS	FAT	CARB	CHOL	SOD
Fruit Salad	1 serv (6 oz)	59	1	14	0	6
Neptune Salad	1 serv	361	34	3	25	659
Spinach Tossed Salad	1 serv (4 oz)	88	6	6	44	147
Spring Salad Bowl	1 serv (4 oz)	22	tr	5	0	21
SOUPS						
Gumbo Chicken	1 serv (8 oz)	92	2	9	22	1033
Gumbo Seafood	1 serv (8 oz)	98	2	10	45	1300
Vegetable	1 serv (8 oz)	49	tr	10	0	998

PIZZA HUT
MAIN MENU SELECTIONS

FOOD	PORTION	CALS	FAT	CARB	CHOL	SOD
Bread Stick	1 (1.3 oz)	130	4	20	0	170
Bread Stick Dipping Sauce	1 serv (1.2 oz)	30	1	5	0	170
Cavatini Pasta	1 serv (12.5 oz)	480	14	66	25	1170
Cavatini Supreme Pasta	1 serv (13.9 oz)	560	19	73	30	1400
Garlic Bread	1 slice (1.3 oz)	150	8	16	0	240
Ham & Cheese Sandwich	1 (9.7 oz)	550	21	19	65	2150
Hot Buffalo Wings	4 pieces (2.1 oz)	210	12	4	130	900
Spaghetti Marinara	1 serv (16.6 oz)	490	6	91	0	730
Spaghetti Meat Sauce	1 serv (16.4 oz)	600	13	98	25	910
Spaghetti Meatballs	1 serv (18.8 oz)	850	24	120	50	1120
Supreme Sandwich	1 (10.2 oz)	640	28	62	85	2150
Wild Buffalo Wings	5 pieces (2.9 oz)	200	12	tr	150	510

PIZZA

FOOD	PORTION	CALS	FAT	CARB	CHOL	SOD
Beef Topping Hand Tossed	1 slice (3.9 oz)	280	10	32	20	860
Beef Topping Pan	1 slice (3.9 oz)	310	14	31	20	720
Beef Topping Stuffed Crust	1 slice (5.6 oz)	410	14	49	30	1270
Beef Topping Thin 'N Crispy	1 slice (3.1 oz)	240	11	22	20	790
Cheese Hand Tossed	1 slice (3.9 oz)	280	10	32	25	770
Cheese Pan	1 slice (3.9 oz)	300	14	30	25	610
Cheese Stuffed Crust	1 slice (5.4 oz)	380	11	49	25	1160
Cheese Thin'N Crispy	1 slice (2.6oz)	210	9	21	20	530
Chicken Supreme Pan	1 slice (4.1 oz)	280	11	32	25	570
Chicken Supreme Stuffed Crust	1 slice (6.4 oz)	390	13	46	40	1130
Chicken Supreme Thin 'N Crispy	1 slice (4.2 oz)	240	6	31	25	660
Dessert Apple	1 slice (2.8 oz)	250	5	48	0	230

FOOD	PORTION	CALS	FAT	CARB	CHOL	SOD
Dessert Cherry	1 slice (2.8 oz)	250	5	47	0	220
Ham Hand Tossed	1 slice (3.4 oz)	230	6	30	25	710
Ham Pan	1 slice (3.4 oz)	250	9	31	10	590
Ham Stuffed Crust	1 slice (5.4 oz)	380	14	43	45	1250
Ham Thin 'N Crispy	1 slice (2.4 oz)	190	6	23	15	560
Italian Sausage Hand Tossed	1 slice (4 oz)	300	12	32	30	780
Italian Sausage Pan	1 slice (4.3 oz)	350	18	31	40	740
Italian Sausage Stuffed Crust	1 slice (5.7 oz)	430	19	46	35	1200
Italian Sausage Thin 'N Crispy	1 slice (3.4 oz)	300	16	34	35	740
Meat Lover's Hand Tossed	1 slice (3.9 oz)	290	11	32	35	820
Meat Lover's Pan	1 slice (4.4 oz)	360	19	30	40	870
Meat Lover's Stuffed Crust	1 slice (6.6 oz)	500	23	47	60	1510
Meat Lover's Thin 'N Crispy	1 slice (3.7 oz)	310	16	25	35	900
Pepperoni Hand Tossed	1 slice (3.4 oz)	260	9	31	30	750
Pepperoni Lover's Hand Tossed	1 slice (4 oz)	320	13	31	35	910
Pepperoni Lover's Pan	1 slice (4.1 oz)	350	17	32	20	800
Pepperoni Lover's Stuffed Crust	1 slice (6.1 oz)	480	22	47	60	1440
Pepperoni Lover's Thin 'N Crispy	1 slice (3.1 oz)	270	12	26	25	780
Pepperoni Pan	1 slice (3.4 oz)	280	12	31	20	640
Pepperoni Stuffed Crust	1 slice (5.3 oz)	410	17	46	40	1250
Pepperoni Thin 'N Crispy	1 slice (2.3 oz)	220	9	22	20	610
Personal Pan Cheese	1 pie (8.1 oz)	630	24	76	45	1160
Personal Pan Pepperoni	1 pie (8.1 oz)	670	29	73	60	1250
Personal Pan Supreme	1 pie (9.5 oz)	710	31	76	60	1380
Pork Topping Hand Tossed	1 slice (3.9 oz)	290	11	33	25	850
Pork Topping Pan	1 slice (3.6 oz)	300	13	31	30	720
Pork Topping Stuffed Crust	1 slice (5.6 oz)	420	16	46	30	1290
Pork Topping Thin 'N Crispy	1 slice (3.2 oz)	270	13	22	25	780
Super Supreme Hand Tossed	1 slice (4.7 oz)	290	10	34	35	830
Super Supreme Pan	1 slice (4.6 oz)	340	16	33	30	790
Super Supreme Stuffed Crust	1 slice (7.2 oz)	470	20	49	50	1440

FOOD	PORTION	CALS	FAT	CARB	CHOL	SOD
Super Supreme Thin 'N Crispy	1 slice (4 oz)	280	13	26	30	810
Supreme Hand Tossed	1 slice (3.9 oz)	270	9	32	25	760
Supreme Pan	1 slice (4 oz)	300	13	32	25	670
Supreme Stuffed Crust	1 slice (6.4 oz)	440	16	51	40	1380
Supreme Thin 'N Crispy	1 slice (3.4 oz)	250	11	24	20	710
Veggie Lover's Hand Tossed	1 slice (4 oz)	240	7	34	20	650
Veggie Lover's Pan	1 slice (3.9 oz)	240	9	31	10	480
Veggie Lover's Stuffed Crust	1 slice (5.9 oz)	390	14	48	25	1140
Veggie Lover's Thin 'N Crispy	1 slice (2.6 oz)	170	6	23	10	460

PONDEROSA
BEVERAGES

FOOD	PORTION	CALS	FAT	CARB	CHOL	SOD
Cherry Coke	6 oz	77	0	20	0	4
Chocolate Milk	8 oz	208	9	26	33	149
Coca-Cola	6 oz	72	0	19	0	7
Coffee Black	6 oz	2	0	tr	0	26
Diet Coke	6 oz	tr	0	tr	0	8
Diet Coke Caffeine Free	6 oz	tr	0	tr	0	8
Diet Sprite	6 oz	2	0	0	0	4
Dr Pepper	6 oz	72	0	19	0	14
Lemonade	6 oz	68	0	19	0	50
Milk	8 oz	159	9	12	34	122
Mr. Pibb	6 oz	71	0	18	0	10
Orange Soda	6 oz	82	0	21	0	0
Root Beer	6 oz	80	0	21	0	9
Sprite	6 oz	72	0	18	0	16
Tea	6 oz	2	0	1	0	0

ICE CREAM

FOOD	PORTION	CALS	FAT	CARB	CHOL	SOD
Ice Milk Chocolate	3.5 oz	152	3	30	22	70
Ice Milk Vanilla	3.5 oz	150	3	30	20	58
Topping Caramel	1 oz	100	1	26	2	72
Topping Chocolate	1 oz	89	tr	24	0	37
Topping Strawberry	1 oz	71	tr	24	0	29
Topping Whippped	1 oz	80	6	5	0	16

MAIN MENU SELECTIONS

FOOD	PORTION	CALS	FAT	CARB	CHOL	SOD
BBQ Sauce	1 tbsp	25	0	5	0	260
Bake 'R Broil Fish	1 serv (5.2 oz)	230	13	10	50	330
Baked Potato	1 (7.2 oz)	145	tr	33	0	6
Beans Baked	1 serv (4 oz)	170	6	21	0	330
Beans Green	1 serv (3.5 oz)	20	0	3	0	391

FOOD	PORTION	CALS	FAT	CARB	CHOL	SOD
Breaded Cauliflower	1 serv (4 oz)	115	1	23	1	446
Breaded Okra	1 serv (4 oz)	124	1	23	1	483
Breaded Onion Rings	1 serv (4 oz)	213	9	30	2	620
Breaded Zucchini	1 serv (4 oz)	102	1	18	1	584
Carrots	1 serv (3.5 oz)	31	tr	7	0	33
Cheese Herb Garlic Spread	1 tbsp	100	10	0	0	120
Cheese Sauce	2 oz	52	2	6	4	355
Chicken Breast	1 serv (5.5 oz)	90	2	1	54	400
Chicken Wings	2	213	9	11	75	610
Chopped Steak	4 oz	225	16	1	80	150
Chopped Steak	5.3 oz	296	22	1	105	296
Corn	1 serv (3.5 oz)	90	tr	21	0	5
Fish Fried	1 serv (3.2 oz)	190	9	17	15	170
Fish Nuggets	1	31	2	2	8	52
French Fries	1 serv (3 oz)	120	4	17	3	39
Gravy Brown	2 oz	25	1	4	0	167
Gravy Turkey	2 oz	25	tr	5	0	228
Halibut Broiled	1 serv (6 oz)	170	2	0	—	68
Hot Dog	1	144	13	1	27	460
Italian Breadsticks	1	100	1	19	0	200
Kansas City Strip	5 oz	138	6	1	76	850
Macaroni And Cheese	4 oz	67	2	18	4	320
Margarine Liquid	1 tbsp	100	11	0	0	110
Mashed Potatoes	1 serv (4 oz)	62	tr	13	20	191
Meatballs	1	58	2	1	11	8
Mini Shrimp	6	47	tr	6	22	125
New York Strip Choice	10 oz	314	15	1	50	1420
New York Strip Choice	8 oz	384	11	2	62	570
Pasta Shells Plain	2 oz	78	tr	16	0	tr
Peas	1 serv (3.5 oz)	67	tr	12	0	120
Porterhouse	13 oz	441	30	1	67	1844
Porterhouse Choice	16 oz	640	31	3	82	1130
Potato Wedges	1 serv (3.5 oz)	130	6	16	—	171
Ribeye	5 oz	219	13	1	75	1130
Ribeye Choice	6 oz	281	14	tr	60	570
Rice Pilaf	1 serv (4 oz)	160	4	26	22	450
Roll Dinner	1	184	3	33	0	311
Roll Sourdough	1	110	1	22	0	230
Roughy Broiled	1 serv (5 oz)	139	5	—	28	88
Salmon Broiled	1 serv (6 oz)	192	3	3	60	72
Sandwich Steak	4 oz	408	11	2	62	850
Scrod Baked	1 serv (7 oz)	120	1	0	65	80
Shrimp Fried	7 pieces	231	tr	31	105	612

FOOD	PORTION	CALS	FAT	CARB	CHOL	SOD
Sirloin Choice	7 oz	241	11	1	63	570
Sirloin Tips Choice	5 oz	473	8	2	72	280
Spaghetti Plain	2 oz	78	tr	16	0	tr
Spaghetti Sauce	4 oz	110	4	17	0	520
Steak Kabobs Meat Only	3 oz	153	5	2	67	280
Stuffing	4 oz	230	11	27	22	800
Sweet/Sour Sauce	1 oz	37	1	8	0	80
Swordfish Broiled	1 serv (6 oz)	271	9	0	85	0
T-Bone	8 oz	176	9	1	71	850
T-Bone Choice	10 oz	444	18	2	80	850
Teriyaki Steak	5 oz	174	3	5	64	1420
Tortilla Chips	1 oz	150	8	16	0	80
Trout Broiled	1 serv (5 oz)	228	4	1	110	51
Winter Mix	1 serv (3.5 oz)	25	0	4	0	33
SALAD DRESSINGS						
Blue Cheese	1 oz	130	13	1	27	266
Cole Slaw	1 oz	150	14	6	31	284
Creamy Italian	1 oz	103	10	3	0	373
Cucumber Reduced Calorie	1 oz	69	6	3	tr	315
Italian Reduced Calorie	1 oz	31	3	1	0	371
Parmesan Pepper	1 oz	150	15	2	9	282
Ranch	1 oz	147	15	1	3	298
Salad Oil	1 tbsp	120	14	0	0	0
Sour Cream	1 tbsp	26	3	1	5	6
Sweet-N-Tangy	1 oz	122	9	9	1	347
Thousand Island	1 oz	113	10	9	1	405
SALADS AND SALAD BARS						
Alfalfa Sprouts	1 oz	10	0	1	0	0
Apple	1	80	1	20	0	1
Apples Canned	4 oz	90	0	22	0	15
Applesauce	4 oz	80	0	20	0	20
Banana	1	87	tr	23	0	1
Banana Chips	0.2 oz	25	1	3	0	tr
Banana Pudding	1 oz	52	2	6	0	29
Bean Sprouts	1 oz	10	tr	2	0	1
Beets Diced	4 oz	55	tr	13	0	307
Breadsticks Sesame	2	35	0	6	0	60
Broccoli	1 oz	9	1	2	0	4
Cabbage Green	1 oz	9	0	2	0	7
Cabbage Red	1 oz	1	0	tr	0	1
Cantaloupe	1 wedge	13	0	3	0	5
Carrots	1 oz	12	tr	3	0	13
Cauliflower	1 oz	8	tr	2	0	4

FOOD	PORTION	CALS	FAT	CARB	CHOL	SOD
Celery	1 oz	4	0	1	0	36
Cheese Imitation Shredded	1 oz	90	7	1	5	420
Cheese Spread	1 oz	98	7	4	26	188
Cherry Peppers	2 pieces	7	tr	1	0	415
Chicken Salad	3.5 oz	212	15	8	42	335
Chow Mein Noodles	0.2 oz	25	1	3	0	42
Cocktail Sauce	1 oz	34	1	6	0	453
Coconut Shredded	0.2 oz	25	2	2	0	14
Cottage Cheese	4 oz	120	5	5	17	330
Croutons	1 oz	115	4	18	0	351
Cucumber	1 oz	4	0	1	0	2
Eggs Diced	2 oz	94	7	1	260	75
Fruit Cocktail	4 oz	97	tr	25	0	7
Garbanzo Beans	1 oz	102	0	17	0	7
Gelatin Plain	4 oz	71	0	17	0	73
Granola	0.2 oz	24	1	3	0	—
Grapes	10	34	tr	9	0	2
Green Onion	1	7	tr	2	0	1
Green Pepper	1 oz	6	tr	1	0	4
Ham Diced	2 oz	120	10	1	76	780
Honeydew	1 wedge	24	tr	6	0	9
Lemon	1 wedge	3	tr	1	0	0
Lettuce	1 oz	5	0	2	0	5
Macaroni Salad	3.5 oz	335	12	49	9	431
Margarine Whipped	1 tbsp	34	1	0	0	65
Meal Mates Sesame Crackers	2	45	2	6	0	95
Melba Snacks	2	18	0	4	0	60
Mousse Chocolate	1 oz	78	4	7	0	18
Mousse Strawberry	1 oz	74	5	6	0	17
Mushrooms	1 oz	8	tr	1	0	4
Olives Black	1	4	tr	tr	0	24
Olives Green	1	3	tr	tr	0	69
Onions Red & Yellow	1 oz	11	0	3	3	3
Orange	1	45	tr	11	0	1
Pasta Salad	3.5 oz	269	12	34	tr	441
Peaches Canned	4 oz	70	0	18	0	10
Peanuts Chopped	0.2 oz	30	2	1	0	—
Pears Canned	4 oz	98	tr	25	0	7
Pickles Dill Spears	0.14 oz	tr	0	tr	0	54
Pickles Sweet Chips	0.14 oz	4	0	1	0	tr
Pineapple Tidbits	4 oz	95	tr	25	0	2
Pineapple Fresh	1 wedge	11	tr	3	0	tr

FOOD	PORTION	CALS	FAT	CARB	CHOL	SOD
Potato Salad	3.5 oz	126	6	16	7	300
Radishes	1 oz	4	0	1	0	5
Ritz	2	40	2	4	0	50
Saltine Crackers	2	25	tr	4	0	38
Spiced Apple Rings	4 oz	100	0	24	0	20
Spinach	1 oz	7	tr	1	0	20
Strawberries	2 oz	14	tr	3	—	61
Strawberry Glaze	1 oz	37	0	10	—	4
Sunflower Seeds	0.2 oz	31	0	1	0	—
Tartar Sauce	1 oz	85	11	11	9	477
Tomatoes	1 oz	6	tr	1	0	1
Turkey Ham Salad	3.5 oz	186	13	10	12	655
Turkey Julienne	1 oz	29	tr	1	15	192
Vanilla Wafer	2	35	1	6	5	25
Watermelon	1 wedge	111	1	27	0	4
Yogurt Fruit	4 oz	115	1	23	5	70
Yogurt Vanilla	4 oz	110	2	18	6	75
Zucchini	1 oz	5	0	1	0	tr

POPEYE'S

FOOD	PORTION	CALS	FAT	CARB	CHOL	SOD
Apple Pie	1 serv (3.1 oz)	290	16	37	10	820
Biscuit	1 serv (2.3 oz)	250	15	26	<5	430
Breast Mild	1 (3.7 oz)	270	16	9	60	660
Breast Spicy	1 (3.7 oz)	270	16	9	60	590
Cajun Rice	1 serv (3.9 oz)	150	5	17	25	1260
Cole Slaw	1 serv (4 oz)	149	11	14	3	271
Corn On The Cob	1 serv (5.2 oz)	127	3	21	0	20
French Fries	1 serv (3 oz)	240	12	31	10	610
Leg Mild	1 (1.7 oz)	120	7	4	40	240
Leg Spicy	1 (1.7 oz)	120	7	4	40	240
Nuggets	1 serv (4.2 oz)	410	32	18	55	660
Nuggets Mild Tender	1 (1.2 oz)	110	7	6	15	160
Nuggets Spicy Tender	1 (1.2 oz)	110	7	6	15	215
Onion Rings	1 serv (3.1 oz)	310	19	31	25	210
Potatoes & Gravy	1 serv (3.8 oz)	100	6	11	<5	460
Red Beans & Rice	1 serv (5.9 oz)	270	17	30	10	680
Shrimp	1 serv (2.8 oz)	250	16	13	110	650
Thigh Mild	1 (3.1 oz)	300	23	9	70	620
Thigh Spicy	1 (3.1 oz)	300	23	9	70	450
Wing Mild	1 (1.6 oz)	160	11	7	40	290
Wing Spicy	1 (1.6 oz)	160	11	7	40	290

PUDGIE'S FAMOUS CHICKEN

FOOD	PORTION	CALS	FAT	CARB	CHOL	SOD
Fried Chicken	3.5 oz	233	13	4	81	440

FOOD	PORTION	CALS	FAT	CARB	CHOL	SOD
QUINCY'S						
BAKED SELECTIONS						
Banana Nut Bread	1 serv (2 oz)	165	7	22	5	195
Biscuit	1 (2.5 oz)	270	15	29	11	610
Cornbread	1 serv (2 oz)	140	5	19	0	340
Yeast Roll	1 (2 oz)	160	4	29	0	285
BREAKFAST SELECTIONS						
Bacon	1 serv (0.25 oz)	35	3	0	5	100
Corned Beef Hash	1 serv (4.5 oz)	210	15	11	45	795
Country Ham	1 serv (1.5 oz)	90	6	1	35	1100
Escalloped Apples	1 serv (3.5 oz)	120	2	26	0	20
Oatmeal	1 serv (1 oz)	175	2	18	0	285
Pancakes	1 (1.5 oz)	95	3	12	30	250
Sausage Gravy	1 serv (4 oz)	70	6	3	10	150
Sausage Links	1 (2 oz)	225	22	0	20	390
Sausage Patties	1 (2 oz)	230	23	0	45	350
Scrambled Eggs	1 serv (2 oz)	95	7	1	215	270
Steak Fingers	1 serv (3.5 oz)	360	25	18	50	690
Syrup	1 oz	75	0	20	0	15
DESSERTS						
Banana Pudding	1 serv (5 oz)	240	12	30	10	240
Brownie Pudding Cake	1 serv (4 oz)	310	5	66	0	395
Caramel Topping	1 serv (1 oz)	105	1	24	0	120
Chocolate Chip Cookies	1 (0.5 oz)	60	8	8	5	35
Cobbler Apple	1 serv (6 oz)	255	8	49	5	285
Cobbler Cherry	1 serv (6 oz)	410	8	55	5	185
Cobbler Peach	1 serv (6 oz)	305	8	50	5	190
Frozen Yogurt	1 serv (4 oz)	135	2	25	5	85
Fudge Topping	1 serv (1 oz)	105	4	15	0	75
Sugar Cookie	1 (0.5 oz)	60	3	8	5	30
MAIN MENU SELECTIONS						
⅓ Pound Hamburger	1 serv (8 oz)	565	33	32	66	603
BBQ Beans	1 serv (4 oz)	114	1	21	0	604
Bacon Cheese Burger	1 (9 oz)	663	41	33	87	997
Baked Potato	1 (6 oz)	115	0	30	0	0
Broccoli	1 serv (4 oz)	34	0	5	0	50
Cheese Sauce	1 serv (1 oz)	58	5	1	11	212
Chopped Steak Steak	1 serv (8 oz)	499	42	0	89	348
Cinnamon Apples	1 serv (4 oz)	172	5	34	0	149
Corn	1 serv (4 oz)	96	1	24	0	271
Country Steak w/ Gravy	1 serv (8 oz)	530	25	44	54	1161
Cowboy Steak	1 serv (14 oz)	580	33	9	176	1308
Filet w/ Bacon	1 serv (8 oz)	340	17	2	124	311

FOOD	PORTION	CALS	FAT	CARB	CHOL	SOD
Green Beans	1 serv (4 oz)	61	4	6	0	796
Grilled Chicken	1 reg serv (5 oz)	120	2	1	55	540
Grilled Chicken Sandwich	1 (9 oz)	324	4	39	55	1183
Grilled Salmon	1 serv (7 oz)	228	4	1	109	112
Homestyle Chicken Fillet	1 serv (3 oz)	217	9	21	25	682
Junior Sirloin Steak	1 serv (5.5 oz)	194	10	0	69	199
Large Sirloin Steak	1 serv (10 oz)	368	20	2	119	390
Mashed Potatoes	1 serv (4 oz)	54	6	11	0	195
NY Strip Steak	1 serv (10 oz)	450	26	1	148	156
Philly Cheese Steak	1 serv (11 oz)	588	30	38	87	1684
Porterhouse Steak	1 serv (17 oz)	683	46	0	154	346
Regular Sirloin Steak	1 serv (8 oz)	285	16	0	71	317
Ribeye Steak	1 serv (10 oz)	452	29	0	116	156
Rice Pilaf	1 serv (4 oz)	119	2	23	0	1283
Roasted BBQ Chicken	1 serv (14 oz)	941	65	21	340	1548
Roasted Herb Chicken	1 serv (14 oz)	875	65	4	340	1238
Sirloin Tips w/ Mushroom Gravy	1 serv (6 oz)	196	7	5	64	578
Sirloin Tips w/ Peppers & Onions	1 serv (5 oz)	203	8	4	63	793
Smothered Steak Sandwich	1 (9 oz)	429	15	36	69	846
Smothered Strip Steak	1 serv (10 oz)	622	41	12	148	239
Southern Breaded Shrimp	1 serv (7 oz)	546	31	47	135	821
Spicy BBQ Chicken Sandwich	1 (10 oz)	368	1	45	55	1608
Steak & Shrimp	1 serv (9 oz)	677	39	33	170	816
Steak Fries	1 serv (4 oz)	358	19	45	0	245
T-Bone Steak	1 serv (13 oz)	521	35	0	118	265
SALAD DRESSINGS						
Blue Cheese	1 serv (1 oz)	155	16	2	10	165
French	1 serv (1 oz)	125	12	4	0	500
Honey Mustard	1 serv (1 oz)	100	6	10	0	220
Italian	1 serv (1 oz)	135	14	3	0	230
Light Creamy Italian	1 serv (1 oz)	65	4	8	0	485
Light French	1 serv (1 oz)	85	4	13	0	285
Light Italian	1 serv (1 oz)	20	2	2	0	485
Light Thousand Island	1 serv (1 oz)	65	4	8	20	340
Parmesan Peppercorn	1 serv (1 oz)	150	14	4	0	280
Ranch	1 serv (1 oz)	110	11	1	10	195

FOOD	PORTION	CALS	FAT	CARB	CHOL	SOD
SOUPS						
Chili With Beans	1 serv (6 oz)	235	11	21	15	920
Clam Chowder	1 serv (6 oz)	180	9	21	0	835
Cream Of Broccoli	1 serv (6 oz)	170	10	18	0	770
Vegetable Beef	1 serv (6 oz)	90	2	14	0	325
RALLY'S						
BEVERAGES						
Coke	1 serv (16 oz)	132	0	35	0	13
Coke	1 serv (20 oz)	177	0	47	0	17
Coke	1 serv (32 oz)	264	0	70	0	26
Coke	1 serv (42 oz)	372	0	99	0	36
Diet Coke	1 serv (20 oz)	1	0	0	0	18
Diet Coke	1 serv (32 oz)	1	0	1	0	27
Diet Coke	1 serv (42 oz)	2	0	0	0	38
Fanta Orange	1 serv (16 oz)	150	0	38	0	11
Fanta Orange	1 serv (20 oz)	202	0	52	0	15
Fanta Orange	1 serv (32 oz)	301	0	77	0	22
Fanta Orange	1 serv (42 oz)	424	0	109	0	32
Mr. Pibb	1 serv (16 oz)	113	0	29	0	16
Mr. Pibb	1 serv (20 oz)	159	0	40	0	22
Mr. Pibb	1 serv (32 oz)	237	0	60	0	33
Mr. Pibb	1 serv (42 oz)	334	0	84	0	46
Root Beer	1 serv (16 oz)	146	0	38	0	16
Root Beer	1 serv (20 oz)	197	0	52	0	22
Root Beer	1 serv (32 oz)	294	0	77	0	33
Root Beer	1 serv (42 oz)	414	0	109	0	46
Shake Banana	1 serv	399	11	70	38	223
Shake Chocolate	1 serv	411	12	73	38	262
Shake Strawberry	1 serv	399	11	70	38	223
Shake Vanilla	1 serv	320	11	49	38	197
Sprite	1 serv (16 oz)	132	0	33	0	29
Sprite	1 serv (20 oz)	161	0	40	0	36
Sprite	1 serv (32 oz)	264	0	66	0	59
Sprite	1 serv (42 oz)	338	0	84	0	76
MAIN MENU SELECTIONS						
Big Buford	1	743	46	35	151	1860
Chicken Fillet Sandwich	1	399	15	43	42	790
Chili w/ Cheese & Onion	1 serv (13 oz)	669	41	37	137	2125
Chili w/ Cheese & Onion	1 serv (7 oz)	360	22	20	74	1144
French Fries	1 extra lg (8 oz)	423	21	52	13	585
French Fries	1 lg (6 oz)	317	16	39	10	439
French Fries	1 reg (4 oz)	211	11	26	7	293
Onion Rings	1 serv	210	2	45	0	855

FOOD	PORTION	CALS	FAT	CARB	CHOL	SOD
Rallyburger	1	433	22	35	63	1176
Rallyburger w/ Cheese	1	488	35	35	27	1376
Spicy Chicken Sandwich	1	437	18	50	40	887
Super Barbecue Bacon	1	593	31	49	88	1709
Super Double Cheeseburger	1	762	48	37	154	1734

RAX
BEVERAGES
Chocolate Shake	1 (11 fl oz)	445	12	77	35	248
Coke	16 fl oz	205	0	53	0	11
Diet Coke	16 fl oz	1	0	0	0	21

DESSERTS
Chocolate Chip Cookie	1 (2 oz)	262	12	36	6	192

MAIN MENU SELECTIONS
Bacon	1 slice (0.1 oz)	14	1	0	2	40
Baked Potato	1 (10 oz)	264	0	61	0	15
Baked Potato w/ 1 Tbsp Margarine	1 (10.5 oz)	364	11	61	0	115
Barbecue Sauce	1 pkg (0.4 oz)	11	0	3	0	158
Beef Bacon 'N Cheddar	1 (6.7 oz)	523	32	37	42	1042
Cheddar Cheese Sauce	1 fl oz	29	tr	4	0	225
Country Fried Chicken Breast Sandwich	1 (7.4 oz)	618	29	49	45	1078
Deluxe Roast Beef	1 (7.9 oz)	498	30	39	36	864
French Fries	1 serv (3.25 oz)	282	14	36	3	75
Grilled Chicken Breast Sandwich	1 (6.9 oz)	402	23	26	69	872
Grilled Chicken Garden Salad w/ French Dressing	1 serv (12.7 oz)	477	31	34	32	1189
Grilled Chicken Garden Salad w/ Lite Italian Dressing	1 serv (12.7 oz)	264	12	22	32	1040
Mushroom Sauce	1 fl oz	16	tr	1	0	113
Philly Melt	1 (8.2 oz)	396	16	40	27	1055
Regular Rax	1 (4.7 oz)	262	10	25	15	707
Swiss Slice	1 slice (0.4 oz)	42	3	0	10	157

SALAD DRESSINGS
French	2 fl oz	275	22	20	0	442
Lite Italian	2 fl oz	63	3	8	0	294

SALADS AND SALAD BARS
Gourmet Garden Salad w/ French Dressing	1 serv (10.7 oz)	409	29	33	10	792

FOOD	PORTION	CALS	FAT	CARB	CHOL	SOD
Gourmet Garden Salad w/ Lite Italian Dressing	1 serv (10.7 oz)	305	10	22	2	643
Gourmet Garden Salad w/o Dressing	1 serv (8.7 oz)	134	6	13	2	350
Grilled Chicken Garden Salad w/o Dressing	1 serv (10.7 oz)	202	9	14	32	747

RED LOBSTER
CHILDREN'S MENU SELECTIONS

FOOD	PORTION	CALS	FAT	CARB	CHOL	SOD
Cheeseburger	1 serv	1040	56	—	130	720
Fried Chicken Fingers	1 serv	680	33	—	35	630
Fried Shrimp	1 serv	650	33	—	80	510
Grilled Chicken Tenders	1 serv	580	24	—	55	400
Hamburger	1 serv	920	47	—	100	550
Popcorn Shrimp	1 serv	650	35	—	120	480
Popcorn Shrimp & Cheesesticks	1 serv	750	41	—	125	680
Spaghetti & Cheesesticks	1 serv	830	39	—	5	950

DESSERTS

FOOD	PORTION	CALS	FAT	CARB	CHOL	SOD
Carrot Cake	1 serv (6.5 oz)	730	31	—	—	—
Cheesecake	1 serv (5.5 oz)	530	41	—	—	—
Fudge Overboard	1 serv	620	23	—	105	110
Ice Cream	1 serv (4.5 oz)	140	7	—	30	60
Key Lime Pie	1 serv (5 oz)	450	15	—	—	—
Raspberry Cobbler	1 serv (3 oz)	530	33	—	—	—
Sensational 7	1 serv	790	41	—	140	690

MAIN MENU SELECTIONS

FOOD	PORTION	CALS	FAT	CARB	CHOL	SOD
Admiral's Feast	1 serv	1060	52	—	265	2400
Appetizer Calamari	1 serv	350	22	—	190	510
Appetizer Chicken Fingers	1 serv	390	18	—	65	770
Appetizer Chilled Shrimp In The Shell	1 serv (6 oz)	110	2	—	235	270
Appetizer Crab & Shrimp Cakes	1 serv	480	24	—	80	1550
Appetizer Crab Add-On	1 serv	60	1	—	55	160
Appetizer Fresh Fried Mushrooms	1 serv	790	51	—	<5	1280
Appetizer Lobster Quesadilla	1 serv	760	47	—	160	1300
Appetizer Lobster Stuffed Mushroom	1 serv	400	26	—	100	960

FOOD	PORTION	CALS	FAT	CARB	CHOL	SOD
Appetizer Mozzarella Cheesesticks	1 serv	730	46	—	50	1570
Appetizer Parmesan Zucchini	1 serv	620	40	—	10	1200
Appetizer Shrimp Cocktail	1 serv	50	1	—	105	120
Appetizer Stuffed Mushrooms	1 serv	420	27	—	90	940
Applesauce	1 serv (4 oz)	90	0	—	0	5
Atlantic Cod	1 lunch serv (5 oz)	110	1	—	60	85
Atlantic Cod	1 serv (8 oz)	200	2	—	105	150
Atlantic Salmon	1 lunch serv (5 oz)	200	9	—	80	60
Atlantic Salmon	1 serv (8 oz)	340	15	—	135	105
Baked Atlantic Cod	1 serv	220	6	—	100	440
Baked Atlantic Haddock	1 serv	220	6	—	100	440
Baked Flounder	1 lunch serv	190	7	—	90	440
Baked Potato	1 (8 oz)	130	0	—	0	10
Broccoli	1 serv (3 oz)	25	0	—	0	10
Broiled Fisherman's Platter	1 serv	600	23	—	250	1660
Broiled Rock Lobster Tail	1 tail	190	6	—	110	750
Broiled Seafarer's Platter	1 serv	450	19	—	190	1100
Caesar Salad w/ Dressing	1 serv	240	21	—	15	490
Catfish	1 lunch serv (5 oz)	130	2	—	75	115
Catfish	1 serv (8 oz)	220	3	—	130	200
Catfish Santa Fe	1 serv	340	9	—	165	890
Catfish Santa Fe	1 lunch serv	180	6	—	85	450
Chicken Fingers	1 lunch serv	390	18	—	64	770
Chicken Fresco	1 lunch serv	660	36	—	120	990
Chicken Fresco	1 serv	1320	73	—	240	1990
Clam Strips	1 lunch serv	360	19	—	15	910
Clam Strips	1 serv	720	39	—	35	1820
Cocktail Sauce	1 oz	30	0	—	0	380
Cole Slaw	1 serv (4 oz)	190	16	—	25	260
Crab Alfredo	1 lunch serv	590	33	—	135	980
Crab Alfredo	1 serv	1170	66	—	270	1970
Fish & Shrimp Combo	1 serv	730	35	—	230	1630
Fish Nuggets	1 lunch serv	320	14	—	95	760
Fish Seasoning Add On For Blackened Dinner	1 serv	70	5	—	0	410

FOOD	PORTION	CALS	FAT	CARB	CHOL	SOU
Fish Seasoning Add On For Blackened Lunch	1 serv	50	4	—	0	280
Fish Seasoning Add On For Broiled Dinner	1 serv	45	5	—	0	300
Fish Seasoning Add On For Broiled Lunch	1 serv	35	4	—	0	240
Fish Seasoning Add On For Grilled Dinner	1 serv	35	4	—	0	30
Fish Seasoning Add On For Grilled Lunch	1 serv	25	3	—	0	25
Fish Seasoning Add On For Lemon Pepper Dinner	1 serv	35	4	—	0	80
Fish Seasoning Add On For Lemon Pepper Lunch	1 serv	30	3	—	0	65
Fish Seasoning Add On For Santa Fe Style Dinner	1 serv	60	4	—	0	330
Fish Seasoning Add On For Santa Fe Style Lunch	1 serv	40	3	—	0	260
Flounder	1 lunch serv (5 oz)	130	2	—	75	115
Flounder	1 serv (8 oz)	220	3	—	130	200
French Fries	1 serv (4 oz)	350	22	—	0	180
Fried Flounder	1 lunch serv	230	10	—	60	590
Fried Shrimp	1 lunch serv	270	15	—	115	460
Fried Shrimp	12 lg	500	27	—	290	950
Garden Salad w/o Dressing	1 serv	50	1	—	0	90
Garlic Cheese Biscuit	1	140	8	—	5	320
Grilled Cheeseburger	1	580	34	—	130	540
Grilled Chicken Breasts	1 serv	230	7	—	105	280
Grilled Chicken Salad w/o Dressing	1 serv	320	10	—	70	910
Grouper	1 lunch serv (5 oz)	130	2	—	50	60
Grouper	1 serv (8 oz)	220	3	—	90	100
Haddock	1 lunch serv (5 oz)	120	1	—	80	95
Haddock	1 serv (8 oz)	210	2	—	140	160
Halibut	1 lunch serv (5 oz)	150	4	—	45	75

FOOD	PORTION	CALS	FAT	CARB	CHOL	SOD
Halibut	1 serv (8 oz)	260	6	—	75	130
King Salmon	1 lunch serv (5 oz)	250	15	—	95	70
King Salmon	1 serv (8 oz)	420	25	—	160	110
Lake Trout	1 lunch serv (5 oz)	200	9	—	80	75
Lake Trout	1 serv (8 oz)	340	16	—	140	125
Lemon Pepper Grilled Maki Mahi	1 serv	240	7	—	130	280
Lobster Shrimp & Scallop Scampi	1 lunch serv	430	16	—	80	450
Lobster Shrimp & Scallop Scampi	1 serv	870	33	—	135	900
Mahi Mahi	1 lunch serv (5 oz)	130	2	—	75	115
Mahi Mahi	1 serv (8 oz)	220	3	—	130	200
Maine Lobster Steamed	1 serv (1.25 lb)	160	1	—	125	670
Maine Lobster Stuffed	1 serv (2 lb)	430	10	—	210	1610
Marinara Sauce	1 serv	50	4	—	0	220
Melted Butter	1 oz	200	22	—	60	240
Neptune's Feast	1 serv	1210	62	—	290	3050
New York Strip Steak	1 serv	560	34	—	180	530
Perch	1 lunch serv (5 oz)	130	2	—	75	120
Perch	1 serv (8 oz)	220	3	—	130	200
Pollack	1 lunch serv (5 oz)	120	2	—	100	120
Popcorn Shrimp	1 lunch serv	380	24	—	235	580
Popcorn Shrimp	1 serv	580	37	—	360	880
Red Rockfish	1 lunch serv (5 oz)	130	2	—	50	85
Red Rockfish	1 serv (8 oz)	230	4	—	85	140
Red Snapper	1 lunch serv (5 oz)	140	2	—	50	65
Red Snapper	1 serv (8 oz)	240	3	—	90	105
Rice Pilaf	1 serv (4 oz)	180	2	—	0	790
Roasted Vegetables	1 lunch serv (4 oz)	80	3	—	0	210
Roasted Vegetables	1 serv (6 oz)	120	4	—	0	310
Sailor's Platter	1 lunch serv	250	12	—	170	440
Sandwich Blackened Catfish	1	340	9	—	85	740
Sandwich Broiled Fish	1	300	8	—	80	690
Sandwich Cajun Grilled Chicken	1	370	14	—	55	740

FOOD	PORTION	CALS	FAT	CARB	CHOL	SO
Sandwich Classic Fish	1	520	23	—	90	1050
Sandwich Grilled Chicken	1	290	7	—	50	430
Sassy Sauce	1 oz	80	6	—	5	140
Seafood Broil	1 lunch serv	310	14	—	110	850
Shrimp & Chicken	1 serv	340	15	—	225	470
Shrimp Caesar Salad w/o Dressing	1 serv	240	11	—	110	580
Shrimp Carbonara	1 lunch serv	650	38	—	155	1060
Shrimp Carbonara	1 serv	1290	76	—	310	2130
Shrimp Combo	1 serv	380	23	—	210	610
Shrimp Feast	1 serv	470	24	—	390	1040
Shrimp Milano	1 lunch serv	590	33	—	170	990
Shrimp Milano	1 serv	1190	65	—	340	1970
Shrimp Scampi	1 lunch serv	110	7	—	100	150
Smothered Chicken	1 serv	530	31	—	170	740
Snow Crab Legs	1 serv	110	2	—	115	320
Sockeye Salmon	1 lunch serv (5 oz)	240	12	—	95	75
Sockeye Salmon	1 serv (8 oz)	410	21	—	165	125
Sole	1 lunch serv (5 oz)	130	2	—	75	115
Sole	1 serv (8 oz)	220	3	—	130	200
Soup Bread Salad w/o Dressing	1 lunch serv	430	18	—	40	1960
Steak & Fried Shrimp	1 serv	780	46	—	340	770
Steak & Rock Lobster Tail	1 serv	570	31	—	220	880
Swordfish	1 lunch serv (5 oz)	170	6	—	70	90
Swordfish	1 serv (8 oz)	290	10	—	115	150
Tartar Sauce	1 oz	160	17	—	15	210
Teriyaki Grilled Chicken Breast	1 serv	240	7	—	105	660
Twice Baked Potato	1	430	23	—	60	1320
Walleye	1 lunch serv (5 oz)	120	2	—	120	70
Walleye	1 serv (8 oz)	210	3	—	205	120
Yellow Lake Perch	1 lunch serv (5 oz)	130	2	—	75	120
Yellow Lake Perch	1 serv (8 oz)	220	3	—	130	200
SALAD DRESSINGS						
Blue Cheese	1 serv	170	18	—	30	200
Buttermilk Ranch	1 serv	110	11	—	15	300

FOOD	PORTION	CALS	FAT	CARB	CHOL	SOD
Caesar	1 serv	170	18	—	10	290
Dijon Honey Mustard	1 serv	140	13	—	20	180
Fat Free Ranch	1 serv	50	0	—	0	310
Lite Red Wine Vinaigrette	1 serv	50	3	—	0	270
SOUPS						
Bayou Style Gumbo	1 serv (6 oz)	120	4	—	65	710
Broccoli Cheese	1 serv	160	9	—	25	800
Clam Chowder	1 serv (6 oz)	130	5	—	20	820

ROY ROGERS
BEVERAGES

FOOD	PORTION	CALS	FAT	CARB	CHOL	SOD
Orange Juice	11 fl oz	140	tr	34	0	5
BREAKFAST SELECTIONS						
3 Pancakes	1 serv (4.8 oz)	280	2	56	15	890
3 Pancakes w/ 1 Sausage	1 serv (6.2 oz)	430	16	56	40	1290
3 Pancakes w/ 2 Bacon	1 serv (5.3 oz)	350	9	56	25	1130
Bagel Cinnamon Raisin	1 (4 oz)	300	1	63	0	490
Bagel Plain	1 (4 oz)	300	2	60	0	520
Big Country Platters w/ Bacon	1 serv (7.6 oz)	740	43	61	305	1800
Big Country Platters w/ Ham	1 serv (9.4 oz)	710	39	67	330	2210
Big Country Platters w/ Sausage	1 serv (9.6 oz)	920	60	61	340	2230
Biscuit	1 (2.9 oz)	390	21	44	0	1000
Biscuit Bacon	1 (3.1 oz)	420	23	44	5	1140
Biscuit Bacon & Egg	1 (4.2 oz)	470	26	44	150	1190
Biscuit Cinnamon 'N' Raisin	1 (2.8 oz)	370	18	48	0	450
Biscuit Ham & Cheese	1 (4.5 oz)	450	24	48	25	1570
Biscuit Ham & Egg	1 (5.1 oz)	460	23	48	165	1395
Biscuit Ham, Egg & Cheese	1 (5.6 oz)	500	27	48	170	1620
Biscuit Sausage	1 (4.1 oz)	510	31	44	25	1360
Biscuit Sausage & Egg	1 (5.2 oz)	560	35	44	170	1400
Hashrounds	1 serv (2.8 oz)	230	14	24	0	560
Sourdough Ham, Egg & Cheese	1 (6.8 oz)	480	24	45	185	1440
DESSERTS						
Strawberry Shortcake	1 serv (6.6 oz)	480	21	39	40	330
ICE CREAM						
a Cream Cone	1 (4.1 oz)	180	4	29	15	80

FOOD	PORTION	CALS	FAT	CARB	CHOL	SOD
Sundae Hot Fudge	1 (6 oz)	320	10	50	25	260
Sundae Strawberry	1 (5.5 oz)	260	6	44	15	95
MAIN MENU SELECTIONS						
¼ Cheeseburger	1 (6 oz)	510	26	44	—	620
¼ Hamburger	1 (5.5 oz)	460	22	44	—	390
¼ Roaster Dark Meat	7.4 oz	490	34	2	225	1120
¼ Roaster Dark Meat w/ Skin Off	4 oz	190	10	1	110	400
¼ Roaster White Meat	8.6 oz	500	29	3	240	1450
¼ Roaster White Meat w/ Skin Off	4.7 oz	190	6	2	100	700
Bacon Cheeseburger	1 (5.9 oz)	520	31	32	—	740
Baked Beans	1 serv (5 oz)	160	2	30	10	560
Baked Potato	1 (3.9 oz)	130	1	27	0	65
Baked Potato w/ Margarine	1 (4.4 oz)	240	13	27	0	220
Baked Potato w/ Margarine & Sour Cream	1 (5.4 oz)	300	19	28	15	230
Cheeseburger	1 (4.2 oz)	300	13	34	25	690
Chicken Fillet Sandwich	1 (8.3 oz)	500	24	49	20	1050
Cole Slaw	1 serv (5 oz)	295	25	16	15	430
Cornbread	1 serv (2.7 oz)	310	17	35	30	260
Fisherman's Fillet	1 (6.5 oz)	490	21	56	15	1040
Fried Chicken Breast	1 (5.2 oz)	370	15	29	75	1190
Fried Chicken Leg	1 (2.4 oz)	170	7	15	45	570
Fried Chicken Thigh	1 (4.2 oz)	330	15	30	60	1000
Fried Chicken Wing	1 (2.3 oz)	200	8	23	30	740
Fry	1 lg (6.1 oz)	430	18	59	0	190
Fry	1 reg (5 oz)	350	15	49	0	150
Gravy	1 serv (1.5 fl oz)	20	tr	3	0	260
Grilled Chicken Sandwich	1 (8.3 oz)	340	11	32	30	910
Hamburger	1 (3.8 oz)	260	9	33	20	460
Mashed Potatoes	1 serv (5 oz)	92	tr	20	0	320
Nuggets	6 (4 oz)	290	18	20	15	610
Nuggets	9 (6.2 oz)	460	29	32	25	970
Pizza	1 serv (4.75 oz)	282	6	44	14	549
Roast Beef Sandwich	1 (5.7 oz)	260	4	30	60	700
Sourdough Bacon Cheeseburger	1 (9.1 oz)	770	50	45	—	1410
Sourdough Grilled Chicken	1 (10.1 oz)	500	21	46	45	1530

FOOD	PORTION	CALS	FAT	CARB	CHOL	SOD
SALADS AND SALAD BARS						
Garden Salad	1 (9.3 oz)	190	14	3	40	280
Grilled Chicken Salad	1 serv (9.8 oz)	120	4	2	60	520
Side Salad	1 (4.9 oz)	20	tr	3	0	20

SCHLOTZSKY'S DELI
PIZZA

FOOD	PORTION	CALS	FAT	CARB	CHOL	SOD
Chicken & Pesto	1	634	18	—	—	—
Onion & Mushroom	1	577	20	—	—	—
Smoked Turkey & Jalapeno	1	589	13	—	—	—
Vegetarian	1	555	17	—	—	—
SALADS AND SALAD BARS						
Chicken Chef	1 serv	192	8	—	—	—
Turkey Club	1 serv	233	10	—	—	—
SANDWICHES						
Chicken Breast	1 sm	514	22	—	—	—
Dijon Chicken Breast	1 sm	469	16	—	—	—
Smoked Turkey	1 sm	510	22	—	—	—
The Original	1 sm	598	33	—	—	—
SOUPS						
Creole Vegetable	1 serv (8 fl oz)	120	3	—	—	—
Red Bean	1 serv (8 fl oz)	110	2	—	—	—
Shrimp & Okra	1 serv (8 fl oz)	100	3	—	—	—
Spicy Chicken	1 serv (8 fl oz)	120	3	—	—	—

SHAKEY'S
MAIN MENU SELECTIONS

FOOD	PORTION	CALS	FAT	CARB	CHOL	SOD
3 Piece Fried Chicken And Potatoes	1 serv	947	56	51	—	2293
5 Piece Fried Chicken And Potatoes	1 serv	1700	90	130	—	5327
Hot Ham And Cheese	1	550	21	56	—	2135
Potatoes	15 pieces	950	36	120	—	3703
Spaghetti With Meat Sauce And Garlic Bread	1 serv	940	33	134	—	1904
PIZZA						
Thick Crust Cheese	1 slice	170	5	22	13	421
Thick Crust Green Pepper, Black Olives, Mushrooms	1 slice	162	4	22	13	418
Thick Crust Pepperoni	1 slice	185	6	22	17	422
Thick Crust Sausage, Mushrooms	1 slice	179	6	22	15	420

FOOD	PORTION	CALS	FAT	CARB	CHOL	SOD
Thick Crust Sausage, Pepperoni	1 slice	177	8	22	19	424
Thick Crust Shakey's Special	1 slice	208	8	22	18	423
Thin Crust Cheese	1 slice	133	5	13	14	323
Thin Crust Onion, Green Pepper, Black Olives, Mushrooms	1 slice	125	5	14	11	313
Thin Crust Pepperoni	1 slice	148	7	13	14	403
Thin Crust Sausage, Mushroom	1 slice	141	6	13	13	336
Thin Crust Sausage, Pepperoni	1 slice	166	8	13	17	397
Thin Crust Shakey's Special	1 slice	171	9	14	16	475

SHONEY'S
BEVERAGES

FOOD	PORTION	CALS	FAT	CARB	CHOL	SOD
Clear Soda	1 lg	105	0	28	0	21
Clear Soda	1 sm	52	0	14	0	10
Coffee Regular & Decaf	1 cup	8	0	1	0	8
Cola	1 lg	139	0	33	0	10
Cola	1 sm	69	0	17	0	5
Creamer	3/8 oz	14	1	1	0	8
Hot Chocolate	1 cup	110	2	20	154	154
Hot Tea	1 cup	0	0	tr	0	19
Milk 2%	1 cup	121	5	12	18	122
Orange Juice	4 oz	54	tr	13	0	1
Sugar	1 pkg	13	0	3	0	0

BREAKFAST SELECTIONS

FOOD	PORTION	CALS	FAT	CARB	CHOL	SOD
100% Natural	1/2 cup	244	11	33	0	45
Ambrosia Salad	1/4 cup	75	3	12	0	167
Apple	1	81	1	21	0	1
Apple Butter	1 tbsp	37	tr	9	0	0
Apple Grape Surprise	1/4 cup	19	0	5	0	2
Apple Ring	1	15	0	4	0	0
Apple Sliced	1 slice	13	tr	3	0	0
Bacon	1 strip	36	3	0	5	101
Beef Stick	1	43	1	5	—	17
Biscuit	1	170	8	22	0	364
Blueberries	1/4 cup	21	tr	5	0	2
Blueberry Muffin	1	107	4	18	17	1
Bread Pudding	1 sq	305	11	44	80	409
Breakfast Ham	1 slice	26	1	tr	14	263

FOOD	PORTION	CALS	FAT	CARB	CHOL	SOD
Brunch Cake Apple	1 sq	160	8	19	0	150
Brunch Cake Banana	1 sq	152	7	21	0	120
Brunch Cake Carrot	1 sq	150	7	20	0	159
Brunch Cake Pineapple	1 sq	147	7	20	0	120
Brunch Cake Sour Cream	1 sq	160	8	21	0	135
Buttered Toast	2 slices	163	5	25	0	296
Cantaloupe Sliced	1 slice	8	tr	2	0	2
Cantaloupe Diced	½ cup	28	tr	7	0	7
Captain Crunch Berry	½ cup	73	2	14	0	122
Cheese Sauce	1 ladle	26	2	4	0	166
Chicken Pieces	1 piece	40	2	2	—	28
Chocolate Pudding	¼ cup	81	2	16	7	81
Cinnamon Honey Bun	1	344	12	54	0	169
Cottage Cheese	1 tbsp	12	tr	1	1	66
Cottage Fries	¼ cup	62	2	10	0	124
Country Gravy	¼ cup	82	7	4	1	255
Croissant	1	260	16	22	2	260
Donut Mini Cinnamon	1 (14 g)	56	3	7	0	65
DoughNugget	1	157	10	15	0	194
Egg Fried	1	159	15	1	274	69
Egg Scrambled	¼ cup	95	7	1	248	155
English Muffin w/ Margarine	1	140	2	18	0	1
Fluff	¼ cup	16	0	3	0	0
French Toast	1 slice	69	3	9	0	157
Fruit Delight	¼ cup	54	2	10	0	2
Fruit Topping All Flavors	1 tbsp	24	0	6	0	3
Glaced Fruit	¼ cup	51	tr	13	0	5
Golden Pound Cake	1 slice	134	5	20	13	144
Grape Jelly	1 tbsp	60	0	16	0	0
Grapefruit Canned	¼ cup	24	tr	6	0	5
Grapes	25	57	1	14	0	2
Grits	¼ cup	57	3	6	0	62
Hashbrowns	¼ cup	43	2	7	0	24
Home Fries	¼ cup	53	2	9	0	24
Honey Bun	1	265	14	32	3	33
Honeydew Sliced	1 slice	13	0	3	0	4
Jelly Packet	1	40	0	10	0	2
Jr. Bun Chocolate	1	141	5	22	0	70
Jr. Bun Honey	1	141	5	22	0	70
Jr. Bun Maple	1	141	5	22	0	70
Kiwi Sliced	1 slice	11	tr	3	0	1
Marble Cake w/ Icing	1 slice	136	5	22	0	149
Mixed Fruit	¼ cup	37	tr	9	0	3

FOOD	PORTION	CALS	FAT	CARB	CHOL	SOD
Mushroom Topping	1 oz	25	2	1	0	323
Oleo Whipped	1 tbsp	70	8	0	0	97
Omelette Topping	1 spoonful	23	2	1	3	99
Orange	1 med	65	tr	16	0	2
Orange Sections	1 section	7	0	2	0	0
Oriental Salad	¼ cup	79	3	13	1	32
Pancake	1	41	tr	9	0	238
Pear	1	98	1	25	0	1
Pineapple Bits	1 tbsp	9	0	2	0	2
Pineapple Fresh Sliced	1 slice	10	tr	3	0	0
Pistachio Pineapple Salad	¼ cup	98	0	20	3	39
Prunes	1 tbsp	19	0	5	0	0
Raisin Bran	½ cup	87	1	22	0	185
Raisin English Muffin w/ Margarine	1	158	4	27	0	280
Sausage Link	1	91	9	tr	13	291
Sausage Patty	1	136	13	1	2	48
Sausage Rice	¼ cup	110	6	10	8	211
Shortcake	1	60	2	13	0	90
Sirloin Steak Charbroiled	6 oz	357	25	0	99	160
Smoked Sausage	1	103	10	1	13	39
Snow Salad	¼ cup	72	4	9	0	18
Strawberries	5	23	tr	5	0	1
Syrup Light	1 ladle	60	0	15	0	0
Syrup Low-Cal	2.2 oz	98	0	24	0	0
Tangerine	1	37	tr	9	0	1
Trix	½ cup	54	tr	13	0	89
Waldorf Salad	¼ cup	81	5	9	2	68
Watermelon Diced	½ cup	50	1	12	0	3
Watermelon Sliced	1 slice	9	tr	2	0	1
Whipped Topping	1 scoop	10	1	1	0	3
CHILDREN'S MENU SELECTIONS						
Jr. Burger All-American	1 serv	234	11	20	30	543
Kid's Chicken Dinner (fried)	1 serv	244	13	11	40	151
Kid's Fish N' Chips (includes fries)	1 serv	337	17	33	41	467
Kid's Fried Shrimp	1 serv	194	12	12	70	633
Kid's Spaghetti	1 serv	247	8	32	27	193
DESSERTS						
Apple Pie A La Mode	1 slice	492	23	67	35	574
Carrot Cake	1 slice	500	26	56	37	476
Strawberry Pie	1 slice	332	17	45	0	247

FOOD	PORTION	CALS	FAT	CARB	CHOL	SOD
Walnut Brownie A La Mode	1	576	34	61	35	435
ICE CREAM						
Hot Fudge Cake	1 slice	522	20	82	27	485
Hot Fudge Sundae	1	451	22	60	60	226
Strawberry Sundae	1	380	19	48	69	145
MAIN MENU SELECTIONS						
All-American Burger	1	501	33	27	86	597
BBQ Sauce	1 souffle cup	41	1	8	0	232
Bacon Burger	1	591	40	29	86	801
Baked Fish	1 serv	170	1	2	83	1641
Baked Fish Light	1 serv	170	1	2	83	1641
Baked Ham Sandwich	1	290	10	28	42	1263
Baked Potato	10 oz	264	tr	61	0	16
Beef Patty Light	1 serv	289	23	0	82	187
Charbroiled Chicken	1 serv	239	7	1	85	592
Charbroiled Chicken Sandwich	1	451	17	28	90	1002
Chicken Fillet Sandwich	1	464	21	39	51	585
Chicken Tenders	1 serv	388	20	17	64	239
Cocktail Sauce	1 souffle cup	36	tr	9	0	260
Country Fried Sandwich	1	588	26	67	29	1501
Country Fried Steak	1 serv	449	27	34	27	1177
Fish N' Chips (includes fries)	1 serv	639	35	50	103	873
Fish N' Shrimp	1 serv	487	26	37	127	644
Fish Sandwich	1	323	13	41	21	740
French Fries	3 oz	189	8	29	0	273
French Fries	4 oz	252	10	39	0	364
Fried Fish Light	1 serv	297	14	22	65	536
Grecian Bread	1 slice	80	2	13	0	94
Grilled Bacon & Cheese Sandwich	1	440	28	28	36	1200
Grilled Cheese Sandwich	1	302	17	25	36	880
Half O'Pound	1 serv	435	34	0	123	280
Ham Club On Whole Wheat	1	642	36	45	78	2105
Hawaiian Chicken	1 serv	262	7	7	85	593
Italian Feast	1 serv	500	20	44	74	369
Lasagna	1 serv	297	10	45	26	870
Liver N' Onions	1 serv	411	23	23	529	321
Mushroom Swiss Burger	1	616	42	29	106	1135
Old-Fashioned Burger	1	470	28	26	82	681
Onion Rings	1	52	3	5	2	102

FOOD	PORTION	CALS	FAT	CARB	CHOL	SOD
Patty Melt	1	640	42	30	171	826
Philly Steak Sandwich	1	673	44	37	103	1242
Reuben Sandwich	1	596	35	32	138	3873
Ribeye	6 oz	605	51	0	141	141
Rice	3.5 oz	137	4	23	1	765
Sauteed Mushrooms	3 oz	75	7	4	0	968
Sauteed Onions	2.5 oz	37	2	4	0	221
Seafood Platter	1 serv	566	28	46	127	893
Shoney Burger	1	498	36	22	79	782
Shrimp Bite-Size	1 serv	387	25	25	140	1266
Shrimp Broiled	1 serv	93	18	0	182	210
Shrimp Charbroiled	1 serv	138	3	3	162	170
Shrimp Sampler	1 serv	412	23	26	217	783
Shrimper's Feast	1 serv	383	22	30	125	216
Shrimper's Feast Large	1 serv	575	33	45	188	324
Sirloin	6 oz	357	25	0	99	160
Slim Jim Sandwich	1	484	24	40	57	1620
Spaghetti	1 serv	496	16	63	55	387
Steak N' Shrimp (charbroiled shrimp)	1 serv	361	23	1	141	198
Steak N' Shrimp (fried shrimp)	1 serv	507	33	15	150	249
Sweet N' Sour Sauce	1 souffle cup	58	0	15	0	5
Tartar Sauce	1 souffle cup	84	8	4	11	177
Turkey Club On Whole Wheat	1	635	33	44	100	1289
SALAD DRESSINGS						
Biscayne Lo-Cal	2 tbsp	62	1	1	0	334
Blue Cheese	2 tbsp	113	13	0	15	109
Creamy Italian	2 tbsp	135	15	1	0	454
French	2 tbsp	124	12	2	12	204
Golden Italian	2 tbsp	141	15	1	0	302
Honey Mustard	2 tbsp	165	17	2	18	5
Ranch	2 tbsp	95	10	0	15	10
Rue French	2 tbsp	122	10	2	0	364
Thousand Island	2 tbsp	130	13	2	12	179
W.W. Italian	2 tbsp	10	0	2	0	615
SALADS AND SALAD BARS						
Ambrosia Salad	¼ cup	75	3	12	0	167
Apple Grape Surprise	¼ cup	19	0	5	0	2
Apple Ring	1	15	0	4	0	3
Bacon Bits	1 spoonful	15	1	1	—	—
Beet Onion Salad	¼ cup	25	1	3	0	167
Broccoli	¼ cup	4	tr	1	0	4

FOOD	PORTION	CALS	FAT	CARB	CHOL	SOD
Broccoli Cauliflower Carrot Salad	¼ cup	53	4	3	1	193
Broccoli Cauliflower Ranch	¼ cup	65	6	2	9	12
Broccoli & Cauliflower	¼ cup	98	9	4	0	478
Carrot	¼ cup	10	tr	2	0	8
Carrot Apple Salad	¼ cup	99	9	4	8	10
Cauliflower	¼ cup	8	tr	2	0	5
Celery	1 tbsp	5	0	tr	0	7
Cheese Shredded	1 tbsp	21	2	tr	2	112
Chocolate Pudding	¼ cup	81	2	16	7	81
Chow Mein Noodles	1 spoonful	13	1	tr	0	0
Cole Slaw	¼ cup	69	5	5	7	106
Cottage Cheese	1 tbsp	12	tr	1	1	66
Croutons	1 spoonful	13	tr	2	0	38
Cucumber	1 tbsp	1	0	tr	0	0
Cucumber Lite	¼ cup	12	tr	3	0	344
Don's Pasta	¼ cup	82	5	9	0	223
Egg Diced	1 tbsp	15	1	tr	54	14
Fruit Delight	¼ cup	54	2	10	0	2
Fruit Topping All Flavors	¼ cup	64	tr	16	0	8
Glaced Fruit	¼ cup	51	tr	13	0	5
Granola	1 spoonful	25	1	3	0	—
Grapefruit	¼ cup	24	tr	6	0	5
Green Pepper	1 tbsp	1	0	tr	0	0
Italian Vegetable	¼ cup	11	tr	3	0	110
Jello	¼ cup	40	0	9	0	26
Jello Fluff	¼ cup	16	tr	3	0	0
Kidney Bean Salad	¼ cup	55	2	7	2	154
Lettuce	1.8 oz	7	tr	1	0	5
Macaroni Salad	¼ cup	207	14	17	14	382
Margarine Whipped	1 tsp	23	3	0	0	32
Melba Toast	2	20	0	4	0	45
Mixed Fruit Salad	¼ cup	37	tr	9	0	3
Mixed Squash	¼ cup	49	4	2	0	230
Mushrooms	1 tbsp	1	0	tr	0	0
Oil	1 tsp	45	5	0	0	0
Olives Black	2	10	1	0	0	38
Olives Green	2	8	1	0	0	162
Onion Sliced	1 tbsp	1	0	tr	0	0
Oriental Salad	¼ cup	79	3	13	1	31
Pea Salad	¼ cup	73	6	4	42	89
Pepperoni	1 tbsp	30	3	0	—	81
Pickle Chips	1 slice	5	0	1	0	30

FOOD	PORTION	CALS	FAT	CARB	CHOL	SOD
Pickle Spear	1 spear	2	0	tr	0	271
Pineapple Bits	1 tbsp	9	0	2	0	2
Pistachio Pineapple Salad	¼ cup	98	3	20	0	39
Prunes	1 tbsp	19	0	5	0	0
Radish	1 tbsp	1	0	tr	0	1
Raisins	1 spoonful	26	0	7	0	1
Rotelli Pasta	¼ cup	78	4	9	0	82
Seign Salad	¼ cup	72	4	8	5	122
Snow Delight	¼ cup	72	4	9	0	18
Spaghetti Salad	¼ cup	81	5	9	0	20
Spinach	¼ cup	1	0	tr	0	4
Spring Pasta	¼ cup	38	3	2	0	162
Summer Salad	¼ cup	114	12	2	0	233
Sunflower Seeds	1 spoonful	40	3	1	0	2
Three Bean Salad	¼ cup	96	5	12	0	189
Trail Mix	1 spoonful	30	0	4	0	0
Turkey Ham	1 tbsp	12	1	tr	1	121
Waldorf	¼ cup	81	5	9	2	68
Wheat Bread	1 slice	71	1	14	0	150
SOUPS						
Bean	6 fl oz	63	1	10	4	479
Beef Cabbage	6 fl oz	86	3	9	13	503
Broccoli Cauliflower	6 fl oz	124	9	12	12	560
Cheddar Chowder	6 fl oz	91	2	14	—	948
Cheese Florentine Ham	6 fl oz	110	8	12	11	890
Chicken Gumbo	6 fl oz	60	2	7	—	1050
Chicken Noodle	6 fl oz	62	1	9	14	127
Chicken Rice	6 fl oz	72	1	13	6	117
Clam Chowder	6 fl oz	94	5	10	0	66
Corn Chowder	6 fl oz	148	5	22	—	510
Cream Of Broccoli	6 fl oz	75	5	11	1	415
Cream Of Chicken	6 fl oz	136	9	14	11	1164
Cream Of Chicken Vegetable	6 fl oz	79	1	13	—	714
Onion	6 fl oz	29	2	2	1	88
Potato	6 fl oz	102	3	17	0	335
Tomato Florentine	6 fl oz	63	1	11	0	683
Tomato Vegetable	6 fl oz	46	tr	10	0	314
Vegetable Beef	6 fl oz	82	2	14	5	1254

SIZZLER
DESSERTS

FOOD	PORTION	CALS	FAT	CARB	CHOL	SOD
Chocolate & Vanilla Soft Serve	4 oz	136	4	24	0	100

FOOD	PORTION	CALS	FAT	CARB	CHOL	SOD
Chocolate Syrup	1 oz	90	0	21	0	15
Strawberry Topping	1 oz	70	0	18	0	5
Whipped Topping	1 tbsp	12	1	1	0	0
HOT BUFFET						
Broccoli Cheese Soup	1 serv (4 oz)	139	9	10	8	355
Chicken Noodle Soup	1 serv (4 oz)	31	1	4	7	495
Chicken Wings	1 oz	73	4	4	20	135
Clam Chowder	1 serv (4 oz)	118	6	11	6	511
Fettucine	2 oz	80	1	15	5	5
Focaccia Bread	2 pieces	108	7	9	1	134
Marinara Sauce	1 oz	13	0	3	0	90
Meatballs	4	157	11	5	30	461
Minestrone Soup	1 serv (4 oz)	36	0	7	1	443
Nacho Cheese Soup	1 serv (4 oz)	120	10	3	30	600
Potato Skins	2 oz	160	8	22	0	463
Refried Beans	¼ cup	62	1	11	5	272
Saltine Crackers	2	25	1	4	2	74
Spaghetti	2 oz	80	0	16	0	1
Taco Filling	2 oz	103	9	3	16	232
Taco Shells	1	50	2	7	0	20
Vegetable Sirloin Soup	1 serv (4 oz)	60	2	6	10	364
MAIN MENU SELECTIONS						
Buttery Dipping Sauce	1 serv (1.5 oz)	330	37	0	0	0
Cheese Toast	1 piece	273	21	16	5	494
Cocktail Sauce	1 serv (1.5 oz)	40	0	8	0	396
Dakota Ranch Steak	1 (6 oz)	316	20	—	101	253
Dakota Ranch Steak	1 (8 oz)	421	27	—	135	337
Dakota Ranch Steak	1 (9.5 oz)	500	32	—	160	400
French Fries	1 serv (4 oz)	358	12	45	0	245
Hamburger	1	626	33	36	142	335
Hibachi Chicken Breast w/ Pineapple	5 oz	193	3	13	65	666
Hibachi Sauce	1 serv (1.5 oz)	57	0	11	0	707
Lemon Herb Chicken Breast	5 oz	140	3	0	65	380
Malibu Chicken Patty	1	310	19	11	75	588
Malibu Sauce	1 serv (1.5 oz)	283	31	0	28	354
Margarine Whipped	1½ tbsp	105	12	0	0	146
Potato Baked Plain	1 (4 oz)	105	0	24	0	6
Rice Pilaf	1 serv (6 oz)	256	5	47	0	866
Salmon	8 oz	110	12	0	41	232
Santa Fe Chicken Breast	5 oz	150	3	0	65	350
Shrimp Broiled	5 oz	150	6	0	218	377
Shrimp Fried	4 pieces	223	2	35	118	706

FOOD	PORTION	CALS	FAT	CARB	CHOL	SOD
Shrimp Mini	4 oz	152	1	24	80	480
Shrimp Scampi	5 oz	143	3	0	150	386
Sour Dressing	2 tbsp	60	6	0	0	30
Swordfish	8 oz	315	14	0	89	331
Tartar Sauce	1 serv (1.5 oz)	170	17	6	14	453
SALAD DRESSINGS						
Blue Cheese	1 oz	111	12	1	8	168
Honey Mustard	1 oz	160	16	4	10	110
Italian Lite	1 oz	14	0	2	0	350
Japanese Rice Vinegar Fat Free	1 oz	10	0	2	0	172
Parmesan Italian	1 oz	100	10	2	0	450
Ranch	1 oz	120	12	2	10	240
Ranch Reduced Calorie	1 oz	90	8	4	10	270
Thousand Island	1 oz	143	15	3	11	125
SALADS AND SALAD BARS						
Alfalfa Sprouts	¼ cup	2	0	0	0	0
Avocado	½	153	15	6	0	11
Bean Sprouts	¼ cup	8	0	2	0	2
Beets	¼ cup	13	0	3	0	117
Bell Peppers	2 oz	8	0	2	0	1
Broccoli	½ cup	12	0	2	0	12
Cabbage Red	¼ cup	5	0	1	0	2
Cantaloupe	½ cup	28	0	7	0	7
Carrot & Raisin Salad	2 oz	130	10	10	10	104
Carrots	¼ cup	12	0	3	0	10
Chinese Chicken Salad	2 oz	54	2	6	10	119
Chives	1 oz	62	6	1	0	181
Cottage Cheese	2 oz	51	1	2	5	230
Cucumber	2 oz	7	0	2	0	1
Eggs	1 oz	44	3	0	122	35
Garbanzo Beans	¼ cup	63	1	11	0	255
Grapes	½ cup	29	0	8	0	1
Guacamole	1 oz	42	4	2	0	425
Honeydew Melon	½ cup	30	0	8	0	9
Iceberg Lettuce	1 cup	7	0	1	0	5
Jicama	2 oz	13	0	3	0	1
Kidney Beans	¼ cup	52	0	10	0	222
Kiwifruit	2 oz	35	0	8	0	3
Mediterranean Minted Fruit Salad	2 oz	29	0	7	0	11
Mexican Fiesta Salad	2 oz	54	1	10	0	99
Mushrooms	¼ cup	4	0	1	0	1
Old Fashioned Potato Salad	2 oz	84	5	10	6	231

FOOD	PORTION	CALS	FAT	CARB	CHOL	SOD
Onions Red	2 tbsp	8	0	2	0	1
Peaches	¼ cup	34	0	9	0	3
Peas	¼ cup	31	0	6	0	35
Pineapple	½ cup	38	0	10	0	1
Real Bacon Bits	1 tbsp	27	2	2	0	165
Red Herb Potato Salad	2 oz	121	9	9	9	271
Romaine Lettuce	1 cup	9	0	1	0	4
Salsa	1 oz	7	0	2	0	156
Seafood Louis Pasta Salad	2 oz	64	2	9	17	139
Seafood Salad	2 oz	56	3	4	7	255
Spicy Jicama Salad	2 oz	16	0	4	0	28
Spinach	½ cup	6	0	1	0	22
Strawberries	½ cup	22	0	5	0	1
Teriyaki Beef Salad	2 oz	49	2	5	7	136
Tomatoes Cherry	¼ cup	12	0	3	0	5
Tuna Pasta Salad	2 oz	133	10	6	10	188
Turkey Ham	1 oz	62	5	0	19	376
Watermelon	½ cup	26	0	6	0	2
Zucchini	¼ cup	5	0	1	0	1

SKIPPER'S
BEVERAGES

FOOD	PORTION	CALS	FAT	CARB	CHOL	SOD
Coke Classic	1 (12 fl oz)	144	0	38	0	14
Coke Diet	1 (12 fl oz)	2	0	0	0	8
Milk Lowfat	1 (12 fl oz)	181	10	32	0	225
Root Beer	1 (12 fl oz)	154	0	42	0	31
Root Beer Float	1 (12 oz)	302	10	33	10	66
Sprite	1 (12 fl oz)	142	0	36	0	45

DESSERTS

FOOD	PORTION	CALS	FAT	CARB	CHOL	SOD
Jell-O	1 serv (2.75 oz)	55	0	12	0	35

MAIN MENU SELECTIONS

FOOD	PORTION	CALS	FAT	CARB	CHOL	SOD
Baked Fish With Margarine & Seasoning	1 serv (4.4 oz)	147	3	0	85	475
Baked Potato	1 (6 oz)	145	0	32	0	6
Captain's Cut	1 piece (2.6 oz)	160	7	14	29	353
Cocktail Sauce	1 tbsp	20	0	5	0	216
Coleslaw	1 serv (5 oz)	289	27	10	50	329
Corn Muffin	1 (2 oz)	91	5	14	16	135
English Style Fish	1 piece (2.4 oz)	187	12	11	—	415
French Fries	1 serv (3.5 oz)	239	12	29	3	57
Green Salad (no dressing)	1 serv (4 oz)	24	0	4	0	8

FOOD	PORTION	CALS	FAT	CARB	CHOL	SOD
Ketchup	1 tbsp	17	0	4	0	213
Margarine	1 serv (0.5 oz)	50	6	0	0	60
Shrimp Fried Cajun	1 serv (4 oz)	342	21	27	64	147
Shrimp Fried Jumbo	1 piece (.65 oz)	51	2	5	9	102
Shrimp Fried Original	1 serv (4 oz)	266	13	25	54	1089
Tartar Original	1 tbsp	65	7	0	4	102
SOUPS						
Clam Chowder	1 cup (6 fl oz)	100	4	14	12	525
Clam Chowder	1 pint (12 fl oz)	200	7	19	24	1050

SONIC DRIVE-IN

FOOD	PORTION	CALS	FAT	CARB	CHOL	SOD
#1 Hamburger	1 (6.6 oz)	409	27	23	58	444
#2 Hamburger	1 (6.6 oz)	323	16	23	50	549
B-L-T Sandwich	1 (6.1 oz)	327	19	27	9	600
Bacon Cheeseburger	1 (7.2 oz)	548	39	23	87	839
Chicken Sandwich Breaded	1 (7.4 oz)	455	25	36	42	755
Chili Pie	1 (3.7 oz)	327	23	20	28	313
Corn Dog	1 (3 oz)	280	15	30	35	700
Extra Long Cheese Coney	1 (8.9 oz)	635	39	45	65	632
Extra Long Cheese Coney w/ Onions	1 (9.4 oz)	640	39	47	65	632
Fish Sandwich	1 (6.1 oz)	277	7	38	6	655
French Fries	1 lg (6.7 oz)	315	11	50	11	67
French Fries	1 reg (5 oz)	233	8	37	8	50
French Fries w/ Cheese	1 lg (7.7 oz)	219	20	51	38	468
Grilled Cheese Sandwich	1 (2.8 oz)	288	17	25	36	841
Grilled Chicken Sandwich w/o Dressing	1 (6.4 oz)	215	4	23	4	716
Hickory Burger	1 (5.1 oz)	314	16	23	50	459
Jalapeno Burger Double Meat & Cheese	1 (9.1 oz)	638	41	22	136	1358
Mini Burger	1 (3.5 oz)	246	11	20	36	510
Mini Cheeseburger	1 (3.9 oz)	281	14	20	45	644
Onion Rings	1 lg (5 oz)	577	38	54	—	532
Onion Rings	1 reg (3.5 oz)	404	27	38	—	372
Regular Cheese Coney	1 (5 oz)	358	15	23	40	341
Regular Cheese Coney w/ Onions	1 (5.3 oz)	361	23	24	40	341
Regular Hot Dog	1 (3.5 oz)	258	15	21	23	241
Steak Sandwich Breaded	1 (3.9 oz)	631	42	46	50	1047
Super Sonic Burger w/ Mustard Double Meat & Cheese	1 (10.1 oz)	644	41	24	136	1128

FOOD	PORTION	CALS	FAT	CARB	CHOL	SOD
Super Sonic Burger w/ Mayo Double Meat & Cheese	1 (10.1 oz)	730	52	24	144	1023
Tater Tots	1 serv (3 oz)	150	7	19	10	330
Tater Tots w/ Cheese	1 serv (3.6 oz)	220	13	19	28	569

STARBUCKS

(FAST FACT: Specialty coffee bars are everywhere, serving a wide variety of drinks. Flavorful plain black coffee is fat and calorie free—add-ons make the difference. Stick with skim or 2% milk; cocoa powder, cinnamon and sugar are fine; go easy on flavored syrups, whipped cream and heavy cream. After regular coffee, the best bets are cappuccino, latte and mocha.)

FOOD	PORTION	CALS	FAT	CARB	CHOL	SOD
Americano Grande	1 serv	10	0	3	0	15
Americano Short	1 serv	5	0	1	0	10
Americano Tall	1 serv	5	0	2	0	10
Cappuccino Grande Lowfat Milk	1 serv	110	4	12	15	110
Cappuccino Grande Nonfat Milk	1 serv	80	0	12	5	115
Cappuccino Grande Whole Milk	1 serv	140	7	12	30	105
Cappuccino Short Lowfat Milk	1 serv	60	2	6	10	55
Cappuccino Short Nonfat Milk	1 serv	40	0	6	0	55
Cappuccino Short Whole Milk	1 serv	70	4	6	15	55
Cappuccino Tall Lowfat Milk	1 serv	80	3	9	15	85
Cappuccino Tall Nonfat Milk	1 serv	60	0	9	5	90
Cappuccino Tall Whole Milk	1 serv	110	6	9	25	85
Cocoa w/ Whipping Cream Grande Lowfat Milk	1 serv	350	20	35	70	190
Cocoa w/ Whipping Cream Grande Nonfat Milk	1 serv	310	15	35	50	190
Cocoa w/ Whipping Cream Grande Whole Milk	1 serv	400	26	34	90	180
Cocoa w/ Whipping Cream Short Lowfat Milk	1 serv	180	11	16	40	85

FOOD	PORTION	CALS	FAT	CARB	CHOL	SOD
Cocoa w/ Whipping Cream Short Nonfat Milk	1 serv	160	8	17	30	85
Cocoa w/ Whipping Cream Short Whole Milk	1 serv	210	14	19	45	80
Cocoa w/ Whipping Cream Tall Lowfat Milk	1 serv	270	15	26	55	140
Cocoa w/ Whipping Cream Tall Nonfat Milk	1 serv	230	11	26	35	140
Cocoa w/ Whipping Cream Tall Whole Milk	1 serv	300	19	26	70	135
Drip Coffee Grande	1 serv	10	0	2	0	15
Drip Coffee Short	1 serv	5	0	1	0	5
Drip Coffee Tall	1 serv	10	0	1	0	10
Espresso Doppio	1 serv	5	0	2	0	0
Espresso Macchiato Doppio Lowfat Milk	1 serv	15	0	3	0	10
Espresso Macchiato Doppio Nonfat Milk	1 serv	15	0	3	0	10
Espresso Macchiato Doppio Whole Milk	1 serv	15	1	3	0	10
Espresso Macchiato Solo Lowfat Milk	1 serv	10	0	2	0	10
Espresso Macchiato Solo Nonfat Milk	1 serv	10	0	2	0	10
Espresso Macchiato Solo Whole Milk	1 serv	15	1	2	0	10
Espresso Solo	1 serv	5	0	1	0	0
Espresso Con Panna Doppio	1 serv	45	4	2	15	5
Espresso Con Panna Solo	1 serv	40	4	1	15	5
Latte Grande Lowfat Milk	1 serv	170	6	18	25	180
Latte Grande Nonfat Milk	1 serv	130	1	19	5	180
Latte Grande Whole Milk	1 serv	220	11	18	45	170
Latte Short Lowfat Milk	1 serv	80	3	8	10	80
Latte Short Nonfat Milk	1 serv	60	0	8	5	80
Latte Short Whole Milk	1 serv	100	5	8	20	75
Latte Tall Lowfat Milk	1 serv	140	5	15	20	150
Latte Tall Nonfat Milk	1 serv	110	1	15	5	150
Latte Tall Whole Milk	1 serv	180	10	14	40	140
Latte Iced Grande Lowfat Milk	1 serv	170	6	18	25	170

FOOD	PORTION	CALS	FAT	CARB	CHOL	SOD
Latte Iced Grande Nonfat Milk	1 serv	130	1	18	5	180
Latte Iced Grande Whole Milk	1 serv	210	11	18	45	170
Latte Iced Short Lowfat Milk	1 serv	90	3	10	15	95
Latte Iced Short Nonfat Milk	1 serv	70	0	10	5	95
Latte Iced Short Whole Milk	1 serv	120	6	9	25	90
Latte Iced Tall Lowfat Milk	1 serv	120	5	13	20	125
Latte Iced Tall Nonfat Milk	1 serv	90	0	13	5	130
Latte Iced Tall Whole Milk	1 serv	150	8	12	35	120
Mocha w/ Whipping Cream Grande Lowfat Milk	1 serv	350	20	35	70	170
Mocha w/ Whipping Cream Grande Nonfat Milk	1 serv	310	15	35	50	180
Mocha w/ Whipping Cream Grande Whole Milk	1 serv	390	25	35	85	170
Mocha w/ Whipping Cream Short Lowfat Milk	1 serv	170	10	16	35	70
Mocha w/ Whipping Cream Short Nonfat Milk	1 serv	150	8	16	30	70
Mocha w/ Whipping Cream Short Whole Milk	1 serv	180	12	16	45	70
Mocha w/ Whipping Cream Tall Lowfat Milk	1 serv	260	15	26	50	125
Mocha w/ Whipping Cream Tall Nonfat Milk	1 serv	230	11	26	35	130
Mocha w/ Whipping Cream Tall Whole Milk	1 serv	290	18	25	65	125
Mocha w/o Whipping Cream Grande Lowfat Milk	1 serv	230	7	33	20	150
Mocha w/o Whipping Cream Grande Nonfat Milk	1 serv	190	3	33	5	150

FOOD	PORTION	CALS	FAT	CARB	CHOL	SOD
Mocha w/o Whipping Cream Grande Whole Milk	1 serv	260	7	33	40	150
Mocha w/o Whipping Cream Short Lowfat Milk	1 serv	120	4	18	15	85
Mocha w/o Whipping Cream Short Nonfat Milk	1 serv	100	2	18	5	90
Mocha w/o Whipping Cream Short Whole Milk	1 serv	150	7	17	25	85
Mocha w/o Whipping Cream Tall Lowfat Milk	1 serv	170	5	24	15	110
Mocha w/o Whipping Cream Tall Nonfat Milk	1 serv	140	2	24	5	110
Mocha w/o Whipping Cream Tall Whole Milk	1 serv	190	9	24	30	105
Mocha Syrup Grande	1 serv (2 oz)	80	3	17	0	0
Mocha Syrup Short	1 serv (1 oz)	40	1	9	0	0
Mocha Syrup Tall	1 serv (1.5 oz)	60	2	13	0	0
Steamed Lowfat Milk Grande	1 serv	180	7	18	30	190
Steamed Lowfat Milk Short	1 serv	90	3	9	15	90
Steamed Lowfat Milk Tall	1 serv	140	5	14	20	150
Steamed Nonfat Milk Grande	1 serv	130	1	18	5	190
Steamed Nonfat Milk Short	1 serv	60	0	9	5	95
Steamed Nonfat Milk Tall	1 serv	100	1	14	5	150
Steamed Whole Milk Grande	1 serv	230	13	17	50	180
Steamed Whole Milk Short	1 serv	110	6	9	25	90
Steamed Whole Milk Tall	1 serv	180	10	14	40	140
Whipping Cream Grande	1 serv (1.1 oz)	110	12	1	45	10
Whipping Cream Short	1 serv (0.7 oz)	70	7	1	25	5
Whipping Cream Tall	1 serv (0.8 oz)	80	9	1	35	10
ICE CREAM						
Biscotte Bliss	½ cup	240	12	30	55	70
Caffe Almond Fudge	½ cup	260	13	30	55	80
Caffe Almond Roast	1 bar	280	18	26	25	45
Dark Roast Expresso Swirl	½ cup	220	10	29	55	60

FOOD	PORTION	CALS	FAT	CARB	CHOL	SOD
Frappuccino Coffee	1 bar	110	2	20	10	50
Italian Roast Coffee	½ cup	230	12	26	65	65
Javachip	½ cup	250	13	29	60	55
Low Fat Latte	½ cup	170	3	31	10	65
Low Fat Mocha Mambo	½ cup	170	3	32	10	75
Vanilla Mochachip	½ cup	270	16	27	75	60

STUFF'N TURKEY

FOOD	PORTION	CALS	FAT	CARB	CHOL	SOD
Chef's Salad	1 serv	288	9	—	58	976
Grilled Turkey Breast	1 serv	244	3	—	23	685
Homemade Turkey Salad	1 serv	651	29	—	110	1079
Real Fresh Roasted Turkey Breast	1 serv	384	5	—	29	628
Rotisserie Turkey Breast	1 serv	251	3	—	48	1026
Thanksgiving Dinner On A Sandwich	1 serv	605	16	—	33	1079
Turkey Barbecue	1 serv	478	6	—	48	782
Turkey Powerhouse	1 serv	482	11	—	50	768

SUBWAY
COOKIES

FOOD	PORTION	CALS	FAT	CARB	CHOL	SOD
Chocolate Chip	1	210	10	29	10	140
Chocolate Chip M&M	1	210	10	29	15	140
Chocolate Chunk	1	210	10	29	10	140
Double Chocolate Brazil Nut	1	230	12	27	10	115
Oatmeal Raisin	1	200	8	29	15	160
Peanut Butter	1	220	12	26	0	180
Sugar	1	230	12	28	20	180
White Chocolate Macadamia Nut	1	230	12	28	10	140

SALAD DRESSINGS

FOOD	PORTION	CALS	FAT	CARB	CHOL	SOD
Creamy Italian	1 tbsp	65	6	2	4	132
Fat Free French	1 tbsp	15	0	4	0	85
Fat Free Italian	1 tbsp	5	0	1	0	152
Fat Free Ranch	1 tbsp	12	0	0	0	177
French	1 tbsp	65	5	5	0	100
Ranch	1 tbsp	87	9	1	1	117
Thousand Island	1 tbsp	65	6	2	7	107

SALADS AND SALAD BARS

FOOD	PORTION	CALS	FAT	CARB	CHOL	SOD
B.L.T.	1 serv	140	8	10	16	672
Bread Bowl	1 serv	330	4	63	0	760
Chicken Taco	1 serv	250	14	15	52	990
Classic Italian B.M.T.	1 serv	274	20	11	56	1379
Cold Cut Trio	1 serv	191	11	11	64	1127

FOOD	PORTION	CALS	FAT	CARB	CHOL	SOD
Ham	1 serv	116	3	11	28	1034
Meatball	1 serv	233	14	16	33	761
Pizza	1 serv	277	20	13	50	1336
Roast Beef	1 serv	117	3	11	20	654
Roasted Chicken Breast	1 serv	162	4	13	48	693
Steak & Cheese	1 serv	212	8	13	70	832
Subway Club	1 serv	126	3	12	26	1067
Subway Melt	1 serv	195	10	12	42	1461
Subway Seafood & Crab	1 serv	244	17	10	34	575
Subway Seafood & Crab w/ Light Mayonnaise	1 serv	161	8	11	32	599
Tuna	1 serv	356	30	10	36	601
Tuna w/ Light Mayonnaise	1 serv	205	13	11	32	654
Turkey Breast	1 serv	102	2	12	19	1117
Turkey Breast & Ham	1 serv	109	3	11	24	1076
Veggie Delight	1 serv	51	1	10	0	308
SANDWICHES						
6 Inch Cold Ham	1	302	5	45	28	1319
6 Inch Cold Tuna w/ Light Mayonnaise	1	391	15	46	32	940
6 Inch Cold Sub B.L.T.	1	327	10	44	16	957
6 Inch Cold Sub Classic Italian B.M.T.	1	460	22	45	56	1664
6 Inch Cold Sub Cold Cut Trio	1	378	13	46	64	1412
6 Inch Cold Sub Roast Beef	1	303	5	45	20	939
6 Inch Cold Sub Subway Club	1	312	5	46	26	1352
6 Inch Cold Sub Subway Seafood & Crab	1	430	19	44	34	860
6 Inch Cold Sub Subway Seafood & Crab w/ Light Mayonniase	1	347	10	45	32	884
6 Inch Cold Sub Tuna	1	542	32	44	36	886
6 Inch Cold Sub Turkey Breast	1	289	4	46	19	1403
6 Inch Cold Sub Turkey Breast & Ham	1	295	5	46	24	1361
6 Inch Cold Sub Veggie Delight	1	237	3	44	0	593
6 Inch Hot Subway Melt	1	382	12	46	42	1746
6 Inch Hot Sub Chicken Taco Sub	1	436	16	49	52	1275

FOOD	PORTION	CALS	FAT	CARB	CHOL	SOD
6 Inch Hot Sub Meatball	1	419	16	51	33	1046
6 Inch Hot Sub Pizza Sub	1	464	22	48	50	1621
6 Inch Hot Sub Roasted Chicken Breast	1	348	6	47	48	978
6 Inch Hot Sub Steak & Cheese	1	398	10	47	70	1117
Bacon	2 strips	45	4	0	8	182
Cheese	2 triangles	41	3	0	10	204
Deli Sandwich Bologna	1	292	12	38	20	744
Deli Sandwich Ham	1	234	4	37	14	773
Deli Sandwich Roast Beef	1	245	4	38	13	638
Deli Sandwich Tuna	1	354	18	37	18	557
Deli Sandwich Tuna w/ Light Mayonnaise	1	279	9	38	16	583
Deli Sandwich Turkey Breast	1	235	4	38	12	944
Light Mayonnaise	1 tsp	18	2	0	2	33
Mayonnaise	1 tsp	37	4	0	3	27
Mustard	2 tsp	8	0	1	0	0
Olive Oil Blend	1 tsp	45	5	0	0	0
Vinegar	1 tsp	1	0	0	0	0

TACO BELL
BEVERAGES

FOOD	PORTION	CALS	FAT	CARB	CHOL	SOD
2% Lowfat Milk	1 serv (8 oz)	110	5	11	15	115
Coffee Black	1 serv (12 oz)	5	0	1	0	5
Diet Pepsi	1 serv (16 oz)	0	0	0	0	47
Dr Pepper	1 serv (16 oz)	208	0	52	0	9
Lipton Iced Tea Sweetened	1 serv (16 oz)	140	0	40	0	60
Lipton Iced Tea Unsweetened	1 serv (16 oz)	0	0	0	0	60
Mountain Dew	1 serv (16 oz)	227	0	61	0	93
Orange Juice	1 serv (6 oz)	80	0	18	0	0
Pepsi Cola	1 serv (16 oz)	200	0	51	0	47
Slice	1 serv (16 oz)	200	0	53	0	73

BREAKFAST MENU SELECTIONS

FOOD	PORTION	CALS	FAT	CARB	CHOL	SOD
Breakfast Quesadilla Cheese	1 (5.5 oz)	380	21	33	280	1010
Breakfast Quesadilla w/ Bacon	1 (6 oz)	450	27	33	290	1200
Breakfast Quesadilla w/ Sausage	1 (6 oz)	430	25	33	285	1090

FOOD	PORTION	CALS	FAT	CARB	CHOL	SOD
Country Breakfast Burrito	1 (4 oz)	270	14	26	195	690
Double Bacon & Egg Burrito	1 (6.25 oz)	480	27	39	405	1240
Fiesta Breakfast Burrito	1 (3.5 oz)	280	16	25	25	580
Grande Breakfast Burrito	1 (6.25 oz)	420	22	43	205	1050
Hash Brown Nuggets	1 serv (3.5 oz)	280	18	29	0	570
MAIN MENU SELECTIONS						
7-Layer Burrito	1 (10 oz)	530	23	66	25	1280
BLT Soft Taco	1 (4.5 oz)	340	23	22	40	610
Bacon Cheeseburger Burrito	1 (8.5 oz)	570	31	46	70	1460
Bean Burrito	1 (7 oz)	380	12	55	10	1100
Big Beef Burrito Supreme	1 (10.5 oz)	520	23	54	55	1520
Big Beef MexiMelt	1 (4.75 oz)	290	15	23	45	850
Big Chicken Burrito Supreme	1 (9 oz)	510	24	52	95	1900
Border Sauce Fire	1 serv (0.3 oz)	0	0	0	0	110
Border Sauce Hot	1 serv (0.3 oz)	0	0	0	0	85
Border Sauce Mild	1 serv (0.3 oz)	0	0	0	0	75
Burger Sauce	1 serv (0.5 oz)	60	5	2	5	110
Burrito Supreme	1 (9 oz)	440	19	51	35	1230
Cheddar Cheese	1 serv (0.25 oz)	30	2	0	5	45
Cheese Quesadilla	1 (4.25 oz)	350	18	32	50	860
Chicken Fajita Wrap	1 (8 oz)	470	22	51	60	1290
Chicken Fajita Wrap Supreme	1 (9 oz)	520	25	53	70	1300
Chicken Quesadilla	1 (6 oz)	410	21	34	90	1170
Chicken Club Burrito	1 (8 oz)	540	32	43	80	1250
Chili Cheese Burrito	1 (5 oz)	330	13	37	35	870
Choco Taco Ice Cream Dessert	1 serv (4 oz)	310	17	37	20	100
Cinnamon Twists	1 serv (1 oz)	140	6	19	0	190
Club Sauce	1 serv (0.5 oz)	80	8	1	10	105
Double Decker Taco	1 (5.75 oz)	340	15	38	25	750
Double Decker Taco Supreme	1 (7 oz)	390	19	40	35	760
Fajita Sauce	1 serv (0.5 oz)	70	7	1	5	130
Green Sauce	1 serv (1 oz)	5	0	1	0	150
Grilled Chicken Burrito	1 (7 oz)	410	15	50	55	1380
Grilled Chicken Soft Taco	1 (4.5 oz)	240	12	21	45	1110
Grilled Steak Soft Taco	1 (4.5 oz)	230	10	20	25	1020
Grilled Steak Soft Taco Supreme	1 (5.75 oz)	290	14	24	35	1040

FOOD	PORTION	CALS	FAT	CARB	CHOL	SOD
Guacamole	1 serv (0.75 oz)	35	3	1	0	80
Mexican Pizza	1 serv (7.75 oz)	570	35	42	45	1040
Mexican Rice	1 serv (4.75 oz)	190	9	23	15	760
Nacho Cheese Sauce	2 serv (2 oz)	120	10	5	5	470
Nachos	1 serv (3.5 oz)	320	18	34	5	570
Nachos Beef Beef Supreme	1 serv (7 oz)	450	24	45	30	810
Nachos Bellgrande	1 serv (11 oz)	770	39	84	35	1310
Picante Sauce	1 serv (0.3 oz)	0	0	0	0	110
Pico De Gallo	1 serv (0.75 oz)	5	0	1	0	65
Pintos 'n Cheese	1 serv (4.5 oz)	190	9	18	15	650
Red Sauce	1 serv (1 oz)	10	0	2	0	320
Soft Taco	1 (3.5 oz)	220	10	21	25	580
Soft Taco Supreme	1 (5 oz)	260	14	23	35	590
Sour Cream	1 serv (0.75 oz)	40	4	1	10	10
Steak Fajita Wrap	1 (8 oz)	470	21	50	40	1190
Steak Fajita Wrap Supreme	1 (9 oz)	510	25	52	50	1200
Taco	1 (2.75 oz)	180	10	12	25	330
Taco Supreme	1 (4 oz)	220	14	14	35	350
Taco Salad w/ Salsa	1 (19 oz)	850	52	65	60	1780
Taco Salad w/ Salsa w/o Shell	1 (16.5 oz)	420	22	32	60	1520
Three Cheese Blend	1 serv (0.25 oz)	25	2	0	5	50
Tostada	1 (6.25 oz)	300	15	31	15	650
Veggie Fajita Wrap	1 (8 oz)	420	19	53	20	980
Veggie Fajita Wrap Supreme	1 (9 oz)	470	22	55	30	990

TACO JOHN'S
CHILDREN'S MENU SELECTIONS

Kid's Meal Softshell Taco	1 serv (8.5 oz)	617	33	64	35	1037
Kids's Meal Crispy Taco	1 serv (8 oz)	579	34	54	35	789

DESSERTS

Choco Taco	1 serv (3.5 oz)	320	17	38	20	100
Churro	1 serv (1.5 oz)	147	8	17	4	160
Flauta Apple	1 serv (2 oz)	84	1	19	0	72
Flauta Cherry	1 serv (2 oz)	143	4	27	0	110
Flauta Cream Cheese	1 serv (2 oz)	181	8	27	10	135
Italian Ice	1 serv (4 oz)	80	0	19	0	5

MAIN MENU SELECTIONS

Bean Burrito	1 (6.5 oz)	387	11	57	18	866
Beans Refried	1 serv (9.5 oz)	357	9	53	17	1032
Beef Burrito	1 (6.5 oz)	449	20	44	52	863

FOOD	PORTION	CALS	FAT	CARB	CHOL	SOD
Chicken Fajita Burrito	1 (6.25)	370	12	45	49	1536
Chicken Fajita Salad w/o Dressing	1 serv (12.25 oz)	557	33	44	56	1541
Chicken Fajita Softshell	1 (4.5 oz)	200	7	21	33	903
Chili	1 serv (9.25 oz)	350	21	19	56	865
Chimichanga Platter	1 serv (18 oz)	979	38	127	59	2341
Combination Burrito	1 (6.5 oz)	418	16	50	35	865
Crispy Tacos	1 serv (3.25 oz)	182	11	12	26	272
Double Enchilada Platter	1 serv (18.25 oz)	967	42	106	89	1921
Meat & Potato Burrito	1 (7.75 oz)	503	24	53	25	1341
Mexi Rolls w/ Nacho Cheese	1 serv (9.75 oz)	863	48	72	54	1392
Mexican Rice	1 serv (8 oz)	567	18	40	0	1293
Nacho Cheese	1 serv (2 oz)	300	10	0	—	600
Nachos	1 serv (3.5 oz)	333	21	27	0	611
Potato Oles	1 lg serv (6.12 oz)	484	30	50	—	1285
Potato Oles	1 serv (4.63 oz)	363	23	38	—	964
Potato Oles Bravo	1 serv (8.88 oz)	579	38	47	7	1550
Potato Oles w/ Nacho Cheese	1 serv (6.63 oz)	483	33	38	—	1564
Ranch Burrito	1 (7 oz)	447	23	44	74	804
Sampler Platter	1 serv (25.5 oz)	1406	61	156	126	2875
Sierra Chicken Fillet Sandwich	1 (8.5 oz)	534	29	40	68	1406
Smothered Burrito Platter	1 serv (19.5 oz)	1031	40	132	70	2351
Softshell Tacos	1 serv (4.25 oz)	230	10	23	26	520
Sour Cream	1 oz	60	5	1	—	15
Super Burrito	1 (8.5 oz)	465	19	53	41	922
Super Nachos	1 serv (13 oz)	919	56	72	48	1484
Taco Bravo	1 serv (6.25 oz)	346	14	39	28	677
Taco Burger	1 (5 oz)	280	12	28	32	576
Taco Salad w/o Dressing	1 (12.4 oz)	584	38	43	46	766

TACOTIME

FOOD	PORTION	CALS	FAT	CARB	CHOL	SOD
Casita Burrito Meat	1 serv (12 oz)	647	31	54	89	1233
Cheddar Cheese	1 serv (0.75 oz)	86	7	0	22	132
Chicken	1 serv (2.5 oz)	109	6	2	33	402
Chips	1 serv (2 oz)	266	12	35	0	461
Crisp Burrito Bean	1 (5.25 oz)	427	18	53	12	453
Crisp Burrito Chicken	1 (4.75 oz)	422	25	32	54	795
Crisp Burrito Meat	1 (5.25 oz)	552	30	39	58	1000

FOOD	PORTION	CALS	FAT	CARB	CHOL	SOD
Crisp Taco	1 (4 oz)	295	17	16	48	609
Crustos	1 serv (3.5 oz)	373	15	47	0	86
Double Soft Bean Burrito	1 (9.5 oz)	506	12	77	22	860
Double Soft Combination Burrito	1 (9.5 oz)	617	23	66	63	1343
Double Soft Meat Burrito	1 serv (6.5 oz)	726	33	55	99	1809
Empanada Cherry	1 (4 oz)	250	9	37	0	46
Enchilada Sauce	1 serv (1 oz)	12	0	3	0	133
Flour Tortilla 10 in	1 (2.75 oz)	213	4	31	0	393
Flour Tortilla 7 in	1 (1.75 oz)	88	1	16	0	42
Flour Tortilla 8 in	1 (1.25 oz)	107	3	16	0	33
Fried Flour Tortilla 10 in	1 (2.75 oz)	318	16	37	0	315
Fried Flour Tortilla 8 in	1 (1.35 oz)	205	11	24	0	203
Guacamole	1 serv (1 oz)	29	2	2	0	94
Hot Sauce	1 serv (1 oz)	10	0	2	0	120
Lettuce	1 serv (0.5 oz)	2	0	0	0	1
Mexi Fries	1 lg (8 oz)	532	34	54	0	1598
Mexi Fries	1 reg (4 oz)	266	17	27	0	799
Mexican Dressing No Fat	1 serv (2 oz)	20	0	5	0	130
Mexican Rice	1 serv (4 oz)	159	2	30	0	530
Nachos	1 serv (10.5 oz)	680	38	61	78	1250
Nachos Deluxe	1 serv (15.25 oz)	1048	57	91	109	2252
Natural Super Taco Meat	1 (11.25 oz)	627	27	60	82	915
Olives	1 serv (0.50 oz)	16	2	1	0	124
Quesadilla Cheese	1 serv (3.25 oz)	205	11	17	30	255
Ranchero Salsa	1 serv (2 oz)	21	1	3	0	192
Refritos	1 serv (2.5 oz)	97	0	18	0	101
Refritos	1 serv (7 oz)	326	10	44	22	525
Rolled Soft Flour Taco	1 (7 oz)	512	23	46	63	1111
Shredded Beef	1 serv (2.5 oz)	70	7	1	—	31
Soft Taco Chicken	1 (7 oz)	387	16	41	48	933
Sour Cream	1 serv (1 oz)	55	5	1	19	11
Sour Cream Dressing	1 serv (1.5 oz)	137	14	2	8	207
Super Shredded Beef Soft Taco	1 (8 oz)	368	11	38	22	556
Taco Cheeseburger	1 (7.5 oz)	633	36	48	66	1291
Taco Meat	1 serv (2.5 oz)	208	11	7	38	576
Taco Salad Chicken w/o Dressing	1 serv (9 oz)	370	21	27	48	861
Taco Salad w/o Dressing	1 serv (7.75 oz)	479	28	30	63	895
Taco Shell 6 in	1 (1.25 oz)	110	6	14	0	48
Thousand Island Dressing	1 serv (1 oz)	160	16	4	10	270

FOOD	PORTION	CALS	FAT	CARB	CHOL	SOD
Tomato	1 serv (0.5 oz)	3	0	1	0	1
Tostada Delight Salad Meat	1 (9.75 oz)	628	33	48	82	1004
Value Soft Bean Burrito	1 (6.75 oz)	380	10	58	15	715
Value Soft Meat Burrito	1 (6.75 oz)	491	21	48	56	1197
Value Soft Taco	1 (5.25 oz)	316	15	23	48	599
Veggie Burrito	1 (11 oz)	491	16	70	24	643
Wheat Tortilla 11 in	1 (3.5 oz)	175	3	33	0	84

TCBY

FOOD	PORTION	CALS	FAT	CARB	CHOL	SOD
Hand Dipped All Flavors 96% Fat Free	½ cup (3 oz)	140	3	26	5	26
Hand Dipped All Flavors Nonfat	½ cup (2.9 oz)	120	0	25	0	60
Lowfat Ice Cream All Flavors No Sugar Added	½ cup (2.6 oz)	110	3	19	10	60
Nonfat Ice Cream All Flavors	½ cup (2.9 oz)	120	0	26	0	55
Soft Serve All Flavors 96% Fat Free	½ cup (3.4 fl oz)	140	3	23	15	60
Soft Serve All Flavors No Sugar Added Nonfat	½ cup (2.8 oz)	80	0	20	<5	35
Soft Serve All Flavors Nonfat	½ cup (3.4 oz)	110	0	23	<5	60
Sorbet All Flavors Nonfat & Nondairy	½ cup (3.4 oz)	100	0	24	0	30

TGI FRIDAY'S

FOOD	PORTION	CALS	FAT	CARB	CHOL	SOD
Chili Yogurt	1 serv	30	—	—	—	—
Corn Salsa	1 serv	175	3	—	—	—
Fresh Vegetable Medley w/ Potato	1 serv	470	8	—	25	—
Fresh Vegetable Medley w/ Rice	1 serv	407	8	—	<2	—
Friday's Gardenburger	1	445	9	—	13	—
Garden Dagwood Sandwich	1 serv	375	11	—	<2	—
Pacific Coast Chicken	1 serv	415	8	—	70	—
Pacific Coast Tuna	1 serv	410	8	—	70	—
Pea Salsa	1 serv (6.4 oz)	175	3	32	0	445
Plum Sauce	1 serv	105	0	—	—	—
Salad & Baked Potato	1 serv	250	5	—	<2	—
Turkey Burger	1 (9.8 oz)	410	19	27	95	780

FOOD	PORTION	CALS	FAT	CARB	CHOL	SOD
T.J. CINNAMONS						
Doughnuts Cake	2	454	22	60	98	582
Doughnuts Raised	2	352	22	32	98	198
Mini-Cinn Plain	1	75	5	7	3	89
Mini-Cinn With Icing	1	80	5	8	3	89
Original Gourmet Cinnamon Roll Plain	1	630	34	75	38	712
Original Gourmet Cinnamon Roll With Icing	1	686	34	89	38	712
Petite Cinnamon Roll Plain	1	185	10	22	11	214
Petite Cinnamon Roll With Icing	1	202	10	26	11	214
Sticky Bun Cinnamon Pecan	1	607	35	69	29	589
Sticky Bun Petite Cinnamon Pecan	1	255	15	29	11	241
Triple Chocolate Classic Roll Plain	1	412	28	35	28	543
Triple Chocolate Classic Roll With Icing	1	462	31	42	28	563
TROPIGRILL						
Banana Tropical	1 serv (7.55 oz)	498	14	90	0	7
Black Beans (combo meal portion)	1 serv (4.78 oz)	153	2	24	0	444
Black Beans (side)	1 serv (8.39 oz)	269	4	43	0	780
Boiled Yuca	1 serv (12 oz)	334	0	81	0	456
Boneless Breast	1 serv (3.14 oz)	140	4	1	83	169
Cheese Potatoes	1 serv (7.42 oz)	177	6	25	10	779
Chicken ¼ Dark Meat	1 serv (4.52 oz)	298	18	1	187	448
Chicken ¼ Dark Meat w/o Skin	1 serv (3.42 oz)	170	7	1	144	312
Chicken ¼ White Meat	1 serv (5.09 oz)	295	14	1	170	894
Chicken ¼ White Meat w/o Skin	1 serv (3.82 oz)	167	3	tr	117	401
Chicken Caesar Sandwich	1 (6.4 oz)	457	20	36	97	931
Chicken Sandwich	1 (7.92 oz)	442	19	35	89	702
Congri	1 serv (7.08 oz)	439	13	69	0	786
Vegetable Kabob	1 (3.07 oz)	106	1	22	0	286
White Rice	1 serv (6.82 oz)	341	6	65	0	239
Yellow Rice	1 serv (7 oz)	294	5	56	0	371
Yucatan Fries	1 serv (5.3 oz)	440	24	54	0	84

FOOD	PORTION	CALS	FAT	CARB	CHOL	SOD

UNO RESTAURANT

FOOD	PORTION	CALS	FAT	CARB	CHOL	SOD
DeepDish Pizza	1 serv	770	38	75	45	1390

VILLAGE INN

FOOD	PORTION	CALS	FAT	CARB	CHOL	SOD
French Toast Cinnamon Raisin	1 serv	809	16	—	9	740
Fruit & Nut Pancakes Low Cholesterol	1 serv	936	19	—	2	754
Omelette Chicken & Cheese	1 serv	721	19	—	120	705
Omelette Fresh Veggie	1 serv	704	18	—	102	883
Omelette Mushroom & Cheese	1 serv	680	18	—	102	688
Turkey & Vegetable Scrambled Sensation	1 serv	726	19	—	124	710

WENDY'S
BEVERAGES

FOOD	PORTION	CALS	FAT	CARB	CHOL	SOD
Coffee Decaffeinated Black	1 cup (6 fl oz)	0	0	1	0	0
Coffee Black	1 cup (6 fl oz)	0	0	1	0	0
Cola	11 oz	130	0	36	0	0
Diet Cola	11 oz	0	0	0	0	15
Hot Chocolate	1 cup (6 fl oz)	80	3	15	0	135
Lemon-Lime Soda	11 oz	130	0	36	0	30
Lemonade	11 oz	130	0	37	0	0
Milk 2%	1 (8 fl oz)	110	4	11	15	115
Tea Hot	1 cup (6 fl oz)	0	0	0	0	0
Tea Iced	1 cup (6 fl oz)	0	0	0	0	0

CHILDREN'S MENU SELECTIONS

FOOD	PORTION	CALS	FAT	CARB	CHOL	SOD
Kid's Meal Cheeseburger	1 (4.3 oz)	320	13	33	45	830
Kid's Meal Hamburger	1 (3.9 oz)	270	10	33	30	610
Kids' Meal Chicken Nuggets	4 pieces (2.1 oz)	190	13	9	25	380

DESSERTS

FOOD	PORTION	CALS	FAT	CARB	CHOL	SOD
Chocolate Chip Cookie	1 (2 oz)	270	13	36	30	120
Frosty Dairy Dessert	1 lg (20 fl oz)	540	14	91	60	320
Frosty Dairy Dessert	1 med (16 fl oz)	440	11	73	50	260
Frosty Dairy Dessert	1 sm (12 oz)	330	8	56	35	200

MAIN MENU SELECTIONS

FOOD	PORTION	CALS	FAT	CARB	CHOL	SOD
¼ lb Hamburger Patty	1 (2.6 oz)	200	14	0	65	290
2 oz Hamburger Patty	1 (1.3 oz)	100	7	0	30	150
American Cheese	1 slice (0.6 oz)	70	5	1	15	320
American Cheese Jr.	1 slice (0.4 oz)	45	4	0	10	220
Bacon	1 strip (4 g)	20	2	0	5	65

FOOD	PORTION	CALS	FAT	CARB	CHOL	SOD
Baked Potato Bacon & Cheese	1 (13.3 oz)	530	18	78	20	1390
Baked Potato Broccoli & Cheese	1 (14.4 oz)	470	14	80	5	470
Baked Potato Cheese	1 (13.4 oz)	570	23	78	30	640
Baked Potato Chili & Cheese	1 (15.4 oz)	630	24	83	40	770
Baked Potato Plain	1 (10 oz)	310	0	71	0	25
Baked Potato Sour Cream & Chives	1 (11 oz)	380	6	74	15	40
Big Bacon Classic	1 (9.9 oz)	580	30	46	100	1460
Breaded Chicken Fillet	1 (3.5 oz)	230	12	10	55	490
Breaded Chicken Sandwich	1 (7.3 oz)	440	18	44	60	840
Cheddar Cheese Shredded	2 tbsp (0.6 oz)	70	6	1	15	110
Chicken Club Sandwich	1 (7.6 oz)	470	20	44	70	970
Chicken Nuggets	5 pieces (2.6 oz)	230	16	11	30	470
Chili	1 lg (12 oz)	310	10	32	45	1190
Chili	1 sm (8 oz)	210	7	21	30	800
French Fries	1 Biggie (5.6 oz)	470	23	61	0	150
French Fries	1 Great Biggie (6.7 oz)	570	27	73	0	180
French Fries	1 med (4.6 oz)	390	19	50	0	120
French Fries	1 sm (3.2 oz)	270	13	35	0	85
Grilled Chicken Fillet	1 (2.9 oz)	110	3	0	60	450
Grilled Chicken Sandwich	1 (6.6 oz)	310	8	35	65	790
Honey Mustard Reduced Calorie	1 tsp (7 g)	25	2	2	0	45
Jr. Bacon Cheeseburger	1 (5.8 oz)	380	19	34	60	850
Jr. Cheeseburger	1 (4.6 oz)	320	13	34	45	830
Jr. Cheeseburger Deluxe	1 (6.3 oz)	360	17	36	50	890
Jr. Hamburger	1 (4.1 oz)	270	10	34	30	610
Kaiser Bun	1 (2.4 oz)	190	3	36	0	340
Ketchup	1 tsp (7 g)	10	0	2	0	75
Lettuce	1 leaf (0.5 oz)	0	0	0	0	0
Mayonnaise	1½ tsp (9 g)	30	3	1	5	60
Mustard	½ tsp (5 g)	5	0	0	0	50
Nuggets Sauce Barbeque	1 pkg (1 oz)	45	0	10	0	160
Nuggets Sauce Honey Mustard	1 pkg (1 oz)	130	12	6	10	220

FOOD	PORTION	CALS	FAT	CARB	CHOL	SOD
Nuggets Sauce Sweet & Sour	1 pkg (1 oz)	50	0	12	0	120
Onion	4 rings (0.5 oz)	5	0	1	0	0
Pickles	4 slices (0.4 oz)	0	0	0	0	140
Pita Dressing Caesar Vinaigrette Reduced Fat Reduced Calorie	1 tbsp (0.6 oz)	70	7	1	0	170
Pita Dressing Garden Ranch Sauce Reduced Fat Reduced Calorie	1 tbsp (0.6 oz)	50	5	1	10	125
Plain Single	1 (4.7 oz)	360	16	31	65	580
Saltines	2 (0.2 oz)	25	1	4	0	80
Sandwich Bun	1 (2 oz)	160	3	29	0	280
Single With Everything	1 (7.7 oz)	420	20	37	70	920
Sour Cream	1 pkt (1 oz)	60	6	1	10	15
Spicy Buffalo Wing Sauce	1 pkg (1 oz)	25	1	4	0	210
Spicy Chicken Fillet	1 (3.6 oz)	210	9	10	60	920
Spicy Chicken Sandwich	1 (7.5 oz)	410	15	43	65	1280
Stuffed Pita Chicken Caesar w/Dressing	1 (8.3 oz)	490	18	48	65	1320
Stuffed Pita Classic Greek w/Dressing	1 (8.2 oz)	440	20	50	35	1050
Stuffed Pita Garden Ranch Chicken w/ Dressing	1 (9.9 oz)	480	18	51	70	1180
Stuffed Pita Garden Veggie w/ Dressing	1 (9 oz)	400	17	52	20	760
Tomatoes	1 slice (0.9 oz)	5	0	1	0	0
Whipped Margarine	1 pkg (0.5 oz)	60	7	0	0	115
SALAD DRESSINGS						
Blue Cheese	2 tbsp (1 oz)	180	19	0	15	180
French	2 tbsp (1 oz)	120	10	6	0	330
French Fat Free	2 tbsp (1 oz)	35	0	8	0	150
Hidden Valley Ranch	2 tbsp (1 oz)	90	10	1	10	220
Hidden Valley Ranch Reduced Fat Reduced Calorie	2 tbsp (1 oz)	60	5	2	10	240
Italian Reduced Fat Reduced Calorie	2 tbsp (1 oz)	40	3	2	0	340
Italian Caesar	2 tbsp (1 oz)	150	16	1	20	240
Salad Oil	1 tbsp (0.5 oz)	120	14	0	0	0
Thousand Island	2 tbsp (1 oz)	90	8	2	10	125
Wine Vinegar	1 tbsp (0.5 oz)	0	0	0	0	0

FOOD	PORTION	CALS	FAT	CARB	CHOL	SOD
SALADS AND SALAD BARS						
Applesauce	2 tbsp (1.4 oz)	30	0	7	0	0
Bacon Bits	2 tbsp (0.5 oz)	45	2	0	10	550
Bananas & Strawberry Glaze	¼ cup (1.6 oz)	30	0	8	0	0
Broccoli	¼ cup (0.5 oz)	0	0	1	0	0
Caesar Side Salad w/o Dressing	1 (3.1 oz)	100	4	8	10	620
Cantaloupe Sliced	1 piece (1.6 oz)	15	0	4	0	0
Carrots	¼ cup (0.6 oz)	5	0	2	0	5
Cauliflower	¼ cup (0.6 g)	0	0	1	0	0
Cheese Shredded Imitation	2 tbsp (0.6 oz)	50	4	1	0	260
Chicken Salad	2 tbsp (1.2 oz)	70	5	2	0	135
Cottage Cheese	2 tbsp (1.1 oz)	30	2	1	5	125
Croutons	2 tbsp (0.2 oz)	25	1	4	0	65
Cucumbers	2 slices (0.5 oz)	0	0	0	0	0
Deluxe Garden Salad w/o Dressing	1 (9.5 oz)	110	6	9	0	350
Eggs Hard Cooked	2 tbsp (0.9 oz)	40	3	0	110	30
Green Peas	2 tbsp (0.7 oz)	15	0	3	0	25
Green Peppers	2 pieces (0.3 oz)	0	0	1	0	0
Grilled Chicken Salad w/o Dressing	1 (11.9 oz)	200	8	9	50	720
Lettuce Iceberg/Romaine	1 cup (2.6 oz)	10	0	2	0	5
Mushrooms	¼ cup (0.5 oz)	0	0	1	0	0
Orange Sliced	2 slices (1.1 oz)	15	0	4	0	0
Parmesan Blend Grated	2 tbsp (0.5 oz)	70	4	5	10	290
Pasta Salad	2 tbsp (1.2 oz)	35	2	4	0	180
Peaches Sliced	1 piece (1 oz)	15	0	4	0	0
Pepperoni Sliced	6 slices (0.2 oz)	30	3	0	5	70
Potato Salad	2 tbsp (1.3 oz)	80	7	5	5	180
Pudding Chocolate	¼ cup (1.8 oz)	70	3	10	0	60
Red Onions	3 rings (0.5 oz)	0	0	1	0	0
Side Salad w/o Dressing	1 (5.4 oz)	60	3	5	0	180
Soft Breadstick	1 (1.5 oz)	130	3	23	5	250
Sunflower Seeds & Raisins	2 tbsp (0.5 oz)	80	5	5	0	0
Taco Chips	15 (1.5 oz)	210	11	24	0	180
Taco Salad w/o Dressing	1 (16.4 oz)	380	19	28	65	1040
Tomatoes Wedged	1 piece (0.9 oz)	5	0	1	0	0
Turkey Ham Diced	2 tbsp (0.8 oz)	50	4	0	25	280
Watermelon Wedged	1 piece (2.2 oz)	20	0	4	0	0

FOOD	PORTION	CALS	FAT	CARB	CHOL	SOD
WHATABURGER						
BAKED SELECTIONS						
Biscuit	1	280	13	37	3	509
Blueberry Muffin	1	239	8	36	0	538
Cinnamon Roll	1	320	16	39	10	190
Cookie Chocolate Chunk	1	247	16	28	36	75
Cookie White Chocolate Macadamia Nut	1	269	16	31	34	80
Fried Apple Turnover	1	215	11	27	0	241
BEVERAGES						
Cherry Coke	1 reg	227	0	60	0	11
Coffee	1 sm	5	0	1	0	5
Coke Classic	1 reg	211	0	56	0	19
Creamer	1 pkg	10	1	1	0	4
Diet Coke	1 reg	2	0	1	0	26
Dr Pepper	1 reg	207	1	52	0	51
Iced Tea	1 reg	5	0	2	0	15
Lemon Juice	1 pkg	1	0	tr	0	1
Milk 2%	1 serv	113	4	11	18	113
Orange Juice	1 serv (10 oz)	140	0	33	0	0
Root Beer	1 reg	237	0	63	0	25
Shake Chocolate	1 junior	364	9	61	36	172
Shake Strawberry	1 junior	352	9	60	35	168
Shake Vanilla	1 junior	325	10	51	37	172
Sprite	1 reg	211	0	48	0	45
Sugar	1 pkg	15	0	4	0	0
Sweet'N Low	1 pkg	4	0	1	0	0
BREAKFAST SELECTIONS						
Biscuit w/ Bacon	1	359	20	37	15	730
Biscuit w/ Bacon Egg & Cheese	1	511	33	38	213	1010
Biscuit w/ Egg & Cheese	1	434	26	38	202	797
Biscuit w/ Sausage	1	446	29	37	37	794
Biscuit w/ Sausage Egg & Cheese	1	601	42	38	236	1081
Biscuit w/ Sausage Gravy	1	479	27	48	20	1253
Breakfast Platter w/ Bacon	1 serv	695	44	54	389	1162
Breakfast Platter w/ Sausage	1 serv	785	53	54	412	1234
Breakfast On A Bun w/ Bacon	1	365	19	29	210	815

FOOD	PORTION	CALS	FAT	CARB	CHOL	SOD
Breakfast On A Bun w/ Sausage	1	455	28	30	232	886
Butter	1 pkg	36	4	0	11	42
Egg Omelette Sandwich	1	288	13	29	198	602
Grape Jelly	1 pkg	45	0	10	0	15
Hashbrown	1 serv	150	9	16	0	228
Honey	1 pkg	25	0	7	0	0
Margarine	1 pkg	25	3	0	0	40
Pancake Syrup	1 pkg	180	0	42	0	50
Pancakes	3	259	6	40	0	842
Pancakes w/ Bacon	1 serv	335	12	40	12	1074
Pancakes w/ Sausage	1 serv	426	21	40	34	1127
Scrambled Eggs	2	189	15	2	374	211
Strawberry Jam	1 pkg	40	0	9	0	15
Taquito Bacon & Egg	1	335	16	32	286	761
MAIN MENU SELECTIONS						
Bacon	1 slice	38	3	0	6	106
Cheese Slice	1 lg	89	7	tr	22	338
Cheese Slice	1 sm	46	4	tr	12	176
Chicken Strips	2	120	5	10	14	420
Club Crackers	1 pkg	30	2	4	0	75
Croutons	1 pkg	30	1	5	0	90
Fajita Beef	1	326	12	34	28	670
Fajita Grilled Chicken	1	272	7	35	33	691
French Fries	1 junior	221	12	25	0	139
French Fries	1 lg	442	24	49	0	227
French Fries	1 reg	332	18	37	0	208
Garden Salad	1	56	1	11	0	32
Grilled Chicken Salad	1 serv	150	1	14	49	434
Grilled Chicken Sandwich	1	442	14	48	66	1103
Grilled Chicken Sandwich on Small Bun w/o Bun Oil w/ Mustard	1	300	3	35	66	994
Grilled Chicken Sandwich w/o Bun Oil & Dressing	1	358	6	46	66	989
Grilled Chicken Sandwich w/o Dressing	1	385	9	46	66	989
Jalapeno Pepper	1	3	tr	1	0	190
Justaburger	1	276	11	30	34	578
Ketchup	1 pkg	30	0	7	0	344

FOOD	PORTION	CALS	FAT	CARB	CHOL	SOD
Onion Rings	1 lg	493	29	51	0	893
Onion Rings	1 reg	329	19	34	0	596
Peppered Gravy	1 serv (3 oz)	75	5	8	0	375
Picante Sauce	1 pkg	5	0	1	0	130
Taquito Potato & Egg	1	446	22	48	281	883
Taquito Sausage & Egg	1	443	26	32	315	790
Texas Toast	1 slice	147	5	22	0	250
Whataburger	1	598	26	61	84	1096
Whataburger Double Meat	1	823	42	62	168	1298
Whataburger Jr.	1	300	12	35	34	583
Whataburger w/o bun oil	1	407	19	34	84	839
Whatacatch Sandwich	1	467	25	43	33	636
Whatachick'n Sandwich	1	501	23	51	40	1122
SALAD DRESSINGS						
Low Fat Ranch	1 pkg	66	3	9	15	607
Low Fat Vinaigrette	1 pkg	37	2	6	0	896
Ranch	1 pkg	320	33	4	50	750
Thousand Island	1 pkg	160	12	12	15	470

WHITE CASTLE

(FAST FACT: E. W. "Billy" Ingram opened the first White Castle restaurant in 1921, selling five-cent hamburgers, coffee and soft drinks.)

FOOD	PORTION	CALS	FAT	CARB	CHOL	SOD
Bun Only	1	74	tr	—	—	—
Cheese Only	0.3 oz	31	2	—	—	—
Cheeseburger	2 (3.6 oz)	310	17	23	30	480
Fish w/o Tartar Sandwich	1	155	5	—	—	—
French Fries	1 reg	301	15	—	—	—
Grilled Chicken Sandwich	2 (4 oz)	250	9	24	20	490
Grilled Chicken Sandwich w/ Sauce	2 (4.8 oz)	290	9	24	20	600
Hamburger	2 (3.2 oz)	270	14	23	20	270
Onion Rings	1 reg	245	13	—	—	—
Sausage Sandwich	1	196	12	—	—	—
Sausage & Egg Sandwich	1	322	22	—	—	—

WINCHELL'S DONUTS

FOOD	PORTION	CALS	FAT	CARB	CHOL	SOD
Apple Fritter	1 (4.25 oz)	580	37	59	—	201
Cinnamon Crumb	1 (2 oz)	240	11	34	—	208
Cinnamon Roll	1 (3 oz)	360	21	39	—	179
Glazed Jelly	1 (3 oz)	300	13	43	—	172
Glazed Round	1 (1.75 oz)	210	12	24	—	100

FOOD	PORTION	CALS	FAT	CARB	CHOL	SOD
Glazed Twist	1 (1.75 oz)	210	11	26	—	100
Iced Chocolate Bar	1 (2 oz)	220	11	28	—	125
Iced Chocolate Cake	1 (2 oz)	230	10	31	—	218
Iced Chocolate Devil's Food	1 (2 oz)	240	12	31	—	221
Iced Chocolate French	1 (1.89 oz)	220	13	23	—	217
Iced Chocolate Raised	1 (1.75 oz)	210	10	26	—	96
Plain	1 (1.58 oz)	200	11	24	—	211
Plain Donut Hole	1 (0.4 oz)	50	3	5	—	13
ZUZU						
Bean & Cheese Burrito Platter	1 serv	475	15	—	15	—
Beans	1 cup	210	6	—	0	—
Cheese Enchilada Platter	1 serv	395	13	—	15	—
Chicken Burrito Platter	1 serv	580	19	—	60	—
Chicken Taco Platter	1 serv	440	13	—	70	—
Chicken Taco w/o Mexican Cream	1	125	4	—	35	—
Frozen Yogurt	1 serv	200	0	—	0	—
Green Salad w/o Dressing or Avocado	1	20	0	—	0	—
Grilled Chicken Salad w/o Dressing	1 serv	305	10	—	70	—
Rice	1 cup	150	2	—	0	—
Salsa Roja Epazote	¼ cup	8	0	—	0	—
Tortilla Corn	1	35	0	—	0	—
Tortilla Flour	1	60	2	—	0	—

PART · TWO

TAKEOUT

NOTES

TAKEOUT describes prepared dishes that you purchase ready-to-eat; those included here serve as a guide to the nutrient values of similar products you may purchase.

Discrepancies in values are due to rounding. All values for calories, fat, carbohydrate, cholesterol and sodium have been rounded to the nearest whole number.

All **fat** values of foods are given in grams (g).

All **carbohydrate** (CARB) values of foods are given in grams.

All **cholesterol** (CHOL) values of foods are given in milligrams (mg).

All **sodium** (SOD) values of foods are given in milligrams.

tr (trace) is the value used when a food contains less than one calorie, less than one gram of fat or carbohydrate, or less than one milligram of cholesterol or sodium.

A dash (—) indicates data was not available.

FOOD	PORTION	CALS	FAT	CARB	CHOL	SOD
ANTELOPE						
roasted	3 oz	127	2	0	107	46
ARTICHOKE						
steamed	1 med (4 oz)	60	tr	13	0	114
ASPARAGUS						
steamed	4 spears	14	tr	3	0	7
BACON						
grilled	3 strips	109	9	tr	16	303
BAGEL						
cinnamon raisin toasted	1 (3½ in)	194	1	39	0	229
egg toasted	1 (3½ in)	197	2	38	17	358
oat bran toasted	1 (3½ in)	181	1	38	0	360
plain toasted	1 (3½ in)	195	1	38	0	379
BASS						
striped baked or grilled	3 oz	105	3	0	87	75
BEANS						
baked beans	½ cup	190	6	27	6	532
barbecue beans	3.5 oz	120	tr	26	0	460
refried beans	½ cup	43	2	5	2	104
three bean salad	¾ cup	230	11	31	0	500
BEEF						
corned beef cooked	3 oz	213	16	tr	83	964
porterhouse steak broiled	3 oz	260	19	0	70	52
prime rib roasted	3 oz	348	30	0	72	54
roast beef medium	2 oz	70	2	0	30	210
roast beef rare	2 oz	70	2	0	30	210
BEEF DISHES						
bubble & squeak	5 oz	186	13	16	—	—
corned beef hash	1 cup (8.3 oz)	440	30	23	100	840
cornish pasty	1 (8 oz)	847	52	79	—	—
irish stew	1 cup (7 oz)	280	16	10	—	—
kebab indian	1 (5.4 oz)	553	40	2	—	—
kheena	6.7 oz	781	71	1	—	—
koftas	5	280	22	3	—	—
roast beef sandwich plain	1	346	14	33	52	792
roast beef sandwich w/ cheese	1	402	18	27	77	1634

FOOD	PORTION	CALS	FAT	CARB	CHOL	SOD
roast beef submarine sandwich w/ tomato lettuce & mayonnaise	1	411	13	44	73	845
samosa	2 (4 oz)	652	62	20	—	—
shepherd's pie	6 oz	196	10	15	—	—
steak & kidney pie w/ top crust	1 slice (5 oz)	400	26	23	—	—
steak sandwich w/ tomato lettuce salt & mayonnaise	1	459	14	52	73	798
stew	6 oz	208	13	6	—	—
stew w/ vegetables	1 cup	220	11	15	71	292
stroganoff	¾ cup	260	19	43	69	503
swiss steak	4.6 oz	214	9	10	61	139
toad in the hole	1 (4.7 oz)	383	29	23	—	—

BEEFALO
roasted	3 oz	160	5	0	49	70

BEETS
pickled	½ cup	75	tr	19	0	301

BISCUIT
buttermilk	1	127	6	17	—	368
plain	1 (35 g)	276	34	13	5	584
w/ egg	1	315	20	24	232	655
w/ egg & bacon	1	457	31	29	353	999
w/ egg & sausage	1	582	39	41	302	1142
w/ egg & steak	1	474	28	37	272	888
w/ egg cheese & bacon	1	477	31	33	261	1261
w/ ham	1	387	18	44	25	1433
w/ sausage	1	485	32	40	34	1071
w/ steak	1	456	26	44	26	795

BISON
roasted	3 oz	122	2	0	70	48

BLINTZE
cheese	2	186	6	18	149	268

BREAD
chapatis as prep w/ fat	1 (2½ oz)	230	9	34	—	—
chapatis as prep w/o fat	1 (2½ oz)	141	1	31	—	—
cornbread	2 in x 2 in (1.4 oz)	107	2	18	28	276
cornstick	1 (1.3 oz)	101	4	13	30	195
focaccia onion	1 piece (4.6 oz)	282	10	43	0	536

FOOD	PORTION	CALS	FAT	CARB	CHOL	SOD
focaccia rosemary	1 piece (3.5 oz)	251	7	40	0	535
focaccia tomato olive	1 piece (4.7 oz)	270	8	42	0	683
french	1 loaf (1 lb)	1270	18	230	0	2633
irish soda bread	1 slice (2 oz)	174	3	34	11	239
italian	1 loaf (1 lb)	1255	4	256	0	2656
naan	1 (6 oz)	571	21	85	—	—
papadums fried	2 (1.5 oz)	81	4	9	—	—
paratha	1 (4.4 oz)	403	18	54	—	—
pita	1 reg (2 oz)	165	1	33	0	322
pita	1 sm (1 oz)	78	tr	16	0	152
stuffed bread broccoli & cheese	½ bread (6 oz)	450	17	54	25	830
white toasted	1 slice	67	1	13	0	136

CABBAGE

coleslaw w/ dressing	¾ cup	147	11	13	5	267
stuffed cabbage	1 (6 oz)	373	22	18	95	1007
sweet & sour red cabbage	4 oz	61	3	8	—	—
vinegar & oil coleslaw	3.5 oz	150	9	16	0	480

CAKE

angelfood	1/12 cake (1 oz)	73	tr	16	0	212
apple crisp	½ cup (5 oz)	230	5	46	0	257
baklava	1 oz	126	9	10	23	78
boston cream pie	1/6 cake (3.3 oz)	293	12	43	43	309
carrot w/ cream cheese icing	1/12 cake (3.9 oz)	484	29	52	60	273
cheesecake w/ cherry topping	1/12 cake (5 oz)	359	23	33	106	254
chocolate w/ chocolate frosting	1/8 cake (2.2 oz)	235	11	35	—	213
coffeecake cheese	1/6 cake (2.7 oz)	258	12	38	—	257
coffeecake crumb topped cheese	1/6 cake (2.7 oz)	258	12	38	—	257
coffeecake crumb topped cinnamon	1/9 cake (2.2 oz)	263	15	29	20	221
cream puff w/ custard filling	1 (4.6 oz)	336	20	30	174	444
eclair w/ chocolate icing & custard filling	1	205	10	—	35	—
fruitcake	1/36 cake (2.9 oz)	302	10	54	24	121
gingerbread	1/9 cake (2.6 oz)	264	12	36	24	242
panettone dal forno	1/9 cake (1.9 oz)	212	8	31	25	120

FOOD	PORTION	CALS	FAT	CARB	CHOL	SOD
pineapple upside down	1/8 cake (4 oz)	367	14	58	25	367
pound	1 slice (1 oz)	120	5	15	32	96
pound fat free	1 oz	80	tr	17	0	96
sheet cake w/ white frosting	1/9 cake	445	14	77	70	275
strudel apple	1 piece (2½ oz)	195	8	29	—	191
tiramisu	1 piece (5.1 oz)	409	30	31	171	79
trifle w/ cream	6 oz	291	16	34	—	—
yellow w/ vanilla frosting	1/8 cake (2.2 oz)	239	9	38	—	220

CALZONE

cheese	1 (12 oz)	1020	54	86	100	1760

CARIBOU

roasted	3 oz	142	4	0	93	51

CATFISH

breaded & fried	3 oz	194	11	7	69	238

CHEESE DISHES

cheese omelette as prep w/ 2 eggs	1 (6.8 oz)	519	44	tr	—	—
fondue	½ cup (3.8 oz)	247	15	4	49	142

CHICKEN

boneless breaded & fried w/ barbecue sauce	6 pieces (4.6 oz)	330	18	25	61	830
boneless breaded & fried w/ honey	6 pieces (4 oz)	339	18	27	61	537
boneless breaded & fried w/ mustard sauce	6 pieces (4.6 oz)	323	17	21	62	791
boneless breaded & fried w/ sweet & sour sauce	6 pieces (4.6 oz)	346	18	29	61	791
breast & wing breaded & fried	2 pieces (5.7 oz)	494	30	20	149	975
chicken breast seasoned lemon pepper	3 oz	90	1	2	55	520
croquettes w/ gravy	2 pieces + ½ cup gravy	282	18	26	—	1040
drumstick breaded & fried	2 pieces (5.2 oz)	430	27	16	165	756
roasted	1 breast (4 oz)	110	3	1	55	500
teriyaki	1 breast (4 oz)	130	3	6	50	650
thigh breaded & fried	2 pieces (5.2 oz)	430	27	16	165	756
w/ skin roasted	½ chicken (10.5 oz)	715	41	0	263	244
wings hot & spicy	4 pieces (5 oz)	230	16	5	85	280

FOOD	PORTION	CALS	FAT	CARB	CHOL	SOD
CHICKEN DISHES						
chicken & dumplings	¾ cup	256	12	12	109	1283
chicken & noodles	1 cup	365	18	26	103	600
chicken a la king	1 cup	470	34	12	221	760
chicken cacciatore	¾ cup	394	24	9	99	671
chicken paprikash	1½ cups	296	10	—	90	—
chicken pie w/ top crust	1 slice (5.6 oz)	472	31	32	—	—
chicken salad	1 oz	70	3	3	15	125
chicken salad light	1 oz	45	2	3	10	95
fillet sandwich plain	1	515	29	39	60	957
fillet sandwich w/ cheese lettuce mayonnaise & tomato	1	632	39	42	76	1238
CHILI						
con carne w/ beans	8.9 oz	254	8	22	133	1008
CLAMS						
breaded & fried	20 sm	379	21	19	115	684
COCOA						
hot cocoa	1 cup	218	9	26	33	123
COD						
baked	3 oz	95	1	0	43	82
roe baked w/ butter & lemon juice	3.5 oz	126	3	2	—	73
COFFEE						

(FAST FACT: Coffee bars provide a new snacking option. You'll find them in malls and tucked in the corner of your local bookstore. An espresso, cappuccino or cafe au lait is a pleasant pick-me-up. The Specialty Coffee Association predicts that in 1999, there will be more than 10,000 coffee bars.)

FOOD	PORTION	CALS	FAT	CARB	CHOL	SOD
cafe au lait	1 cup (8 fl oz)	77	4	6	17	62
cafe brulot	1 cup (4.8 fl oz)	48	0	3	0	2
cappuccino	1 cup (8 fl oz)	77	4	6	17	62
coffee con leche	1 cup (8 fl oz)	77	4	6	17	62
espresso	1 cup (3 fl oz)	2	0	tr	0	2
irish coffee	1 serv (9 fl oz)	107	3	3	12	25
mocha	1 mug (9.6 fl oz)	202	15	17	40	28
COOKIES						
biscotti with nuts chocolate dipped	1 (1.3 oz)	117	6	16	18	33

FOOD	PORTION	CALS	FAT	CARB	CHOL	SOD
CORN						
creamed corn	½ cup	110	1	25	0	370
fritters	1 (1 oz)	62	2	9	12	126
on-the-cob w/ butter cooked	1 ear	155	3	32	6	30
scalloped	½ cup	258	7	43	47	246
w/ butter	½ cup	90	2	19	5	170
CORNISH HEN						
w/ skin roasted	1 hen (8 oz)	595	42	0	299	146
CORNMEAL						
hush puppies	5 (2.7 oz)	256	12	35	135	965
COTTAGE CHEESE						
creamed	4 oz	117	5	3	17	457
creamed w/ fruit	4 oz	140	4	15	13	457
COUSCOUS						
pilaf	1 cup	200	tr	40	0	480
CRAB						
baked	1 (3.8 oz)	160	2	4	184	550
cake	1 (2 oz)	160	10	5	82	492
soft-shell fried	1 (4.4 oz)	334	18	31	45	1118
CROISSANT						
w/ egg & cheese	1	369	25	24	216	551
w/ egg cheese & bacon	1	413	28	24	215	889
w/ egg cheese & ham	1	475	34	24	213	1080
w/ egg cheese & sausage	1	524	38	25	216	1115
CUCUMBER						
cucumber salad	3.5 oz	50	tr	11	0	480
CUSTARD						
baked	½ cup (5 oz)	148	7	15	123	109
flan	½ cup (5.4 oz)	220	6	35	140	86
zabaione	½ cup (57.2 g)	135	5	13	213	9
DANISH PASTRY						
almond	1 (4¼ in) (2.3 oz)	280	16	30	30	236
apple	1 (4¼ in) (2.5 oz)	264	13	34	—	251
cheese	1 (4¼ in) (2.5 oz)	266	16	26	—	319
cheese	1 (3 oz)	353	25	29	20	320

FOOD	PORTION	CALS	FAT	CARB	CHOL	SOD
cinnamon	1 (4¼ in) (2.3 oz)	262	15	29	—	241
cinnamon	1 (3 oz)	349	17	47	28	326
cinnamon nut	1 (4¼ in) (2.3 oz)	280	16	30	30	236
fruit	1 (3.3 oz)	335	16	45	19	333
lemon	1 (4¼ in) (2.5 oz)	264	13	34	—	251
raisin	1 (4¼ in) (2.5 oz)	264	13	34	—	251
raisin nut	1 (4¼ in) (2.3 oz)	280	16	30	30	236
raspberry	1 (4¼ in) (2.5 oz)	264	13	34	—	251
strawberry	1 (4¼ in) (2.5 oz)	264	13	34	—	251

EEL
smoked	3.5 oz	330	28	0	—	—

EGG
hard cooked	1	77	5	1	213	62
poached	1	74	5	1	212	140
scrambled plain	2	200	15	2	400	211
scrambled w/ whole milk & margarine	1 cup	365	27	5	774	616

EGG DISHES
deviled	2 halves	145	13	1	280	180
salad	½ cup	307	28	2	562	565
sandwich w/ cheese	1	340	19	26	291	804
sandwich w/ cheese & ham	1	348	16	31	245	1005
scotch egg	1 (4.2 oz)	301	21	16	—	—
sunny side up	1	91	7	1	211	162

EGG ROLLS
lobster	1 (4.8 oz)	270	7	43	0	460
meat & shrimp	1 (4.8 oz)	320	12	41	10	470
pork & shrimp	1 (5 oz)	300	10	41	15	890
shrimp	1 (3 oz)	170	5	24	<5	420
spicy pork	1 (3 oz)	200	9	23	5	410
vegetable	1 (3 oz)	170	4	28	0	520

EGGPLANT
baba ghannouj	¼ cup	55	4	5	0	95

FOOD	PORTION	CALS	FAT	CARB	CHOL	SOD
caponata	2 tbsp (1 oz)	30	2	3	0	115
indian eggplant runi	1 serv	180	14	13	0	228
slices grilled	4 (7 oz)	38	0	0	0	—

ELK
roasted	3 oz	124	2	0	62	52

ENGLISH MUFFIN
plain toasted	1	133	1	26	0	262
toasted w/ butter	1	189	6	30	13	386
w/ cheese & sausage	1	394	24	29	58	1036
w/ egg cheese & bacon	1	487	31	31	274	1135
w/ egg cheese & canadian bacon	1	383	20	31	234	785

FALAFEL
falafel	1 (1.2 oz)	57	3	5	0	50

FISH
breaded fillet	1 (2 oz)	155	7	14	64	332
fish cake	1 (4.7 oz)	166	7	6	—	—
jamaican brown fish stew	1 serv	426	22	9	84	419
kedgeree	5.6 oz	242	11	15	—	—
sandwich w/ tartar sauce	1	431	55	41	—	615
sandwich w/ tartar sauce & cheese	1	524	29	48	68	939
stew	1 cup (7.9 oz)	157	4	10	—	—
taramasalata	3.5 oz	446	46	4	—	—

FLOUNDER
battered & fried	3.2 oz	211	11	15	31	484
breaded & fried	3.2 oz	211	11	15	31	484
broiled	1 fillet (4.5 oz)	148	2	0	86	133

FRENCH TOAST
w/ butter	2 slices	356	19	36	117	513

FROG'S LEGS
frog leg as prep w/ seasoned flour & fried	1 (0.8)	70	5	15	12	—

GEFILTE FISH
sweet	1 piece (1.5 oz)	35	1	3	12	220

GOAT
roasted	3 oz	122	3	0	64	73

FOOD	PORTION	CALS	FAT	CARB	CHOL	SOD
GOOSE						
w/ skin roasted	6.6 oz	574	41	0	172	132
GRAPE LEAVES						
grape leaves stuffed w/ rice	6 pieces (4.9 oz)	180	8	22	0	870
HALIBUT						
broiled	½ fillet (5.6 oz)	223	5	0	65	110
HAM						
patties grilled	1 patty (2 oz)	203	18	—	43	—
steak	4 oz	229	15	tr	61	1566
HAM DISHES						

(FAST FACT: Since the 1940s ham and cheese sandwiches have topped the list of favorite sandwiches.)

FOOD	PORTION	CALS	FAT	CARB	CHOL	SOD
croquettes	1 (3.1 oz)	217	14	11	77	475
salad	½ cup	287	23	5	237	671
sandwich w/ cheese	1	353	15	33	58	772
HAMBURGER						

(FAST FACT: More hamburgers are ordered in restaurants than any other food. Americans eat over 5 billion a year—that's about 20 for every man, woman and child.)

FOOD	PORTION	CALS	FAT	CARB	CHOL	SOD
double patty w/ bun	1 reg	544	28	43	99	554
double patty w/ cheese & bun	1 reg	457	28	22	110	635
double patty w/ cheese & double bun	1 reg	461	22	44	80	892
double patty w/ cheese ketchup mayonnaise onion pickle tomato & bun	1 reg	416	21	35	60	1051
double patty w/ ketchup mayonnaise onion pickle tomato & bun	1 reg	649	35	53	94	920
double patty w/ ketchup cheese mayonnaise mustard pickle tomato & bun	1 lg	706	44	40	141	1149
double patty w/ ketchup mustard mayonnaise onion pickle tomato & bun	1 lg	540	27	40	122	791
double patty w/ ketchup mustard onion pickle & bun	1 reg	576	32	39	102	742

FOOD	PORTION	CALS	FAT	CARB	CHOL	SOD
single patty w/ bacon ketchup cheese mustard onion pickle & bun	1 lg	609	37	37	112	1044
single patty w/ bun	1 lg	400	23	25	71	474
single patty w/ bun	1 reg	275	12	31	36	387
single patty w/ cheese & bun	1 lg	608	33	47	96	1589
single patty w/ cheese & bun	1 reg	320	15	32	50	500
single patty w/ ketchup cheese ham mayonnaise pickle tomato & bun	1 lg	745	48	38	122	1713
single patty w/ ketchup mustard mayonnaise onion pickle tomato & bun	1 reg	279	13	27	26	504
triple patty w/ cheese & bun	1 lg	769	51	27	161	1211
triple patty w/ ketchup mustard pickle & bun	1 lg	693	41	29	142	713

HERRING

FOOD	PORTION	CALS	FAT	CARB	CHOL	SOD
atlantic kippered	1 fillet (1.4 oz)	87	5	0	33	367
atlantic pickled	½ oz	39	3	1	2	131

HOT DOG

FOOD	PORTION	CALS	FAT	CARB	CHOL	SOD
corndog	1	460	19	56	79	972
w/ bun chili	1	297	13	31	51	480
w/ bun plain	1	242	15	18	44	671

HUMMUS

FOOD	PORTION	CALS	FAT	CARB	CHOL	SOD
hummus	⅓ cup	140	7	17	0	200

ICE CREAM AND FROZEN DESSERTS

FOOD	PORTION	CALS	FAT	CARB	CHOL	SOD
cone vanilla light soft serve	1 (4.6 oz)	164	6	24	28	92
gelato chocolate hazelnut	½ cup (5.3 oz)	370	29	26	92	49
gelato vanilla	½ cup (3 oz)	211	15	18	151	78
sundae caramel	1 (5.4 oz)	303	9	49	25	195
sundae hot fudge	1 (5.4 oz)	284	9	48	21	182
sundae strawberry	1 (5.4 oz)	269	8	45	21	92

KNISH

FOOD	PORTION	CALS	FAT	CARB	CHOL	SOD
cheese & blueberry	1 (7 oz)	378	13	40	40	—

FOOD	PORTION	CALS	FAT	CARB	CHOL	SOD
cheese & cherry	1 (7 oz)	378	13	40	40	—
everything	1 (7 oz)	221	8	34	0	—
kashe	1 (7 oz)	270	8	45	0	—
potato	1 lg (7 oz)	332	12	49	72	470
potato	1 med (3.5 oz)	166	6	25	36	235
potato w/ broccoli & cheese	1 (7 oz)	312	15	33	24	—
potato w/ spinach & mushroom	1 (7 oz)	214	8	32	0	—
LAMB						
rib chop broiled	3 oz	307	25	0	84	64
LAMB DISHES						
curry	¾ cup	345	17	22	89	258
moussaka	5.6 oz	312	21	16	—	—
stew	¾ cup	124	5	11	29	140
LENTILS						
indian sambar	1 serv	236	5	37	10	189
LOBSTER						
newburg	1 cup	485	27	13	455	127
steamed	1 (5.7 oz)	233	3	5	146	370
MONKFISH						
baked	3 oz	82	2	0	27	20
MOOSE						
roasted	3 oz	114	1	0	66	58
MOUSSE						
chocolate	½ cup (7.1 oz)	447	33	33	299	87
crab	¼ cup	364	20	—	136	—
MUSHROOMS						
breaded	7 (2.8 oz)	90	1	16	0	390
NOODLE DISHES						
noodle pudding	½ cup	132	7	11	27	222
ONION						
fried	½ cup (7.5 oz)	176	11	17	—	—
rings breaded & fried	8 to 9	275	16	31	14	430
ORIENTAL FOOD						
chicken teriyaki	¾ cup	399	27	7	92	2190
chicken teriyaki w/ rice	1 serv (11 oz)	430	6	77	25	1210
chop suey w/ beef & pork	1 cup	300	17	13	68	1053

FOOD	PORTION	CALS	FAT	CARB	CHOL	SOD
chop suey w/ pork	1 cup	375	29	29	62	1378
chow mein chicken	1 cup	255	10	10	75	718
chow mein pork	1 cup	425	24	21	89	1673
chow mein shrimp	1 cup	221	10	21	55	1658
chow mein vegetable	1 serv (8 oz)	90	3	15	0	1010
fried rice	6.6 oz	249	6	48	—	—
fried rice w/ egg	6.7 oz	395	20	49	—	—
spring roll deep fried	3.5 oz	202	9	24	—	—
sweet & sour pork	1 serv (8 oz)	250	8	37	30	1500
szechuan chicken w/ lo mein	1 cup (5.3 oz)	190	1	35	5	560
wonton fried	½ cup (1 oz)	111	8	8	31	147
wonton soup	1 cup	205	3	26	89	322

OYSTERS

battered & fried	6 (4.9 oz)	368	18	40	109	677
breaded & fried	6 (4.9 oz)	368	18	40	109	677
oysters rockefeller	3 oysters	66	2	5	38	80
steamed	1 med	41	1	2	—	53
stew	1 cup	278	18	15	100	928

PANCAKES

blueberry	1 (4 in diam)	84	4	11	21	157
buckwheat	1 (4 in diam)	55	2	6	20	125
potato	1 (4 in diam)	78	6	4	60	238
w/ butter & syrup	3	519	14	91	57	1103

PASTA DINNERS

lasagna	1 piece (2.5 in x 2.5 in)	374	21	25	107	668
macaroni & cheese	1 cup	230	10	26	24	730
manicotti	¾ cup (6.4 oz)	273	12	28	77	414
rigatoni w/ sausage sauce	¾ cup	260	12	28	59	106
spaghetti w/ meatballs & cheese	1 cup	407	19	38	104	696

PASTA SALAD

elbow macaroni salad	3.5 oz	160	5	26	0	590
italian style pasta salad	3.5 oz	140	7	15	0	480
mustard macaroni salad	3.5 oz	190	10	23	0	560
pasta salad w/ vegetables	3.5 oz	140	4	21	0	210

PEAS

pea & potato curry	1 serv (7 oz)	284	22	19	—	—
pea curry	1 serv (4.4 oz)	438	42	11	—	—

FOOD	PORTION	CALS	FAT	CARB	CHOL	SOD
PIE						
apple	⅛ of 9 in pie (5.4 oz)	411	19	58	0	327
banana cream	⅛ of 9 in pie (5.2 oz)	398	20	49	75	355
blueberry	⅛ of 9 in pie (5.2 oz)	360	18	49	0	272
cherry	⅛ of 9 in pie (6.3 oz)	486	22	69	0	343
coconut custard	⅙ of 8 in pie (3.6 oz)	271	14	32	36	348
custard	⅙ of 9 in pie	330	17	36	169	436
lemon meringue	⅛ of 9 in pie (4.5 oz)	362	16	50	68	307
mince	⅛ of 9 in pie (5.8 oz)	477	18	79	0	419
pecan	⅙ of 8 in pie (4 oz)	452	21	65	36	480
pumpkin	⅙ of 8 in pie (3.8 oz)	229	10	30	22	308
PIEROGI						
pierogi	¾ cup (4.4 oz)	307	19	24	49	369
PIG'S EARS AND FEET						
feet pickled	1 lb	923	73	tr	419	—
PIZZA						

(FAST FACT: Ten percent of all restaurants in the United States are pizzerias. America's favorite topping is pepperoni, followed by extra cheese.)

FOOD	PORTION	CALS	FAT	CARB	CHOL	SOD
cheese	⅛ of 12 in pie	140	3	21	9	336
cheese	12 in pie	1121	26	164	74	2680
cheese deep dish individual	1 (5.5 oz)	460	24	47	20	750
cheese meat & vegetables	⅛ of 12 in pie	184	5	21	21	382
cheese meat & vegetables	12 in pie	1472	43	170	165	3054
pepperoni	⅛ of 12 in pie	181	7	20	14	267
pepperoni	12 in pie	1445	56	157	115	2133
PLANTAINS						
ripe fried	2.8 oz	214	7	38	—	—
POLENTA						
polenta	½ cup (5 oz)	110	0	24	0	470

FOOD	PORTION	CALS	FAT	CARB	CHOL	SOD
POMPANO						
florida cooked	3 oz	179	10	0	54	65
POPOVER						
popover	1 (1.4 oz)	90	3	11	47	82
PORK						
center loin chop broiled	1 (3.1 oz)	275	24	0	84	61
center loin chop roasted	1 chop (3.1 oz)	268	19	—	80	—
spareribs	3 oz	338	26	0	103	79
PORK DISHES						
pork roast	2 oz	70	3	0	40	390
tourtiere	1 piece (4.9 oz)	451	34	21	—	—
POT PIE						
beef	⅓ of 9 in pie (7.4 oz)	515	30	39	42	596
chicken	⅓ of 9 in pie (8.1 oz)	545	31	42	56	594

POTATO

(FAST FACT: Most French fry lovers wouldn't think of eating them without ketchup. The average person eats two fourteen-ounce bottles of ketchup a year. The good news is that studies show that the pigment "lycopene" in tomato ketchup (and other tomato products) is good for you and protects against cancer and heart attacks.)

FOOD	PORTION	CALS	FAT	CARB	CHOL	SOD
au gratin w/ cheese	½ cup	178	10	17	18	548
baked topped w/ cheese sauce	1	475	29	47	19	381
baked topped w/ cheese sauce & bacon	1	451	26	44	30	973
baked topped w/ cheese sauce & broccoli	1	402	14	47	20	484
baked topped w/ cheese sauce & chili	1	481	22	56	31	701
baked topped w/ sour cream & chives	1	394	22	50	23	182
curry	1 serv (6 oz)	292	16	36	—	—
french fried in beef tallow	1 lg	358	19	44	20	187
french fried in beef tallow	1 reg	237	12	29	13	124
french fried in vegetable oil	1 lg	355	19	44	0	187

FOOD	PORTION	CALS	FAT	CARB	CHOL	SOD
french fried in vegetable oil	1 reg	235	12	29	0	124
hash brown	½ cup	163	11	17	—	19
indian yogurt potatoes	1 serv	315	9	52	18	216
mashed	½ cup	111	4	18	2	309
mustard potato salad	3.5 oz	120	6	16	0	393
o'brien	1 cup	157	3	30	7	421
potato dumpling	3½ oz	334	1	74	—	1
potato pancakes	1 (1.3 oz)	101	7	11	35	188
potato salad	½ cup	179	10	14	86	661
potato salad	⅓ cup	108	6	13	57	312
potato salad w/ vegetables	3.5 oz	120	3	20	0	390
scalloped	½ cup	127	5	18	7	435

PUDDING

FOOD	PORTION	CALS	FAT	CARB	CHOL	SOD
blancmange	1 serv (4.7 oz)	154	5	25	—	—
bread pudding	½ cup (4.4 oz)	212	7	31	83	291
bread w/ raisins	½ cup	180	5	31	77	185
chocolate	½ cup (5.5 oz)	206	4	41	9	157
queen of puddings	1 serv (4.4 oz)	266	10	41	—	—
rice pudding	1 serv (3 oz)	110	4	17	—	—
rice w/ raisins	½ cup	246	6	42	136	270
tapioca	½ cup (5.3 oz)	189	7	26	124	288
vanilla	½ cup (4.3 oz)	130	4	20	17	113

QUICHE

FOOD	PORTION	CALS	FAT	CARB	CHOL	SOD
cheese	1 slice (3 oz)	283	20	16	—	—
lorraine	1 slice (3 oz)	352	25	18	—	—
mushroom	1 slice (3 oz)	256	18	17	—	—

RABBIT

FOOD	PORTION	CALS	FAT	CARB	CHOL	SOD
roasted meat only	3 oz	167	7	0	70	40
wild rabbit stewed meat only	3 oz	147	3	0	104	38

RICE

FOOD	PORTION	CALS	FAT	CARB	CHOL	SOD
brown rice	½ cup	109	tr	23	0	5
pilaf	½ cup	84	3	11	22	362
risotto	6.6 oz	426	18	65	—	—
spanish	¾ cup	363	27	19	35	1339
sticky rice	½ cup	116	tr	25	0	6
white rice	½ cup	131	tr	28	0	2

ROUGHY

FOOD	PORTION	CALS	FAT	CARB	CHOL	SOD
orange roughy baked	3 oz	75	1	0	22	69

FOOD	PORTION	CALS	FAT	CARB	CHOL	SOD
SABLEFISH						
smoked	1 oz	72	6	0	18	206
SALAD						
caesar	2 cups (5 oz)	235	20	11	10	440
chef w/o dressing	1½ cups	386	28	9	244	279
tossed w/o dressing	1½ cups	32	tr	7	0	53
tossed w/o dressing	¾ cup	16	0	3	0	27
tossed w/o dressing w/ cheese & egg	1½ cups	102	6	5	98	119
tossed w/o dressing w/ chicken	1½ cups	105	2	4	72	209
tossed w/o dressing w/ pasta & seafood	1½ cups (14.6 oz)	380	21	32	50	1572
tossed w/o dressing w/ shrimp	1½ cups	107	2	7	180	487
waldorf	½ cup	79	6	6	8	49
SALMON						
baked	½ fillet (5.4 oz)	286	12	0	76	91
lox	2 oz	80	3	1	30	1150
salmon cake	1 (3 oz)	241	15	6	104	602
smoked	1 oz	33	1	0	7	220
SANDWICH						
submarine w/ salami ham cheese lettuce tomato onion & oil	1	456	19	51	35	1650
SAUSAGE						
pork	1 link (0.5 oz)	48	4	tr	11	168
pork	1 patty (1 oz)	100	8	tr	22	349
SAUSAGE DISHES						
sausage roll	1 (2.3 oz)	311	24	22	—	—
SCALLOP						
breaded & fried	6 (5 oz)	386	19	38	107	919
SCONE						
cheese	1 (1.75 oz)	182	9	22	—	—
fruit	1 (1.75 oz)	158	5	27	—	—
plain	1 (1.75 oz)	181	7	27	—	—
SHAD						
roe baked w/ butter & lemon	3.5 oz	126	3	2	—	73

FOOD	PORTION	CALS	FAT	CARB	CHOL	SOD
SHARK						
batter-dipped & fried	3 oz	194	12	5	50	103
SHRIMP						
breaded & fried	6 to 8 (6 oz)	454	25	40	201	1447
jambalaya	¾ cup	188	5	26	50	83
steamed	4 large	22	tr	0	43	49
SNAPPER						
grilled	1 fillet (6 oz)	217	3	0	80	96
SOLE						
battered & fried	3.2 oz	211	11	15	31	484
breaded & fried	3.2 oz	211	11	15	31	484
broiled	1 fillet (4.5 oz)	148	2	0	86	133
SOUFFLE						
cheese	3.5 oz	253	20	10	—	—
spinach	1 cup	218	18	3	184	763
SOUP						
beef stew soup	1 cup (8.8 oz)	221	5	20	60	461
black bean turtle soup	1 cup	241	1	45	0	6
brunswick stew soup	1 cup (8.5 oz)	232	6	17	71	438
corn & cheese chowder	¾ cup	215	12	21	66	386
gazpacho	1 cup	46	tr	5	0	63
greek	¾ cup	63	2	7	83	386
hot & sour	1 serv (14 oz)	173	8	8	87	475
oxtail	5 oz	64	3	7	—	—
pasta e fagioli	1 cup (8.8 oz)	194	5	30	3	790
ratatouille	1 cup (7.5 oz)	266	25	12	0	329
SOYBEANS						
sprouts stir fried	1 cup	125	7	9	0	14
SPAGHETTI SAUCE						
alfredo	½ cup (4.2 fl oz)	400	38	8	80	510
bolognese	5 oz	195	15	4	—	—
marinara	½ cup (4.4 fl oz)	80	4	8	0	470
olive oil w/ garlic & grated cheese	¼ cup (2.1 oz)	370	36	3	20	540
SPANISH FOOD						
burrito w/ apple	1 lg (5.4 oz)	484	20	73	7	443
burrito w/ apple	1 sm (2.6 oz)	231	10	35	3	211
burrito w/ beans	2 (7.6 oz)	448	14	71	5	986

FOOD	PORTION	CALS	FAT	CARB	CHOL	SOD
burrito w/ beans & cheese	2 (6.5 oz)	377	12	55	27	1166
burrito w/ beans & chili peppers	2 (7.2 oz)	413	15	58	33	1043
burrito w/ beans & meat	2 (8.1 oz)	508	18	66	48	1335
burrito w/ beans cheese & beef	2 (7.1 oz)	331	13	40	125	990
burrito w/ beans cheese & chili peppers	2 (11.8 oz)	663	23	85	158	2060
burrito w/ beef	2 (7.7 oz)	523	21	59	65	1492
burrito w/ beef & chili peppers	2 (7.1 oz)	426	17	49	54	1116
burrito w/ beef cheese & chili peppers	2 (10.7 oz)	634	25	64	170	2091
burrito w/ cherry	1 lg (5.4 oz)	484	20	73	7	443
burrito w/ cherry	1 sm (2.6 oz)	231	10	35	3	211
chimichanga w/ beef	1 (6.1 oz)	425	20	43	9	910
chimichanga w/ beef & cheese	1 (6.4 oz)	443	23	39	51	956
chimichanga w/ beef & red chili peppers	1 (6.7 oz)	424	19	46	9	1169
chimichanga w/ beef cheese & red chili peppers	1 (6.3 oz)	364	18	38	50	895
enchilada eggplant	1	142	5	—	7	—
enchilada w/ cheese	1 (5.7 oz)	320	19	29	44	784
enchilada w/ cheese & beef	1 (6.7 oz)	324	18	30	40	1320
enchirito w/ cheese beef & beans	1 (6.8 oz)	344	16	34	49	1251
frijoles w/ cheese	1 cup (5.9 oz)	226	8	29	36	882
nachos w/ cheese	6 to 8 (4 oz)	345	19	36	18	816
nachos w/ cheese & jalapeno peppers	6 to 8 (7.2 oz)	607	34	60	83	1736
nachos w/ cheese beans ground beef & peppers	6 to 8 (8.9 oz)	568	31	56	21	1800
nachos w/ cinnamon & sugar	6 to 8 (3.8 oz)	592	36	63	39	439
taco	1 sm (6 oz)	370	21	27	57	802
taco salad	1½ cups	279	15	24	44	763
taco salad w/ chili con carne	1½ cups	288	13	27	4	886
tostada w/ beans & cheese	1 (5.1 oz)	223	10	27	30	543

FOOD	PORTION	CALS	FAT	CARB	CHOL	SOD
tostada w/ beans beef & cheese	1 (7.9 oz)	334	17	30	75	870
tostada w/ beef & cheese	1 (5.7 oz)	315	16	23	41	896
tostada w/ guacamole	2 (9.2 oz)	360	23	32	39	789

SPINACH
indian saag	1 serv	28	2	2	0	44
spanakopita spinach pie	1 cup (6 oz)	196	3	35	30	590
steamed	½ cup	21	tr	3	0	63

SQUASH
acorn squash mashed	½ cup	41	tr	11	0	3
butternut baked	½ cup	41	tr	11	0	4
spaghetti cooked	½ cup	23	tr	5	0	14

SQUID
calamari fried	3 oz	149	6	7	221	260

STUFFING/DRESSING
bread	½ cup	251	15	25	tr	627

SUSHI
california roll	1 piece (0.8 oz)	28	1	4	1	37
kim chi	⅓ cup (5.8 oz)	18	tr	4	0	2143
sashimi	1 serv (6 oz)	198	7	4	63	718
tuna roll	1 piece (0.7 oz)	23	tr	3	3	33
vegetable roll	1 piece (1.2 oz)	27	1	5	0	47
vinegared ginger	⅓ cup (1.6 oz)	48	tr	12	0	6
wasabi	2 tsp (0.3 oz)	5	tr	1	0	124
yellowtail roll	1 piece (0.6 oz)	25	1	3	0	32

SWEET POTATO
baked	1 (3½ oz)	118	tr	28	0	12
candied	3½ oz	144	3	29	0	73

SWORDFISH
broiled	3 oz	132	4	0	43	98

TILEFISH
grilled	½ fillet (5.3 oz)	220	7	0	—	88

TOFU
fresh fried	1 piece (0.5 oz)	35	3	1	0	2

TOMATO
stewed	1 cup	80	3	13	0	460

TROUT
rainbow grilled	3 oz	129	4	0	62	29
seatrout baked	3 oz	113	4	0	90	63

FOOD	PORTION	CALS	FAT	CARB	CHOL	SOD
TUNA						
grilled	3 oz	118	1	0	49	40
TUNA DISHES						
tuna salad	1 cup	383	19	19	27	824
tuna salad submarine sandwich w/ lettuce & oil	1	584	28	55	47	1294
VEAL DISHES						
parmigiana	4.2 oz	279	18	6	136	545
VEGETABLES MIXED						
caponata	¼ cup	28	1	—	0	—
curry	1 serv (7.7 oz)	398	33	22	—	—
gyoza potstickers vegetable	8 (4.9 oz)	210	4	34	0	500
pakoras	1 (2 oz)	108	5	12	—	—
ratatouille	8.8 oz	190	16	10	—	—
samosa	2 (4 oz)	519	46	25	—	—
succotash	½ cup	111	1	23	0	16
VENISON						
roasted	3 oz	134	3	0	95	46
WAFFLES						
plain	1 (7 in diam)	218	11	25	52	383
WHITEFISH						
smoked	1 oz	39	tr	0	9	285
WILD RICE						
cooked	½ cup	83	tr	18	0	3
ZUCCHINI						
indian paalkora	1 serv	46	2	7	1	141
slices grilled	½ cup	14	tr	4	0	2

PART · THREE

SNACKS

NOTES

Discrepancies in values are due to rounding. All values for calories, fat, carbohydrate, cholesterol and sodium have been rounded to the nearest whole number.

All **fat** values of foods are given in grams (g).

All **carbohydrate** (CARB) values of foods are given in grams.

All **cholesterol** (CHOL) values of foods are given in milligrams (mg).

All **sodium** (SOD) values of foods are given in milligrams.

tr (trace) is the value used when a food contains less than one calorie, less than one gram of fat or carbohydrate, or less than one milligram of cholesterol or sodium.

A dash (—) indicates data was not available.

Fast Fact

More Americans are snacking, instead of eating "three squares" a day. According to a recent survey, only 24 percent of those polled ate three meals a day without snacks. This percentage is expected to drop to 21 percent by the year 2000.

FOOD	PORTION	CALS	FAT	CARB	CHOL	SOD
ALMONDS						
Planters						
Honey Roasted	1 oz	160	14	7	0	190
APPLE						
Dole						
Fresh	1	80	1	18	0	0
Sonoma						
Dried Pieces	10-12 pieces (1.4 oz)	110	0	29	0	0
Tastee						
Candy Apple	1 (3 oz)	160	5	26	0	20
Caramel Apple	1 (3 oz)	160	5	26	0	20
APPLE JUICE						
After The Fall						
Organic	1 bottle (10 oz)	110	0	28	0	25
Minute Maid						
Box	8.45 fl oz	120	0	29	0	30
Tree Top						
Cider	6 oz	90	0	22	0	10
APPLESAUCE						
Mott's						
Fruit Snacks Apple Spice	4 oz	70	0	18	0	0
Fruit Snacks Cinnamon	4 oz	90	0	23	0	0
Fruit Snacks Strawberry	4 oz	80	0	19	0	5
Fruit Snacks Sweetened	4 oz	90	0	22	0	0
APRICOT JUICE						
Libby						
Nectar	1 can (11.5 fl oz)	220	0	52	0	10
APRICOTS						
fresh	3	51	tr	12	0	1
Del Monte						
Sun Dried	⅓ cup (1.4 oz)	80	0	25	0	5
BANANA						
banana chips	1 oz	147	10	17	0	2
fresh	1	105	tr	27	0	1

FOOD	PORTION	CALS	FAT	CARB	CHOL	SOD
Rainforest Farms						
Dried Slices	5 slices (1.3 oz)	60	0	12	0	10

BANANA JUICE
Libby

FOOD	PORTION	CALS	FAT	CARB	CHOL	SOD
Nectar	1 can (11.5 fl oz)	190	0	47	0	35

BEER AND ALE

FOOD	PORTION	CALS	FAT	CARB	CHOL	SOD
ale brown	10 oz	77	0	8	—	—
ale pale	10 oz	88	0	12	—	—
beer light	12 oz can	100	0	5	0	10
beer regular	12 oz can	146	0	13	0	19
lager	10 oz	80	0	4	—	—
pilsener lager beer	7 fl oz	85	tr	13	—	4
stout	10 oz	102	0	6	—	—
Amstel						
Light	12 oz	95	0	—	0	—
Anheuser Busch						
Natural Light	12 oz	110	0	—	0	—
Bud						
Light	12 oz	108	0	—	0	—
Coors						
Beer	12 oz	132	0	30	0	10
Extra Gold	12 oz	147	0	32	0	10
Light	12 oz	101	0	13	0	10
Guiness						
Kaliber Nonalcoholic	12 oz	43	0	—	0	—
Hamm's						
Beer	12 oz	137	0	12	0	—
Nonalcoholic	12 oz	55	0	12	0	—
Killian's						
Beer	12 oz	212	0	29	0	10
Kingsbury						
Nonalcoholic	12 fl oz	60	0	—	0	—
Michelob						
Light	12 oz	134	0	—	0	—
Miller						
Lite	12 oz	96	0	—	0	—
Molson						
Light	12 oz	109	0	—	0	—
Old Milwaukee						
Beer	12 oz	145	0	13	0	25
Light	12 oz	122	0	9	0	18

FOOD	PORTION	CALS	FAT	CARB	CHOL	SOD
Olympia						
Beer	12 oz	143	0	12	0	—
Pabst						
Beer	12 oz	143	0	12	0	—
Nonalcoholic	12 oz	55	0	12	0	—
Piels						
Light	12 oz	136	0	—	0	—
Schaefer						
Beer	12 oz	138	0	13	0	23
Light	12 oz	111	0	8	0	16
Schlitz						
Beer	12 oz	145	0	13	0	23
Light	12 oz	99	0	3	0	9
Schmidts						
Light	12 oz	96	0	—	0	—
Signature						
Beer	12 oz	150	0	13	0	21
Spirit						
Nonalcoholic	12 oz	80	0	16	0	—
Strohs						
Beer	12 oz	142	0	13	0	23
Light	12 oz	115	0	7	0	11
Winterfest						
Beer	12 oz	167	0	38	0	11

BREADSTICKS

FOOD	PORTION	CALS	FAT	CARB	CHOL	SOD
plain	1	41	1	7	0	66
plain	1 sm	25	1	4	0	66

BREAKFAST BAR

FOOD	PORTION	CALS	FAT	CARB	CHOL	SOD
Carnation						
Chewy Chocolate Chip	1 (1.26 oz)	150	6	22	0	80
Chewy Peanut Butter Chocolate Chip	1 (1.26 oz)	140	5	21	0	90
Glenny's						
Sunrise Bee Pollen	1 (1.5 oz)	190	8	22	—	—
Sunrise Ginseng	1 (1.5 oz)	160	7	24	—	—
Sunrise Spirulina	1 (1.5 oz)	140	5	21	—	—
Nutri-Grain						
Apple Cinnamon	1 (1.3 oz)	140	3	27	0	60
Blueberry	1 (1.3 oz)	140	3	27	0	60
Peach	1 (1.3 oz)	140	3	27	0	60
Raspberry	1 (1.3 oz)	140	3	27	0	60
Strawberry	1 (1.3 oz)	140	3	27	0	60

FOOD	PORTION	CALS	FAT	CARB	CHOL	SOD

BREAKFAST DRINKS

Carnation

FOOD	PORTION	CALS	FAT	CARB	CHOL	SOD
Instant Breakfast Cafe Mocha	1 can (10 fl oz)	220	3	35	5	210
Instant Breakfast Cafe Mocha	1 pkg	130	1	28	<5	100
Instant Breakfast Cafe Mocha	1 pkg + skim milk (9 fl oz)	220	1	39	6	216
Instant Breakfast Classic Chocolate Malt	1 pkg	130	2	26	<5	130
Instant Breakfast Classic Chocolate Malt	1 pkg + skim milk (9 fl oz)	220	1	39	6	240
Instant Breakfast Creamy Milk Chocolate	1 can (10 fl oz)	220	3	37	5	230
Instant Breakfast Creamy Milk Chocolate	1 pkg	130	1	28	<5	100
Instant Breakfast Creamy Milk Chocolate	1 pkg + skim milk (9 fl oz)	220	1	39	8	240
Instant Breakfast Creamy Milk Chocolate	8 fl oz	220	3	36	10	220
Instant Breakfast French Vanilla	1 pkg	130	0	27	<5	110
Instant Breakfast French Vanilla	1 pkg + skim milk	220	1	39	6	240
Instant Breakfast No Sugar Added Classic Chocolate	1 pkg	70	2	11	<5	120
Instant Breakfast No Sugar Added Classic Chocolate	1 pkg + skim milk (9 fl oz)	160	2	24	6	240
Instant Breakfast No Sugar Added Creamy Milk Chocolate	1 pkg	70	1	12	<5	90
Instant Breakfast No Sugar Added Creamy Milk Chocolate	1 pkg + skim milk (9 fl oz)	160	1	24	6	216

FOOD	PORTION	CALS	FAT	CARB	CHOL	SOD
Carnation (CONT.)						
Instant Breakfast No Sugar Added French Vanilla	1 pkg	70	0	12	<5	90
Instant Breakfast No Sugar Added French Vanilla	1 pkg + skim milk (9 fl oz)	150	1	24	6	216
Instant Breakfast No Sugar Added Strawberry Creme	1 pkg	70	0	12	<5	90
Instant Breakfast No Sugar Added Strawberry Creme	1 pkg + skim milk (9 fl oz)	150	1	24	6	216
Instant Breakfast Strawberry Creme	1 pkg	130	0	28	<5	160
Instant Breakfast Strawberry Creme	1 pkg + skim milk	220	1	39	6	288
Pillsbury						
Instant Breakfast Chocolate Malt as prep w/ milk	1 serv	290	9	38	—	310
Instant Breakfast Chocolate as prep w/ milk	1 serv	290	9	38	—	310
Instant Breakfast Strawberry as prep w/ milk	1 serv	290	9	39	—	300
Instant Breakfast Vanilla as prep w/ whole milk	1 serv	300	9	41	—	330
BROWNIE						
plain	1 lg (2 oz)	227	9	36	10	175
Greenfield						
Brownie HomeStyle	1 (1.4 oz)	120	0	29	0	65
Hostess						
Brownie Bites	5 (2 oz)	260	14	32	50	125
Brownie Bites Walnut	5 (2 oz)	270	15	31	50	140
Lance						
Brownie	1 pkg (78 g)	320	12	52	5	210
Little Debbie						
Fudge	1 pkg (2.1 oz)	270	13	39	15	170
Fudge	1 pkg (2.5 oz)	310	15	44	15	190
Fudge	1 pkg (2.9 oz)	360	17	52	15	230

FOOD	PORTION	CALS	FAT	CARB	CHOL	SOD
Little Debbie (CONT.)						
Fudge	1 pkg (3.6 oz)	450	21	65	20	280
Sweet Rewards						
Double Fudge	1 (1.1 oz)	110	0	25	0	100
Fat Free Brownie	1 bar (1 oz)	90	0	21	0	90
Tastykake						
Brownie	1 (85 g)	340	14	53	20	220
CAKE						
angelfood	1 cake (11.9 oz)	876	3	197	0	2548
carrot w/cream cheese icing	1 cake (10 in diam)	6175	328	775	1183	4470
cheesecake	1 cake (9 in diam)	3350	213	317	2053	2464
cheesecake	1/6 cake (2.8 oz)	256	18	20	44	165
coffeecake fruit	1/8 cake (1.8 oz)	156	5	26	—	192
eccles cake	1 slice (2 oz)	285	16	36	—	—
eclair	1 (1.4 oz)	149	10	15	—	—
fruitcake dark	1 cake (7½ in x 2¼ in)	5185	228	738	640	2123
pound cake	1 loaf (8½ in x 3½ in)	1935	94	265	1100	1645
pound cake	1/10 cake (1 oz)	117	6	15	66	119
pound cake fat free	1 cake (12 oz)	961	4	208	0	1158
sheet cake w/ white frosting	1 cake (9 in sq)	4020	129	694	636	2488
sheet cake w/o frosting	1 cake (9 in sq)	2830	108	434	552	2331
sheet cake w/o frosting	1/9 cake	315	12	48	61	258
sponge	1/12 cake (1.3 oz)	110	1	23	39	93
tiramisu	1 cake (4.4 lbs)	5732	421	439	2395	1107
yellow cake w/ chocolate frosting	1/8 cake (2.2 oz)	242	11	36	35	216
Baby Watson						
Cheesecake	1 slice (3.8 oz)	390	30	23	142	330
Cheesecake Light	1/16 cake (3.9 oz)	280	16	24	33	270
Baker Maid						
Creole Royal Pineapple Apricot	1 slice (1.7 oz)	90	1	20	5	75
Creole Royal Pineapple Apricot	3 slices (5 oz)	270	3	61	20	230
Carousel						
New York Cheese Cake	1 cake (3 oz)	250	19	16	95	180

FOOD	PORTION	CALS	FAT	CARB	CHOL	SOD
Drake's						
Coffee Cake	1 (1.1 oz)	140	6	18	10	90
Coffee Cake Chocolate Crumb	1 (2.5 oz)	245	9	38	18	206
Coffee Cake Cinnamon Crumb	1/12 cake (1.3 oz)	150	6	22	10	110
Coffee Cake Small	1 (2 oz)	220	9	33	15	160
Devil Dog	1 (1.5 oz)	160	6	24	0	135
Funny Bones	1 (1.25 oz)	150	8	18	0	110
Light & Fruity Apple	1 (1.2 oz)	90	1	20	0	110
Light & Fruity Blueberry	1 (1.2 oz)	90	1	20	0	95
Light & Fruity Cinnamon Raisin	1 (1.2 oz)	90	1	19	0	105
Mini Coffee Cakes	4 (1.83 oz)	220	9	33	18	140
Pound Cake	1	110	5	16	25	70
Ring Ding	1 (1.5 oz)	180	10	23	0	115
Ring Ding Mint	1 (1.5 oz)	190	11	22	0	115
Sunny Doodle	1 (1 oz)	100	3	16	10	100
Yankee Doodle	1 (1 oz)	100	4	16	0	110
Yodel's	1 (1 oz)	150	9	16	5	65
Entenmann's						
Apple Puffs	1 (3 oz)	280	13	39	—	320
Apple Strudel Old Fashioned	1 serv (1.5 oz)	120	5	17	—	110
Cheese Topped Buns	1 (2.3 oz)	240	12	29	—	240
Cinnamon Buns	1 (2.1 oz)	230	10	31	—	200
Cinnamon Filbert Ring	1 serv (1.5 oz)	190	12	19	—	160
Coffee Cake Cheese	1 serv (1.6 oz)	150	7	20	—	140
Coffee Cake Cheese Filled Crumb	1 serv (1.4 oz)	130	6	18	—	140
Coffee Cake Crumb	1 serv (1.3 oz)	160	7	21	—	160
Danish Ring	1 serv (1.5 oz)	180	10	18	—	160
Danish Ring Pecan	1 serv (1.5 oz)	190	12	19	—	130
Danish Ring Walnut	1 serv (1.5 oz)	190	12	19	—	130
Danish Twist Lemon	1 serv (1.2 oz)	140	7	17	—	140
Danish Twist Raspberry	1 serv (1.2 oz)	140	7	18	—	120
Devil's Food Cake Fudge Iced	1 serv (1.2 oz)	130	5	19	—	120
French Crumb Cake All Butter	1 serv (1.6 oz)	180	8	26	—	220
Louisiana Crunch Cake	1 serv (1.7 oz)	180	8	27	—	180

FOOD	PORTION	CALS	FAT	CARB	CHOL	SOD
Entenmann's (CONT.)						
Pound Loaf All Butter	1 serv (1 oz)	110	5	15	—	150
Pound Loaf Sour Cream	1 serv (1 oz)	120	7	14	—	90
Thick Fudge Golden Cake	1 serv (1.2 oz)	130	6	20	—	120
Freihofer's						
Angel Food	⅕ cake (2 oz)	150	0	35	0	410
Cinnamon Swirl Buns	1 (2.8 oz)	290	9	47	30	250
Coffee Cake Cinnamon Pecan	⅛ cake (2 oz)	220	9	33	25	160
Crumb	⅛ cake (2 oz)	240	11	33	15	260
Homestyle Golden Loaf	⅛ cake (1.8 oz)	200	9	28	50	190
Pound	⅕ cake (2.8 oz)	330	17	41	65	330
Greenfield						
Blondie Apple Spice	1 (1.4 oz)	120	0	28	0	65
Blondie Chocolate Chip	1 (1.4 oz)	120	0	29	0	65
Hostess						
Angel Food Ring	⅙ cake (1.6 oz)	150	3	29	<5	220
Apple Twist	1 (2.5 oz)	220	4	42	15	270
Baseball Yellow Cakes	1 (1.6 oz)	160	3	32	<5	160
Choco Licious	1 (1.5 oz)	170	6	28	10	190
Choco-Diles	1 (1.8 oz)	210	10	31	20	160
Cinnaminis Original	5 (2.4 oz)	300	17	37	20	230
Cinnamon Roll	1 (2.3 oz)	220	6	39	25	260
Crumb Cake	1 (1.9 oz)	210	8	33	15	135
Crumb Cake Light	1 (1.8 oz)	150	1	35	0	190
Cup Cakes Chocolate	1 (1.6 oz)	170	5	28	<5	160
Cup Cakes Chocolate Light	1 (1.4 oz)	120	2	26	0	170
Cup Cakes Orange	1 (1.5 oz)	160	5	28	10	160
Ding Dongs	1 (1.3 oz)	160	9	21	5	110
Fruit Cake Holiday	⅙ cake (5.3 oz)	490	14	93	10	410
Fruit Loaf	1 (3.8 oz)	350	10	67	5	290
Ho Ho's	1 (1 oz)	130	6	17	10	75
Holiday Cakes	1 (1.6 oz)	160	3	32	<5	160
Honey Bun Glazed	1 (2.7 oz)	320	19	35	15	90
Honey Bun Iced	1 (3.4 oz)	390	20	49	15	220
Hopper Cakes	1 (1.6 oz)	160	3	32	<5	160
Lil Angels	1 (1 oz)	90	2	17	<5	130
Pecan Spinners	1 (1 oz)	110	5	15	0	65
Pound Cake	⅕ cake (3.2 oz)	350	16	48	55	360

FOOD	PORTION	CALS	FAT	CARB	CHOL	SOD
Hostess (cont.)						
Sno Balls	1 (1.6 oz)	160	5	29	0	180
Suzy Q's	1 (2 oz)	220	9	35	10	270
Suzy Q's Banana	1 (2 oz)	220	10	32	25	280
Swirls Caramel Pecan	1 (2 oz)	140	15	25	15	55
Tiger Tails	1 (1.5 oz)	160	6	26	15	150
Twinkies	1 (1.4 oz)	140	4	25	15	180
Twinkies Banana	2 (2.7 oz)	300	13	42	35	370
Twinkies Devil Food	2 (2.7 oz)	300	12	47	15	360
Twinkies Lights	1 (1.4 oz)	120	2	24	0	200
Twinkies Strawberry Fruit 'n Creme	1 (1.6 oz)	150	3	30	20	200
Kellogg's						
Pop-Tarts Apple Cinnamon	1 (1.8 oz)	210	5	38	0	170
Pop-Tarts Blueberry	1 (1.8 oz)	210	7	36	0	210
Pop-Tarts Brown Sugar Cinnamon	1 (1.8 oz)	220	9	32	0	210
Pop-Tarts Cherry	1 (1.8 oz)	200	5	37	0	220
Pop-Tarts Chocolate Graham	1 (1.8 oz)	210	6	36	0	220
Pop-Tarts Frosted Blueberry	1 (1.8 oz)	200	5	37	0	210
Pop-Tarts Frosted Brown Sugar Cinnamon	1 (1.8 oz)	210	7	34	0	180
Pop-Tarts Frosted Cherry	1 (1.8 oz)	200	5	37	0	220
Pop-Tarts Frosted Chocolate Vanilla Creme	1 (1.8 oz)	200	5	37	0	230
Pop-Tarts Frosted Chocolate Fudge	1 (1.8 oz)	200	5	37	0	220
Pop-Tarts Frosted Grape	1 (1.8 oz)	200	5	38	0	200
Pop-Tarts Frosted Raspberry	1 (1.8 oz)	210	6	37	0	210
Pop-Tarts Frosted S'mores	1 (1.8 oz)	200	5	37	0	200
Pop-Tarts Frosted Strawberry	1 (1.8 oz)	200	5	38	0	170
Pop-Tarts Minis Frosted Chocolate	1 pkg (1.5 oz)	170	4	30	0	200
Pop-Tarts Minis Frosted Grape	1 pkg (1.5 oz)	170	4	32	0	180

FOOD	PORTION	CALS	FAT	CARB	CHOL	SOD
Kellogg's (CONT.)						
Pop-Tarts Minis Frosted Strawberry	1 pkg (1.5 oz)	170	4	32	0	180
Pop-Tarts Strawberry	1 (1.8 oz)	200	5	37	0	180
Rice Krispies Treats	1 (0.8 oz)	90	2	18	0	75
Lance						
Apple Oatmeal	1 pkg (51 g)	200	9	35	10	210
Dunking Sticks	1 (39 g)	190	10	22	5	130
Fig Cake	1 pkg (60 g)	210	3	43	0	90
Honey Buns	1 (85 g)	330	14	48	0	210
Oatmeal Cake	1 (57 g)	240	11	35	0	250
Pecan Twirls	1 pkg (57 g)	220	8	34	0	190
Raisin Cake	1 (57 g)	230	10	35	0	200
Little Debbie						
Apple Delights	1 pkg (1.2 oz)	140	5	24	5	115
Apple-Roos	1 pkg (1.5 oz)	150	3	32	0	80
Banana Nut Muffin Loaves	1 pkg (1.9 oz)	210	9	30	10	210
Banana Twins	1 pkg (2.2 oz)	250	10	40	10	180
Be My Valentine	1 pkg (2.2 oz)	280	14	39	0	150
Cherry Cordials	1 pkg (1.3 oz)	160	8	23	0	100
Choc-o-Jel	1 pkg (1.2 oz)	150	7	21	0	95
Choco-Cakes	1 pkg (2.1 oz)	250	13	35	0	170
Choco-Cakes	1 pkg (2.2 oz)	240	12	35	0	180
Chocolate	1 pkg (3 oz)	360	17	52	0	220
Chocolate Chip	1 pkg (2.4 oz)	290	15	42	0	190
Chocolate Twins	1 pkg (2.4 oz)	240	9	42	20	280
Christmas Tree Cakes	1 pkg (1.5 oz)	190	9	27	0	90
Coconut	1 pkg (2.1 oz)	270	13	38	5	180
Coconut	1 pkg (2.4 oz)	300	14	42	5	200
Coconut Rounds	1 pkg (1.2 oz)	140	7	22	0	85
Coffee Cake Apple	1 pkg (1.9 oz)	220	7	36	10	190
Coffee Cake Apple Streusel	1 pkg (2 oz)	220	7	37	10	200
Devil Cremes	1 pkg (1.6 oz)	190	8	28	0	160
Devil Cremes	1 pkg (3.2 oz)	380	17	57	5	310
Devil Squares	1 pkg (2.2 oz)	260	13	39	0	180
Easter Basket Cakes	1 pkg (2.5 oz)	310	15	44	0	180
Fancy Cakes	1 pkg (2.4 oz)	300	15	42	0	160
Fudge Crispy	1 pkg (1.1 oz)	170	10	20	0	50
Fudge Round	1 pkg (2.5 oz)	290	12	49	5	170
Fudge Round	1 pkg (3 oz)	350	14	59	5	210
Fudge Rounds	1 pkg (1.2 oz)	140	5	23	5	80

FOOD	PORTION	CALS	FAT	CARB	CHOL	SOD
Little Debbie (CONT.)						
Golden Cremes	1 pkg (1.5 oz)	170	7	25	0	180
Golden Cremes	1 pkg (3 oz)	330	15	50	10	350
Holiday Cake Chocolate	1 pkg (2.4 oz)	290	14	43	0	180
Holiday Cake Vanilla	1 pkg (2.5 oz)	310	15	44	0	180
Honey Bun	1 pkg (3 oz)	380	23	39	0	190
Honey Bun	1 pkg (4 oz)	510	31	53	0	250
Jelly Rolls	1 pkg (2.1 oz)	230	7	41	15	160
Lemon Stix	1 pkg (1.5 oz)	210	10	30	0	45
Marshmallow Supremes	1 pkg (1.1 oz)	130	5	22	0	70
Mint Sprints	1 pkg (1.5 oz)	230	13	28	0	70
Nutty Bar	1 pkg (2 oz)	290	17	34	0	115
Pecan Twins	1 pkg (2 oz)	220	9	32	0	200
Pumpkin Delights	1 pkg (1.1 oz)	130	5	21	5	115
Smiley Faces Cherry	1 pkg (1.2 oz)	140	5	23	5	115
Smiley Faces Pumpkin	1 pkg (1 oz)	130	5	20	5	215
Snack Cake Chocolate	1 pkg (2.5 oz)	300	15	43	0	180
Snack Cake Vanilla	1 pkg (2.6 oz)	320	16	45	0	180
Spice	1 pkg (2.5 oz)	300	15	43	10	230
Star Crunch	1 pkg (1.1 oz)	140	6	21	0	85
Star Crunch	1 pkg (2.6 oz)	330	14	51	0	240
Swiss Rolls	1 pkg (2.1 oz)	250	12	38	15	160
Swiss Rolls	1 pkg (2.7 oz)	320	15	47	15	210
Swiss Rolls	1 pkg (3.2 oz)	380	18	57	20	250
Teddy Berries	1 pkg (1.2 oz)	130	4	23	5	105
Vanilla	1 pkg (3 oz)	370	18	53	0	210
Vanilla Cremes	1 pkg (1.4 oz)	170	7	25	0	125
Zebra Cakes	1 pkg (2.6 oz)	150	16	45	0	180
Nabisco						
Frosted Strawberry	1 (1.7 oz)	190	5	35	0	190
Pepperidge Farm						
Apple Turnover	1	300	17	34	—	210
Boston Cream Supreme	1 piece (2⅞ oz)	290	14	39	50	190
Toaster Tart Apple Cinnamon	1	170	7	25	0	120
Toaster Tart Cheese	1	190	10	22	14	180
Toaster Tart Strawberry	1	190	7	28	0	120
Perugina						
Pannettone Au Beurre	⅙ cake (2.9 oz)	310	12	47	110	140

FOOD	PORTION	CALS	FAT	CARB	CHOL	SOD
Pillsbury						
Apple Turnovers	1	170	8	23	0	330
Cherry Turnovers	1	170	8	23	0	320
Coffee Cake Cinnamon Swirl	⅛ of cake	180	9	22	0	170
Coffee Cake Pecan Struesel	⅛ of cake	180	9	21	0	170
Sara Lee						
Cheesecake Original Strawberry	1 slice (3.2 oz)	222	8	34	—	171
Cheesecake Original Plain	1 slice (2.8 oz)	230	11	27	—	153
Coffee Cake Cheese Reduced Fat	⅙ cake (2 oz)	180	6	28	20	230
Pound All Butter Family Size	1 slice (1 oz)	130	7	14	—	85
Pound All Butter Original	1 slice (1 oz)	130	7	14	—	85
Pound Free & Light	1 slice (1 oz)	70	0	17	0	105
Sinbad						
Baklava	1 piece (2 oz)	337	20	44	10	153
Tastykake						
Butter Cream Cream Filled Cupcake	1 (32 g)	120	4	20	5	120
Chocolate Cream Filled Cupcake	1 (34 g)	130	5	21	5	130
Chocolate Cupcake	1 (30 g)	100	3	19	5	120
Honeybun Glazed	1 pkg (92 g)	360	20	42	0	220
Honeybun Iced	1 pkg (92 g)	350	15	50	50	250
Junior Chocolate	1 pkg (94 g)	340	12	57	60	220
Junior Coconut	1 pkg (94 g)	300	6	60	50	300
Junior Lemon	1 pkg (94 g)	310	7	75	75	330
Junior Orange	1 pkg (94 g)	340	9	61	50	240
Kandy Kake Chocolate	1 (19 g)	80	3	13	0	35
Kandy Kake Coconut	1 (19 g)	80	4	11	0	40
Kandy Kake Peanut Butter	1 (19 g)	90	4	11	5	40
Koffee Kake Cream Filled	1 (29 g)	110	4	18	15	80
Koffee Kake Junior	1 pkg (71 g)	260	8	44	40	210
Kreme Kup	1 (25 g)	90	3	15	5	115
Krimpet Butterscotch	1 (28 g)	100	1	19	19	85
Krimpet Jelly	1 (28 g)	90	1	19	20	80
Krimpet Strawberry	1 (28 g)	100	2	20	20	85

FOOD	PORTION	CALS	FAT	CARB	CHOL	SOD
Tastykake (CONT.)						
Pastry Pocket Apple	1 (85 g)	320	18	38	10	220
Pastry Pocket Cheese	1 (85 g)	330	19	38	10	230
Pastry Pocket Cherry	1 (85 g)	330	17	41	10	230
Pecan Twirls	1 (28 g)	110	1	17	—	75
Royale Chocolate Cupcake	1 (46 g)	170	7	28	5	130
Tasty Too Chocolate Cream Filled Cupcake	1 (32 g)	100	1	21	0	115
Tasty Too Vanilla Cream Filled Cupcake	1 (32 g)	100	1	21	0	120
Tasty Twists	1 (4 g)	18	1	3	—	—
Thomas'						
Date Nut Loaf	1 oz	90	2	18	<5	170
Toast-R-Cakes						
Blueberry	1	110	3	18	—	158
Bran	1	103	3	18	—	163
Corn	1	120	4	19	—	142
Toastettes						
Frosted Blueberry	1 (1.7 oz)	190	5	45	0	190
Frosted Brown Sugar Cinnamon	1 (1.7 oz)	190	5	35	0	180
Frosted Cherry	1 (1.7 oz)	190	5	35	0	190
Frosted Fudge	1 (1.7 oz)	190	5	34	0	280
Strawberry	1 (1.7 oz)	190	5	35	0	200
Weight Watchers						
Brownie Cheesecake	1 cake (3.5 oz)	200	6	33	5	220
Caramel Fudge A La Mode	1 cake (6.07 oz)	180	3	34	0	170
Chocolate Eclair	1 (2.1 oz)	150	5	24	0	150
Coffee Cake Cinnamon Streusel	1 (2.25 oz)	190	2	35	0	190
Double Fudge	1 piece (2.75 oz)	190	4	36	0	200
Strawberry Cheesecake	1 (3.9 oz)	190	5	28	15	230
Strawberry Shortcake A La Mode	1 (6.49 oz)	180	2	39	5	160
Toasted Almond Amaretto Cheesecake	1 (3 oz)	170	5	24	5	160
Triple Chocolate Cheesecake	1 (3.15 oz)	200	5	32	10	200

FOOD	PORTION	CALS	FAT	CARB	CHOL	SOD
Well-Bred Loaf						
Banana Bread	1 slice (3.5 oz)	330	11	52	60	380
Banana Nut	1 slice (4.3 oz)	440	19	59	85	350
Blueberry	1 slice (4.3 oz)	440	16	69	110	330
Carrot	1 slice (4.3 oz)	480	24	64	125	125
Carrot Traditional	1 slice (4.3 oz)	440	16	71	40	280
Chocolate Chip	1 slice (4.3 oz)	490	19	74	105	320
Cinnamon Walnut	1 slice (4.3 oz)	480	18	72	110	340
Coconut Rum	1 slice (4.3 oz)	490	23	64	95	330
Cranberry	1 slice (4.3 oz)	460	15	77	100	320
Marble	1 slice (4.3 oz)	530	18	83	115	390
Pound All Butter	1 slice (4.3 oz)	470	17	73	115	360
Pound Mandarin Orange	1 slice (4 oz)	460	18	68	70	310
Raisin	1 slice (4.3 oz)	460	15	76	105	310

CANDY

FOOD	PORTION	CALS	FAT	CARB	CHOL	SOD
boiled sweets	¼ lb	327	0	87	—	—
butterscotch	1 oz	112	1	27	3	12
butterscotch	1 piece (6 g)	24	tr	6	1	3
candied cherries	1 (4 g)	12	tr	3	0	—
candied citron	1 oz	89	tr	23	0	82
candied lemon peel	1 oz	90	tr	23	0	14
candied orange peel	1 oz	90	tr	23	0	14
candied pineapple slice	1 slice (2 oz)	179	tr	45	0	—
candy corn	1 oz	105	0	27	0	57
caramels	1 piece (8 g)	31	1	6	1	20
caramels	1 pkg (2.5 oz)	271	6	55	5	174
caramels chocolate	1 bar (2.3 oz)	231	2	56	0	—
caramels chocolate	1 piece (6 g)	22	tr	6	0	—
carob bar	1 (3.1 oz)	453	28	42	—	—
crisped rice bar almond	1 bar (1 oz)	130	6	18	0	66
crisped rice bar chocolate chip	1 bar (1 oz)	115	4	21	0	79
dark chocolate	1 oz	150	10	16	0	5
divinity home recipe	1 (11 g)	38	0	10	0	5
divinity home recipe	1 recipe 48 pieces (19 oz)	1891	tr	486	0	247
fondant chocolate coated	1 lg (1.2 oz)	128	3	28	0	9
fondant chocolate coated	1 sm (0.4 oz)	40	1	9	0	3
fondant home recipe	1 piece (0.6 oz)	57	0	15	0	6
fondant home recipe	1 recipe 60 pieces (32.6 oz)	3327	tr	863	0	374

FOOD	PORTION	CALS	FAT	CARB	CHOL	SOD
fondant mint	1 oz	105	0	27	0	57
fruit pastilles	1 tube (1.4 oz)	101	0	25	—	—
fudge brown sugar w/ nuts home recipe	1 piece (0.5 oz)	56	1	11	1	14
fudge brown sugar w/ nuts home recipe	1 recipe 60 pieces (30.7 oz)	3453	88	676	49	852
fudge chocolate home recipe	1 piece (0.6 oz)	65	1	14	2	10
fudge chocolate home recipe	1 recipe 48 pieces (29 oz)	3161	70	660	120	511
fudge chocolate marshmallow home recipe	1 piece (0.7 oz)	84	3	14	5	21
fudge chocolate marshmallow home recipe	1 recipe (43.1 oz)	5182	207	880	304	1273
fudge chocolate marshmallow w/ nuts home recipe	1 piece (0.8 oz)	96	4	15	5	21
fudge chocolate marshmallow w/ nuts home recipe	1 recipe 60 pieces (43.1 oz)	5182	207	880	304	1273
fudge chocolate marshmallow w/ nuts home recipe	1 recipe 60 pieces (46.1 oz)	5742	258	903	291	1234
fudge chocolate w/ nuts home recipe	1 piece (0.7 oz)	81	3	14	3	11
fudge chocolate w/ nuts home recipe	1 recipe 48 pieces (32.7 oz)	3967	150	678	130	562
fudge peanut butter home recipe	1 piece (0.6 oz)	59	1	13	1	12
fudge peanut butter home recipe	1 recipe 36 pieces (20.4 oz)	2161	38	456	25	424
fudge vanilla home recipe	1 piece (0.6 oz)	59	1	13	3	11
fudge vanilla home recipe	1 recipe 48 pieces (27.5 oz)	2893	42	644	125	525
fudge vanilla w/ nuts home recipe	1 piece (0.5 oz)	62	2	11	2	9

FOOD	PORTION	CALS	FAT	CARB	CHOL	SOD
fudge vanilla w/ nuts home recipe	1 recipe 60 pieces (31 oz)	3666	117	665	125	538
gumdrops	10 lg (3.8 oz)	420	0	108	0	48
gumdrops	10 sm (0.4 oz)	135	0	35	0	15
hard candy	1 oz	106	0	28	0	11
jelly beans	10 lg (1 oz)	104	tr	26	0	7
jelly beans	10 sm (0.4 oz)	40	tr	10	0	3
lollipop	1 (6 g)	22	0	6	0	2
marzipan	3½ oz	497	25	57	—	5
milk chocolate	1 bar (1.55 oz)	226	14	26	10	36
milk chocolate crisp	1 bar (1.45 oz)	203	11	28	8	59
milk chocolate w/ almonds	1 bar (1.45 oz)	215	14	22	8	30
nougat nut cream	3½ oz	342	31	58	—	—
peanut bar	1 (1.4 oz)	209	14	19	—	91
peanut brittle home recipe	1 oz	128	5	20	4	128
peanut brittle home recipe	1 recipe (17.6 oz)	2288	95	347	66	2269
peanuts chocolate covered	1 cup (5.2 oz)	773	50	74	13	61
peanuts chocolate covered	10 (1.4 oz)	208	13	20	4	16
praline home recipe	1 piece (1.4 oz)	177	10	24	0	24
praline home recipe	1 recipe 23 pieces (31.8 oz)	4116	220	562	0	559
pretzels chocolate covered	1 (0.4 oz)	50	2	8	—	10
pretzels chocolate covered	1 oz	130	5	20	—	—
sesame crunch	1 oz	146	9	14	0	—
sesame crunch	20 pieces (1.2 oz)	181	12	18	0	—
sweet chocolate	1 bar (1.45 oz)	201	14	25	0	7
sweet chocolate	1 oz	143	10	17	0	5
taffy home recipe	1 piece (0.5 oz)	56	1	14	1	13
taffy home recipe	1 recipe 48 pieces (25 oz)	2677	24	651	63	636
toffee home recipe	1 piece (0.4 oz)	65	4	8	13	22
toffee home recipe	1 recipe 48 pieces (19.4 oz)	2997	182	356	580	1036

FOOD	PORTION	CALS	FAT	CARB	CHOL	SOD
truffles home recipe	1 piece (0.4 oz)	59	4	5	6	8
truffles home recipe	1 recipe 49 pieces (21.5 oz)	2985	210	275	318	433
100 Grand						
Bar	1 bar (1.5 oz)	200	8	30	10	75
3 Musketeers						
Bar	1 (2.1 oz)	260	8	46	5	110
Bar	2 fun size (1.2 oz)	140	4	25	5	60
5th Avenue						
Bar	1 (2.1 oz)	290	13	39	5	140
After Eight						
Dark Chocolate Wafer Thin Mints	1	35	1	6	—	0
Almond Joy						
Bar	1 (1.76 oz)	250	14	28	0	70
Baby Ruth						
Bar	1 (2.1 oz)	280	12	38	—	135
Fun Size	2 pieces	200	9	27	—	95
Bar None						
Candy	1 (1.5 oz)	240	14	23	10	50
Bit-O-Honey						
Candy	1.7 oz	200	4	39	—	125
Bits O Brickle						
Candy	1 tbsp (0.5 oz)	80	5	9	5	85
Bonus						
Bar	1 bar (2.1 oz)	290	16	34	0	140
Breath Savers						
Sugar Free Mint Cinnamon	1 piece (2 g)	10	0	2	—	0
Sugar Free Peppermint	1 piece (2 g)	10	0	2	—	0
Sugar Free Spearmint	1 piece (2 g)	10	0	2	—	0
Sugar Free Wintergreen	1 piece (2 g)	10	0	2	—	0
Brock						
Butterscotch Discs	3 pieces (0.6 oz)	70	0	17	0	80
Candy Corn	21 pieces (1.4 oz)	150	0	37	0	85
Candy Rolls	2 rolls (0.5 oz)	50	0	12	0	0
Caramel Dots	3 pieces (1.3 oz)	140	3	25	—	50

FOOD	PORTION	CALS	FAT	CARB	CHOL	SOD
Brock (CONT.)						
Cinnamon Discs	3 pieces (0.6 oz)	70	0	17	0	5
Circus Peanuts	11 pieces (2.5 oz)	260	0	65	0	25
Coconut Mountains	4 pieces (1.4 oz)	170	6	29	—	80
Fruit Basket	3 pieces (0.6 oz)	60	0	15	0	0
Fruit Kisses	3 pieces (0.6 oz)	70	0	17	0	5
Glitters	2 pieces (0.5 oz)	50	0	13	0	15
Gummy Bears	5 pieces (1.4 oz)	130	0	30	0	15
Gummy Squirms	5 pieces (1.3 oz)	120	0	28	0	15
Jelly Beans	12 pieces (1.4 oz)	140	0	36	0	15
Lemon Drops	3 pieces (0.5 oz)	60	0	14	0	5
Orange Slices	4 pieces (1.5 oz)	140	0	36	0	20
Party Mints	9 pieces (0.5 oz)	60	0	15	0	0
Peanut Butter Crunch	3 pieces (0.6 oz)	80	2	15	—	45
Pops Assorted	2 (0.5 oz)	60	0	15	0	5
Sour Balls	3 pieces (0.6 oz)	70	0	17	0	5
Sour Sharks	23 pieces (2.5 oz)	30	3	60	—	45
Spearmint Starlights	3 pieces (0.6 oz)	60	0	16	0	5
Spice Drops	12 pieces (1.4 oz)	130	0	33	0	20
Starlight Mints	3 pieces (0.6 oz)	60	0	16	0	5
Toffee	6 pieces (1.5 oz)	170	5	31	—	45
Butterfinger						
BB's	1 pkg (1.7 oz)	230	10	34	0	90
Bar	1 (2.1 oz)	280	11	41	0	120
Fun Size	2 bars (1.6 oz)	200	8	30	—	85

FOOD	PORTION	CALS	FAT	CARB	CHOL	SOD
Caramello						
Candy	1 (1.6 oz)	220	11	28	10	60
Cellas						
Dark Chocolate Covered Cherries	2 pieces (1 oz)	100	4	—	—	—
Milk Chocolate Covered Cherries	2 pieces (1 oz)	110	4	18	0	15
Certs						
Breath Mints	1 piece (1.67 g)	6	0	2	0	—
Mini Sugar Free	1 piece (0.365 g)	1	0	tr	0	—
Sugar Free	1 piece (1.67 g)	7	0	2	0	—
Charleston Chew						
Candy	1 pkg (1.9 oz)	230	7	—	—	—
Chocolate	½ bar	120	3	—	—	—
Strawberry	½ bar	120	3	—	—	—
Vanilla	½ bar	120	3	—	—	—
Charms						
Blow Pop	1 (0.7 oz)	80	0	—	0	—
Pop	1 (0.6 oz)	70	0	—	0	—
Chuckles						
Candy	4 pieces (1.4 oz)	140	0	34	0	15
Chunky						
Bar	1 (1.4 oz)	200	11	22	<5	20
Clorets						
Mints	1 piece (1.67 g)	6	0	2	0	—
Crunch						
Fun Size	4 bars (1.5 oz)	200	10	25	5	55
Dove						
Dark Chocolate	1 bar (1.3 oz)	200	12	22	5	0
Dark Chocolate	¼ bar (1.5 oz)	230	14	26	5	0
Dark Chocolate Miniatures	7 (1.5 oz)	220	14	26	5	0
Milk Chocolate	1 bar (1.3 oz)	200	12	22	5	25
Milk Chocolate	¼ bar (1.5 oz)	230	13	25	10	30
Milk Chocolate Miniatures	7 (1.5 oz)	230	13	25	10	30
Truffles	3 (1.2 oz)	200	13	19	5	15
Dream						
Caramel & Nougat In Milk Chocolate	1 bar (1 oz)	90	3	21	<5	70
Estee						
Caramels Chocolate & Vanilla No Sugar Added	5 (1.3 oz)	150	5	26	0	65

FOOD	PORTION	CALS	FAT	CARB	CHOL	SOD
Estee (CONT.)						
Dark Chocolate	½ bar (1.4 oz)	200	14	23	10	10
Gum Drops Assorted Fruit Sugar Free	23 (1.4 oz)	140	0	36	0	0
Gum Drops Licorice	23 (1.4 oz)	140	0	36	0	0
Gummy Bears Sugar Free	16 (1.4 oz)	140	0	31	0	0
Hard Candies Assorted Fruit Sugar Free	5 (0.5 oz)	60	0	16	0	0
Hard Candies Assorted Mint Sugar Free	5 (0.5 oz)	60	0	16	0	0
Hard Candies Butterscotch Sugar Free	2 (0.4 oz)	50	0	12	0	50
Hard Candies Peppermint Swirls Sugar Free	3 (0.5 oz)	60	0	14	0	0
Hard Candies Tropical Fruit Sugar Free	5 (0.5 oz)	60	0	16	0	0
Lollipops Assorted Fruit Sugar Free	2 (0.5 oz)	60	0	16	0	0
Milk Chocolate	½ bar (1.4 oz)	230	17	17	20	65
Milk Chocolate With Almonds	½ bar (1.4 oz)	230	17	16	20	65
Milk Chocolate With Crisp Rice	1 bar (2.3 oz)	370	26	29	30	110
Milk Chocolate With Fruit & Nuts	½ bar (1.4 oz)	220	16	18	20	65
Mint Chocolate	½ bar (1.4 oz)	200	14	23	10	10
Peanut Brittle No Sugar Added	⅓ box (1.5 oz)	210	9	28	10	115
Peanut Butter Cups	1 (0.3 oz)	40	3	3	0	0
Peanut Butter Cups	5 (1.3 oz)	200	12	19	5	70
Toffee Sugar Free	5 (0.5 oz)	60	0	16	0	0
Ferrero Rocher						
Candy	2 pieces (0.9 oz)	150	10	11	0	24
Franklin						
Crunch 'N Munch Candied	1.25 oz	170	7	28	0	200
Crunch 'N Munch Caramel	1.25 oz	160	5	28	13	130

FOOD	PORTION	CALS	FAT	CARB	CHOL	SOD
Franklin (CONT.)						
Crunch 'N Munch Maple Walnut	1.25 oz	160	6	28	6	180
Crunch 'N Munch Toffee	1.25 oz	160	5	28	6	210
Glenny's						
Brown Rice Treats Carob & Mint With Oat Bran	1 bar (1.75 oz)	180	2	37	—	20
Brown Rice Treats Cinnamon & Raisin	1 bar (1.75 oz)	170	1	38	—	30
Brown Rice Treats Peanut & Raisin	1 bar (2 oz)	210	5	39	—	29
Brown Rice Treats Plain & Fancy	1 bar (1.25 oz)	120	1	28	—	29
Brown Rice Treats Raisin Bran	1 bar (1.75 oz)	170	1	38	—	17
Brown Rice Treats Toasted Almond With Oat Bran	1 bar (1.75 oz)	200	5	34	—	20
Fruit Drops Black Cherry	1	6	tr	1	—	tr
Fruit Drops Gentle Mint	1	6	tr	1	—	tr
Fruit Drops Mandarin Orange	1	6	tr	1	—	tr
Fruit Drops Mixed Fruit	1	6	tr	1	—	tr
Fruit Drops Twist Of Lemon	1	6	tr	1	—	tr
Hard Candies Fruit	1	19	tr	4	—	tr
Hard Candies Peppermint	1	19	tr	4	—	tr
Lollipops C Pops	1	35	tr	8	—	tr
Lollipops Fruit	1	21	tr	5	—	tr
Moist & Chewy Coconut Almondine Bar	1 bar (1.5 oz)	190	10	22	—	20
Moist & Chewy Oatmeal Raisin Bar	1 bar (1.5 oz)	160	3	30	—	25
Moist & Chewy Peanut Bar	1 bar (1.5 oz)	180	7	24	—	20
Moist & Chewy Sunflower Bar	1 bar (1.5 oz)	180	7	24	—	15

FOOD	PORTION	CALS	FAT	CARB	CHOL	SOD
Glenny's (CONT.)						
Snack Bar Fat-Free Apple-Cinnamon	1 (125 oz)	120	1	28	—	15
Snack Bar Fat-Free Caramel	1 (1.25 oz)	120	tr	29	—	70
Snack Bar Fat-Free Chocolate	1 (1.25 oz)	120	tr	28	—	10
Snack Bar Fat-Free Raspberry	1 (1.25 oz)	120	tr	29	—	15
Godiva						
Almond Butter Dome	3 pieces (1.5 oz)	240	17	19	5	20
Bouchee Au Chocolat	1 piece (1.5 oz)	210	11	25	5	40
Bouchee Ivory Raspberry	1 piece (1 oz)	160	9	17	5	25
Gold Ballotin	3 pieces (1.5 oz)	210	10	27	5	15
Truffle Amaretto Di Saronno	2 pieces (1.5 oz)	210	12	24	5	25
Truffle Deluxe Liqueur	2 pieces (1.5 oz)	210	13	23	5	25
Golden Almond						
Bar	½ bar	260	17	20	5	35
Golden III						
Bar	½ bar	250	15	26	10	40
Goldenberg's						
Peanut Chews	3 pieces (1.3 oz)	180	9	22	0	40
Goo Goo Supreme						
With Pecans	1 pkg (1.5 oz)	188	5	34	0	51
Goobers						
Peanuts	1 pkg (1.38 oz)	210	13	19	<5	20
Good & Fruity						
Candy	1 box (1.8 oz)	140	1	35	—	75
Good & Plenty						
Snacksize	3 boxes (1.5 oz)	140	0	34	0	80
Heath						
Bar	1 (1.4 oz)	210	13	25	20	180
Hershey						
Amazin'Fruit Gummy Candy	2 snack pkg (1.4 oz)	130	0	30	0	45
Bar	1 (1.55 oz)	240	14	25	10	40
Bar With Almonds	1 (1.45 oz)	230	14	20	15	55

FOOD	PORTION	CALS	FAT	CARB	CHOL	SOD
Hershey (CONT.)						
Kisses	9 pieces (1.46 oz)	220	13	23	10	35
Special Dark Sweet Chocolate Bar	1 (1.45)	220	12	25	0	5
Jolly Rancher						
Candies	3 pieces (0.6 oz)	60	0	14	0	5
Joyva						
Halvah	1.5 oz	240	16	16	0	80
Halvah Chocolate Covered	1 bar (2 oz)	380	23	20	0	95
Jells Raspberry	3 pieces (1.6 oz)	200	3	25	0	15
Joys Raspberry	1 (1.6 oz)	200	3	25	0	15
Marshmallow Twists Chocolate Covered	2 (1.5 oz)	190	4	21	0	20
Rings Orange & Raspberry	3 pieces (1.5 oz)	190	3	23	0	15
Sesame Crunch	3 pieces (0.5)	80	4	7	0	25
Sticks Orange	3 pieces (1.6 oz)	200	3	25	0	15
Twists Vanilla & Cherry	2 pieces (1.5 oz)	190	4	21	0	20
Juicefuls						
Candy	3 pieces (0.5 oz)	60	0	15	0	0
Junior Mints						
Candies	1 pkg (1.6 oz)	190	4	—	—	—
Just Born						
Jelly Beans	1 oz	108	tr	—	—	—
Sugar Coated	1½ oz	148	tr	—	—	—
Toasted Coconut	1⅜ oz	140	2	—	—	—
Kit Kat						
Bar	1 (1.625 oz)	250	13	29	10	60
Krackel						
Bar	1 (1.55 oz)	230	13	27	10	80
Laffy Taffy						
Apple Chews	1 oz	110	1	26	—	55
Banana Chews	1 oz	110	1	26	—	55
Grape Chews	1 oz	110	1	26	—	60
Passion Punch Chews	1 oz	110	1	26	—	50
Strawberry Chews	1 oz	110	1	26	—	55
Sweet & Sour Cherry Chews	1 oz	110	1	26	—	55

FOOD	PORTION	CALS	FAT	CARB	CHOL	SOD
Laffy Taffy (CONT.)						
Watermelon Chews	1 oz	110	1	26	—	55
Lance						
Chocolaty Peanut Bar	1 (57 g)	320	18	29	0	40
Peanut Bar	1 pkg (50 g)	260	14	24	0	80
Popscotch	1 pkg (35 g)	160	6	24	0	120
Lifesavers						
Big Tablet Candy Cane	4 pieces (0.5 oz)	60	0	16	0	0
Cards 'N Candy	4 pieces (0.4 oz)	40	0	10	0	0
Christmas Tin	4 pieces (0.5 oz)	60	0	16	0	20
Egg-Sortment	1 roll (0.4 oz)	40	0	10	0	0
Fruit Juicers Lollipops	1	40	0	10	0	0
Gummi Bunnies	3 pkg (1.6 oz)	140	0	34	0	0
Gummi Savers Five Flavor	1 pkg (1.8 oz)	160	0	38	0	0
Gummi Savers Five Flavor	1 roll (1.5 oz)	130	0	32	0	0
Gummi Savers Mixed Berry	1 pkg (1.8 oz)	160	0	38	0	0
Gummi Savers Mixed Berry	1 roll (1.5 oz)	130	0	32	0	0
Gummi Savers Tangy Fruits	1 pkg (1.8 oz)	160	0	38	0	0
Gummi Savers Tangy Fruits	1 roll (1.5 oz)	130	0	32	0	0
Gummi Savers Variety	2 pkg (1.3 oz)	120	0	27	0	0
Gummi Savers Wacky Frootz	1 pkg (1.8 oz)	160	0	38	0	0
Gummi Savers Wacky Frootz	1 roll (1.5 oz)	130	0	32	0	0
Holes Five Flavor	20 pieces (5 g)	20	0	5	0	0
Holes Island Fruit	20 pieces (5 g)	20	0	5	0	0
Holes Sour 'N Sweet	16 pieces (5 g)	20	0	5	0	0
Holes Sunshine Fruits	20 pieces (0.2 oz)	20	0	5	0	0
Holes Super Tart	20 pieces (5 g)	20	0	5	0	0
Holes Tangerine	1 candy	2	0	1	0	0
Holes Wild Fruits	20 pieces (5 g)	20	0	5	<5	0
Lollipops Candy Cane	1 (0.4 oz)	40	0	10	0	0
Lollipops Christmas	1 (0.4 oz)	40	0	10	0	0
Lollipops Easter	1 (0.4 oz)	40	0	10	0	0

FOOD	PORTION	CALS	FAT	CARB	CHOL	SOD
Lifesavers (CONT.)						
Lollipops Fruit Flavors	1 (0.4 oz)	45	0	11	0	0
Lollipops Swirled Flavors	1 (0.4 oz)	40	0	10	0	0
Lollipops Valentine	1 (0.4 oz)	40	0	10	0	0
Roll Butter Rum	2 pieces (5 g)	20	0	5	0	20
Roll Candy Cane	4 pieces (0.4 oz)	40	0	10	0	0
Roll Cryst-O-Mint	2 pieces (5 g)	20	0	5	0	0
Roll Five Flavor	2 pieces (5 g)	20	0	5	0	0
Roll Fruits On Fire	2 pieces (5 g)	20	0	5	0	0
Roll Pep-O-Mint	3 pieces (5 g)	20	0	5	0	0
Roll Spear-O-Mint	3 pieces (5 g)	20	0	5	0	0
Roll Sunshine Fruits	2 pieces (5 g)	20	0	5	0	0
Roll Tangy Fruit Swirl	2 pieces (5 g)	20	0	5	0	0
Roll Tangy Fruit Watermelon	1 pieces (5 g)	20	0	5	0	0
Roll Tangy Fruits	2 pieces (5 g)	20	0	5	0	0
Roll Tropical Fruits	2 pieces (5 g)	20	0	5	0	0
Roll Wild Cherry	1 piece (5 g)	20	0	5	0	0
Roll Wild Flavors	2 pieces (5 g)	20	0	5	0	0
Roll Wild Sour Berries	2 pieces (5 g)	20	0	5	0	0
Roll Wint-O-Green	3 pieces (5 g)	20	0	5	0	0
Sack'it Butter Rum	4 pieces (0.5 oz)	60	0	15	0	65
Sack'it Five Flavor	4 pieces (0.5 oz)	60	0	16	0	0
Sack'it Holiday Tin	4 pieces (0.5 oz)	60	0	16	0	65
Sack'it Pep-O-Mint	4 pieces (0.5 oz)	60	0	16	0	0
Sack'it Tangy Fruits	4 pieces (0.5 oz)	60	0	16	0	0
Sack'it Wild Cherry	4 pieces (0.5 oz)	60	0	16	0	0
Sack'it Wint-O-Green	4 pieces (0.5 oz)	60	0	16	0	0
Sugar Free Iced Mint	1 piece (2 g)	10	0	2	0	0
Sugar Free Vanilla Mint	1 piece (2 g)	10	0	2	0	0
Valentine Book	2 pieces (5 g)	20	0	5	0	20
M&M's						
Almond	1 pkg (1.3 oz)	200	11	21	5	20
Almond	1.5 oz	220	12	24	5	20

FOOD	PORTION	CALS	FAT	CARB	CHOL	SOD
M&M's (CONT.)						
Mint	1 pkg (1.7 oz)	230	10	34	10	35
Mint	1.5 oz	200	9	30	5	30
Peanut	1 fun size (0.7 oz)	110	5	13	5	10
Peanut	1 pkg (1.7 oz)	250	13	30	5	25
Peanut	1.5 oz	220	11	25	5	20
Peanut	½ bag king size (1.6 oz)	240	12	28	5	25
Peanut Butter	1 fun size (0.7 oz)	110	6	12	0	45
Peanut Butter	1 pkg (1.6 oz)	240	13	27	5	100
Peanut Butter	1.5 oz	220	12	25	5	90
Plain	1 pkg (1.7 oz)	230	10	34	6	35
Plain	1 pkg fun size (0.7 oz)	100	4	15	5	15
Plain	1.5 oz	200	9	30	5	30
Plain	½ pkg king size (1.6 oz)	220	9	32	5	30
Mars						
Almond Bar	1 bar (1.8 oz)	240	13	31	5	70
Almond Bar	2 fun size (1.3 oz)	190	10	23	5	55
Mayfair						
Mints	5 pieces (1.3 oz)	180	9	26	0	5
Milk Duds						
Pieces	1 box (1.8 oz)	230	8	38	0	120
Snack Size	4 boxes (1.3 oz)	160	5	26	0	85
Milkshake						
Bar	1 bar (1.8 oz)	220	7	38	0	120
Milky Way						
Bar	1 (2.1 oz)	280	11	43	5	90
Bar	⅓ king size (1.2 oz)	160	6	24	5	50
Bar	2 fun size (1.4 oz)	180	7	28	5	60
Dark	1 bar (1.8 oz)	220	8	36	5	85
Dark	1 fun size (0.7 oz)	90	3	14	0	35
Miniature	5 (1.5 oz)	190	7	30	5	65
Mounds						
Bar	1 (1.9 oz)	260	14	31	0	85

FOOD	PORTION	CALS	FAT	CARB	CHOL	SOD
Mr. Goodbar						
Candy	1 (1.75 oz)	290	19	23	15	20
NECCO						
Mint	1 piece	12	tr	—	0	—
Natural Touch						
Caroby Almond Bar	4 sections (28 g)	150	10	12	—	50
Caroby Milk Bar	4 sections (28 g)	150	9	13	—	55
Caroby Milk Free Bar	4 sections (28 g)	160	11	11	—	25
Caroby Mint Bar	4 sections (28 g)	150	9	13	—	55
Nestle						
Areo Bar	1 bar (1.45 oz)	210	13	26	10	20
Buncha Crunch	1 pkg (1.4 oz)	90	10	26	5	95
Crunch	1 bar (1.55 oz)	230	12	28	5	60
Milk Chocolate	1 bar (1.45 oz)	220	13	23	10	30
Turtles Pecan Caramel Candy	2 pieces (1.2 oz)	160	9	20	<5	30
Newman's Own						
Organics Espresso Sweet Dark Chocolate	1 bar (1.2 oz)	190	12	19	0	10
Nips						
Butter Rum	2 pieces (0.5 oz)	60	2	12	—	35
Caramel	2 pieces (0.5 oz)	60	2	12	—	40
Chocolate Mint	2 pieces (0.5 oz)	60	2	11	—	40
Chocolate Parfait	2 pieces (0.5 oz)	60	2	11	—	35
Peanut Butter Parfait	2 pieces (0.5 oz)	60	2	11	—	40
Ocean Spray						
Fruit Waves Assorted	3 pieces (0.3 oz)	35	0	9	0	0
Oh Henry!						
Bar	1 (1.8 oz)	230	9	32	<5	125
PayDay						
Bar	1 (1.85 oz)	240	12	28	0	170
Pearson						
Licorice	2 pieces (0.5 oz)	60	2	12	—	40

FOOD	PORTION	CALS	FAT	CARB	CHOL	SOD
Pez						
Candy	1 roll (0.3 oz)	30	0	8	0	0
Sugar Free	1 roll (0.3 oz)	30	0	8	0	0
Planters						
Original Peanut Bar	1 pkg (1.6 oz)	230	14	22	0	70
Pom Pom						
Candies	1 pkg (1.6 oz)	200	6	—	—	—
Raisinets						
Raisins	1 pkg (1.58 oz)	200	8	31	<5	15
Reese's						
Peanut Butter Cups	1 (1.8 oz)	280	17	26	10	180
Pieces	1.85 oz	260	11	32	5	90
Riesen						
Candy	5 pieces (1.4 oz)	180	7	29	<5	30
Rolo						
Caramels In Milk Chocolate	8 pieces (1.93 oz)	270	12	37	15	110
Russell Stover						
Assorted Creams	3 pieces (1.4 oz)	180	7	29	<5	50
Pecan Roll	1 (2 oz)	300	20	26	5	95
Skittles						
Original	1 pkg (2.8 oz)	250	3	55	0	10
Original	1.5 oz	170	2	38	0	5
Original	½ king size (1.3 oz)	150	2	34	0	5
Original	2 pkg fun size (1.6 oz)	180	2	41	0	5
Tropical	1 bag (2.2 oz)	250	3	56	0	10
Tropical	1.5 oz	170	2	38	0	5
Tropical	2 bags fun size (1.4 oz)	160	2	36	0	5
Wild Berry	1 bag (2.2 oz)	250	3	56	0	10
Wild Berry	1.5 oz	170	2	38	0	5
Wild Berry	2 bags fun size (1.4 oz)	160	2	36	0	5
Skor						
Toffee Bar	1 (1.4 oz)	220	14	22	25	125
Smucker's						
Jelly Beans	1 pkg (0.7 oz)	70	0	18	0	10
Snickers						
Bar	1 bar (2.1 oz)	280	14	36	10	150
Bar	⅓ king size (1.2 oz)	170	8	21	5	85

FOOD	PORTION	CALS	FAT	CARB	CHOL	SOD
Snickers (CONT.)						
Bar	2 bars fun size (1.4 oz)	190	9	24	5	100
Miniatures	4 (1.3 oz)	170	8	22	5	90
Munch Bar	1 (1.4 oz)	230	15	17	10	150
Peanut Butter	1 bar (2 oz)	310	20	28	5	150
Sno-Caps						
Candies	1 pkg (2.3 oz)	300	13	48	—	0
Solitaires						
Candies	½ bag	260	17	20	5	25
Sour Punch						
Candy Straws Sour Apple	6 pieces (1.4 oz)	130	1	31	0	10
Spice Stix						
And Drops	14 pieces (1.6 oz)	140	0	35	0	15
Starburst						
California Fruits	1 stick (2.1 oz)	240	5	48	2	35
California Fruits	8 pieces (1.4 oz)	160	3	33	0	20
Original Fruits	⅓ king size (1.2 oz)	140	3	28	0	20
Original Fruits	8 pieces (1.4 oz)	160	3	33	0	20
Orignal Fruits	1 stick (2.1 oz)	240	5	48	0	35
Strawberry Fruits	1 stick (2.1 oz)	240	5	48	0	35
Strawberry Fruits	8 pieces (1.4 oz)	160	3	33	0	20
Tropical Fruits	1 stick (2.1 oz)	240	5	48	0	35
Tropical Fruits	8 pieces (1.4 oz)	160	3	33	0	20
Sugar Babies						
Candies	1 pkg (1.7 oz)	190	2	—	—	—
Tidbits	1 pkg	180	2	—	—	—
Sugar Daddy						
Candies	1 pkg (1.7 oz)	200	3	—	—	—
Swedish Red Fish						
Candy	19 pieces (1.4 oz)	150	1	35	0	20
Sweet Escapes						
Triple Chocolate Wafer Bars	1 (0.7 oz)	80	3	14	0	30
Switzer						
Cherry Bites	12 pieces (1.6 oz)	50	0	11	0	25

FOOD	PORTION	CALS	FAT	CARB	CHOL	SOD
Switzer (CONT.)						
Licorice Bites	12 pieces (1.6 oz)	46	0	11	0	56
Symphony						
Almond/ Butterchips	1 (1.4 oz)	220	14	20	—	40
Milk Chocolate	1 (1.4 oz)	220	13	22	10	35
Terry's						
Orange Milk Chocolate	5 pieces (1.5 oz)	240	14	26	10	40
Tootsie Roll						
Candy	1 (1 oz)	110	2	—	—	—
Dots	12 (1.5 oz)	160	0	—	0	—
Midgees	6 (1.4 oz)	160	3	—	—	—
Pop	1 (0.6 oz)	60	0	—	0	—
Twix						
Caramel	1 (1 oz)	140	7	19	0	60
Caramel	1 fun size (0.5 oz)	80	4	10	0	30
Caramel	1 king size (0.8 oz)	120	6	15	0	45
Caramel	1 pkg (2 oz)	280	14	37	5	115
Peanut Butter	1 (0.9 oz)	130	8	13	0	70
Twizzlers						
Candy	4 pieces (1.4 oz)	130	1	30	—	95
Pull-N-Peel Cherry	1 piece (1.1 oz)	110	0	23	0	80
Velamints						
Cocoamint	1 piece (1.7 g)	5	0	2	0	0
Peppermint	1 piece (1.7 g)	5	0	2	0	0
Spearmint	1 piece (1.7 g)	5	0	2	0	0
Wintergreen	1 piece (1.7 g)	5	0	2	0	0
Very Special						
Chocolate Bottles Liquor Filled	3 pieces (1 oz)	150	6	24	0	10
Whatchamacallit						
Bar	1 (1.8 oz)	260	13	30	10	130
Whitman's						
Assorted	3 pieces (1.4 oz)	190	8	27	5	50
Dark Chocolate	3 pieces (1.4 oz)	200	10	25	<5	55
Little Ambassadors	7 pieces (1.4 oz)	190	9	26	5	50
Pecan Delight	1 bar (2 oz)	310	20	27	10	75

FOOD	PORTION	CALS	FAT	CARB	CHOL	SOD
Whitman's (CONT.)						
Pecan Roll	1 bar (2 oz)	300	20	26	5	95
Sampler	3 pieces (1.4 oz)	200	11	25	5	60
Whoppers						
Candy	1 pkg (1.8 oz)	230	10	36	0	130
Y&S						
Bites Cherry	1 oz	100	1	23	0	85
York						
Peppermint Patty	1 (1.5 oz)	180	4	34	0	20
Peppermint Patty	1 snack size (0.5 oz)	57	1	11	0	3
Zero						
Bar	2 pieces (1.4 oz)	170	6	28	0	85
CANTALOUPE						
fresh half	½	94	1	22	0	23
CARROT JUICE						
Odwalla						
Juice	8 fl oz	70	0	18	0	200
CARROTS						
fresh	1 (2.5 oz)	31	tr	7	0	25
CASHEWS						
Beer Nuts						
Cashews	1 pkg (1 oz)	170	13	8	0	65
Fisher						
Honey Roasted Halves	1 oz	150	13	7	0	—
Planters						
Fancy Oil Roasted	1 pkg (2 oz)	340	29	16	0	240
Honey Roasted	1 pkg (2 oz)	310	24	23	0	240
CAVIAR						
black	1 tbsp	40	3	1	94	240
red	1 tbsp	40	3	1	94	240
CHAMPAGNE						
sekt german champagne	3.5 fl oz	84	0	5	0	—
Andre						
Blush	1 fl oz	22	0	1	0	1
Brut	1 fl oz	21	0	1	0	1
Cold Duck	1 fl oz	25	0	2	0	1
Extra Dry	1 fl oz	23	0	1	0	1

FOOD	PORTION	CALS	FAT	CARB	CHOL	SOD
Ballatore						
Spumante	1 fl oz	23	0	2	0	2
Eden Roc						
Brut	1 fl oz	21	0	1	0	1
Brut Rose	1 fl oz	22	0	2	0	1
Extra Dry	1 fl oz	21	0	1	0	1
Tott's						
Blanc de Noir	1 fl oz	22	0	2	0	1
Brut	1 fl oz	20	0	tr	0	1
Extra Dry	1 fl oz	21	0	1	0	1

CHEESE

FOOD	PORTION	CALS	FAT	CARB	CHOL	SOD
Alouette						
Brie Baby	1 oz	110	9	2	30	180
Brie Baby With Herbs	1 oz	110	9	2	30	180
BabyBel						
Mini Light	1 (0.7 oz)	45	3	0	5	180
Frigo						
String	1 oz	80	5	1	10	190
String Lite	1 oz	60	2	1	8	140
Handi-Snacks						
Cheez'n Breadsticks	1 pkg (1.1 oz)	130	7	11	14	340
Cheez'n Crackers	1 pkg (1.1 oz)	130	8	10	15	340
Cheez'n Pretzels	1 pkg (1 oz)	110	6	11	15	420
Mozzarella String Cheese	1 stick (1 oz)	80	6	tr	20	240
Healthy Choice						
Mozzarella String Cheese	1 stick (1 oz)	45	0	1	<5	200
Pizza String	1 stick (1 oz)	45	0	1	<5	200
Kraft						
String With Jalapeno Peppers	1 oz	80	5	1	20	230
Laughing Cow						
Assorted Wedge	1 (1 oz)	70	6	1	20	370
Babybel	1 oz	90	7	0	10	230
Babybel Mini	1 (0.7 oz)	70	6	0	15	170
Bonbel Mini	1 (0.7 oz)	70	6	0	15	170
Cheesebits	6 pieces (1 oz)	70	6	1	20	370
Gouda Mini	1 (0.7 oz)	80	6	0	20	170
Original Wedge	1 (1 oz)	70	6	1	20	370
Wedge Light	1 (1 oz)	50	3	1	10	370
Polly-O						
String Lite	1 piece (1 oz)	60	3	tr	10	230

FOOD	PORTION	CALS	FAT	CARB	CHOL	SOD
Sargento						
MooTown Snackers Cheddar	1 piece (0.8 oz)	100	8	1	25	130
MooTown Snackers Cheddar Mild Light	1 piece (0.8 oz)	60	4	tr	10	170
MooTown Snackers Cheese & Pretzels	1 pkg (1 oz)	90	3	12	10	320
MooTown Snackers Cheese & Sticks	1 pkg (1 oz)	100	4	13	10	260
MooTown Snackers Colby-Jack	1 piece (0.8 oz)	90	8	tr	20	160
MooTown Snackers Pizza Cheese & Sticks	1 pkg (1 oz)	100	4	13	10	260
MooTown Snackers String	1 piece (0.8 oz)	70	5	tr	15	170
MooTown Snackers String Light	1 piece (0.8 oz)	60	3	tr	10	200
CHERRIES						
fresh	10	49	1	11	0	0
CHERRY JUICE						
After The Fall						
Black Cherry	1 can (12 oz)	170	0	42	0	20
CHESTNUTS						
roasted	2 to 3 (1 oz)	70	1	15	0	1
CHEWING GUM						
bubble gum	1 block (8 g)	27	0	8	0	0
stick	1 (3 g)	10	0	3	0	0
Bazooka						
Fruit Chunk	1 piece (6 g)	25	0	5	0	0
Fruit Soft	1 piece (6 g)	25	0	5	0	0
Gum	1 piece (4 g)	15	0	4	0	0
Gum	1 piece (6 g)	25	0	5	0	0
Beech-Nut						
Peppermint	1 stick (3 g)	10	0	2	0	0
Spearmint	1 stick (3 g)	10	0	2	0	0
Big Red						
Stick	1	10	tr	2	0	0
Brock						
Bubble Gum	1 piece (0.2 oz)	20	0	4	0	0
Bubble Yum						
Bananaberry Split	1 piece (0.3 oz)	25	0	6	0	0

FOOD	PORTION	CALS	FAT	CARB	CHOL	SOD
Bubble Yum (CONT.)						
Cotton Candy	1 piece (0.3 oz)	25	0	6	0	0
Grape	1 piece (0.3 oz)	25	0	6	0	0
Luscious Lime	1 piece (0.3 oz)	25	0	6	0	0
Regular	1 piece (0.3 oz)	25	0	6	0	0
Sour Apple	1 piece (0.3 oz)	25	0	6	0	0
Sour Cherry	1 piece (0.3 oz)	25	0	6	0	0
Sugarless	1 piece (0.2 oz)	15	0	3	—	0
Sugarless Grape	1 piece (0.2 oz)	15	0	3	—	0
Sugarless Peppermint	1 piece (0.2 oz)	15	0	3	—	0
Sugarless Strawberry	1 piece (0.2 oz)	15	0	3	—	0
Sugarless Variety	1 piece (0.2 oz)	15	0	3	—	0
Variety Pack	1 piece (0.3 oz)	25	0	6	0	0
Watermelon	1 piece (0.3 oz)	25	0	6	0	0
Wild Strawberry	1 piece (0.3 oz)	25	0	6	0	0
Bubblicious						
Gum	1 piece (7.9 g)	25	0	6	0	—
*Care*Free*						
Sugarless Bubble Gum	1 stick (3 g)	10	0	2	—	0
Sugarless Cinnamon	1 piece (3 g)	5	0	2	—	0
Sugarless Peppermint	1 piece (3 g)	5	0	2	—	0
Sugarless Spearmint	1 piece (3 g)	5	0	2	—	0
Sugarless Wild Cherry	1 stick (3 g)	10	0	2	—	0
Chiclets						
Original	1 piece (1.59 g)	6	0	2	0	—
Tiny Size	8 pieces (0.13 g)	tr	0	tr	0	—
Clorets	1 piece (1.59 g)	6	0	2	0	—
Dentyne						
Cinn-A-Burst	1 piece (3.2 g)	9	0	2	0	—
Gum	1 piece (1.88 g)	6	0	1	0	—
Sugar Free	1 piece (1.88 g)	5	0	1	0	—
Doublemint						
Chewing Gum	1 piece	10	tr	2	0	0
Extra Sugar Free						
Cinnamon	1 piece	8	tr	tr	0	0
Spearmint & Peppermint	1 stick	8	tr	tr	0	0
Winter Fresh	1 piece	8	tr	tr	0	0
Freedent						
Spearmint Peppermint & Cinnamon	1 stick	10	tr	3	0	0

FOOD	PORTION	CALS	FAT	CARB	CHOL	SOD
Freshen-Up						
Gum	1 piece (4.2 g)	13	0	3	0	—
Fruit Stripe						
Bubble Gum Jumbo Pack	1 stick (3 g)	10	0	2	0	0
Variety Pack Chewing & Bubble Gum	1 stick (3 g)	10	0	2	0	0
Hubba Bubba						
Bubble Gum Cola	1 piece	23	tr	6	0	0
Bubble Gum Sugarfree Grape	1 piece	13	tr	tr	0	0
Bubble Gum Sugarfree Original	1 piece	14	tr	tr	0	0
Original	1 piece	23	tr	6	0	0
Strawberry Grape Raspberry	1 piece	23	tr	6	0	0
Juicy Fruit						
Stick	1	10	tr	2	0	0
Rain-Blo						
Bubble Gum Balls	1 piece (2 g)	5	0	2	0	0
Stick*Free						
Sugarless Peppermint	1 stick (3 g)	10	0	2	—	0
Sugarless Spearmint	1 stick (3 g)	10	0	2	—	0
Swell						
Bubble Gum	1 piece (3 g)	10	0	2	0	0
Trident						
Gum	1 piece (1.88 g)	5	0	1	0	—
Soft Bubble Gum	1 piece (3.3 g)	9	0	2	0	—
Wrigley's						
Spearmint	1 stick	10	tr	2	0	0

CHICKEN DISHES

FOOD	PORTION	CALS	FAT	CARB	CHOL	SOD
Croissant Pocket						
Stuffed Sandwich Chicken Broccoli & Cheddar	1 piece (4.5 oz)	300	11	37	35	640
Hillshire						
Lunch 'N Munch Smoked Chicken/ Monterey Jack	1 pkg (4.5 oz)	350	20	19	—	1260
Lunch 'N Munch Smoked Chicken/ Monterey/ Snickers	1 pkg (4.25 oz)	400	23	31	—	1080

FOOD	PORTION	CALS	FAT	CARB	CHOL	SOD
Hot Pocket						
Stuffed Sandwich Chicken & Cheddar With Broccoli	1 (4.5 oz)	300	12	37	30	620
Jimmy Dean						
Grilled Breast Sandwich	1 (5.5 oz)	330	11	27	70	730
Lean Pockets						
Stuffed Sandwich Chicken Fajita	1 (4.5 oz)	260	8	36	40	770
Stuffed Sandwich Chicken Parmesan	1 (4.5 oz)	260	8	34	25	630
Stuffed Sandwich Glazed Chicken Supreme	1 (4.5 oz)	240	7	34	30	600
Oscar Mayer						
Lunchables Chicken/ Monterey Jack	1 pkg (4.5 oz)	350	21	20	75	1690
Lunchables Deluxe Chicken/Turkey	1 pkg (5.1 oz)	380	22	24	70	1840
Lunchables Dessert Chocolate Pudding/ Chicken/ Jack	1 pkg (6.2 oz)	370	18	33	55	1490
Ovenstuffs						
Chicken Turnover	1 (4.75 oz)	350	16	36	—	690
Tyson						
Microwave Breast Sandwich	4.25 oz	328	14	33	—	520
Weight Watchers						
Chicken, Broccoli & Cheese Pocket Sandwich	1 (5 oz)	250	6	40	25	310
Grilled Chicken Sandwich	1 (4 oz)	210	5	24	20	420
White Castle						
Grilled Chicken Sandwich	2 (4 oz)	250	9	24	20	490
Grilled Chicken Sandwich w/ Sauce	2 (4.8 oz)	290	9	33	20	600

CHIPS

FOOD	PORTION	CALS	FAT	CARB	CHOL	SOD
corn barbecue	1 bag (7 oz)	1036	65	111	0	1511
corn barbecue	1 oz	148	9	16	0	216
corn onion	1 oz	142	6	19	0	278

FOOD	PORTION	CALS	FAT	CARB	CHOL	SOD
corn plain	1 bag (7 oz)	1067	66	113	0	1248
corn plain	1 oz	153	10	16	0	179
corn cones nacho	1 oz	152	9	17	—	270
corn cones plain	1 oz	145	8	18	0	290
corn puffs cheese	1 bag (8 oz)	1256	78	122	9	2383
corn puffs cheese	1 oz	157	10	15	1	298
corn twists cheese	1 bag (8 oz)	1256	78	122	9	2383
corn twists cheese	1 oz	157	10	15	1	298
potato	1 bag (8 oz)	1217	79	120	0	1347
potato	1 oz	152	10	15	0	168
potato barbecue	1 oz	139	9	15	0	213
potato barbecue	1 bag (7 oz)	971	64	105	0	1486
potato cheese	1 bag (6 oz)	842	46	98	—	1348
potato cheese	1 oz	140	8	16	—	225
potato light	1 bag (6 oz)	801	35	114	0	836
potato light	1 oz	134	6	19	0	139
potato sour cream & onion	1 oz	150	10	15	2	177
potato sour cream & onion	1 bag (7 oz)	1051	67	102	14	1237
potato sticks	1 oz	148	10	15	0	71
potato sticks	1 pkg (1 oz)	148	10	15	0	71
potato sticks	½ cup (0.6 oz)	94	6	10	0	45
taro	1 oz	141	7	19	0	97
taro	10 (0.8 oz)	115	6	16	0	79
tortilla	1 bag (7.5 oz)	1067	56	134	0	1124
tortilla	1 oz	142	7	18	0	150
tortilla nacho	1 bag (8 oz)	1131	58	142	0	1606
tortilla nacho	1 oz	141	7	18	0	201
tortilla nacho light	1 bag (6 oz)	757	26	122	0	1705
tortilla nacho light	1 oz	126	4	20	0	284
tortilla ranch	1 bag (7 oz)	969	47	128	1	1212
tortilla ranch	1 oz	139	7	18	0	174
tortilla taco	1 bag (8 oz)	1089	55	143	—	1788
tortilla taco	1 oz	136	7	18	—	223
Barrel O' Fun						
Potato Chips	1 oz	150	9	15	0	160
Potato Chips Barbecue	1 oz	145	9	16	0	250
Potato Chips Sour Cream & Onion	1 oz	150	9	15	0	230
Tortilla Nacho	1 oz	140	6	19	0	160
Tortilla White	1 oz	140	6	20	0	50
Tostada Yellow	1 oz	140	6	19	0	40

FOOD	PORTION	CALS	FAT	CARB	CHOL	SOD
Butterfield						
Potato Sticks	1 pkg (1.7 oz)	250	15	26	1	150
Potato Sticks	⅔ cup (1 oz)	150	9	16	0	90
Cape Cod						
Potato Chips	19 chips (1 oz)	150	8	17	0	110
Cottage Fries						
Potato Chips No Salt Added	1 oz	160	11	14	0	5
Doritos						
Tortilla Lightly Salted	16 chips (1 oz)	150	7	18	0	135
Wow Nacho Cheesier	1 pkg (0.75 oz)	70	1	13	0	180
Eden						
Vegetable Chips	50 (1 oz)	130	4	24	0	260
Wasabi Chip Hot & Spicy	50 (1 oz)	130	4	24	0	260
Energy Food Factory						
Corn Pops Fat Free	½ oz	50	0	11	0	110
Corn Pops Nacho	½ oz	50	1	12	0	150
Corn Pops Original	½ oz	50	1	11	0	110
Potato Pops Au Gratin	½ oz	60	2	12	<5	110
Potato Pops Fat Free	½ oz	50	0	13	0	110
Potato Pops Herb & Garlic	½ oz	50	1	11	0	110
Potato Pops Mesquite	½ oz	50	1	12	0	110
Potato Pops Original	½ oz	50	1	11	0	110
Potato Pops Salt N' Vinegar	½ oz	50	1	11	0	110
Frito Lay						
Tortilla Salsa 'N Cheese	16 (1 oz)	150	8	17	0	180
Fritos						
Chili Cheese	34 pieces (1 oz)	160	10	15	0	300
Chips	34 pieces (1 oz)	150	10	16	0	220
Crisp 'N Thin	18 pieces (1 oz)	160	10	16	0	240
Dip Size	13 pieces (1 oz)	150	10	16	0	240
Non-Stop Nacho Cheese	34 pieces (1 oz)	150	9	16	tr	220
Rowdy Rustlers Bar-B-Q	34 pieces (1 oz)	150	9	17	0	300
Wild 'N Mild	32 pieces (1 oz)	160	9	16	0	240
Guiltless Gourmet						
Tortilla Baked	22-26 chips (1 oz)	110	1	21	0	119

FOOD	PORTION	CALS	FAT	CARB	CHOL	SOD
Hain						
Carrot Chips	1 oz	150	9	16	—	160
Carrot Chips Barbecue	1 oz	140	8	16	—	160
Carrot Chips No Salt Added	1 oz	150	7	16	0	30
Taco Style	1 oz	160	11	15	<5	320
Tortilla Sesame	1 oz	140	7	19	0	190
Tortilla Sesame Cheese	1 oz	160	8	20	<5	270
Tortilla Sesame No Salt Added	1 oz	140	7	19	0	<5
Health Valley						
Carrot Lites	0.5 oz	75	4	9	0	5
Corn Chips	1 oz	160	11	13	0	90
Corn Chips No Salt Added	1 oz	160	11	13	0	1
Corn Chips w/ Cheddar Cheese	1 oz	160	10	15	2	120
Potato Chips Country Ripple	1 oz	160	10	15	0	60
Potato Chips Country Ripple No Salt Added	1 oz	160	10	15	0	1
Potato Chips Natural	1 oz	160	10	15	0	60
Potato Chips Natural No Salt Added	1 oz	160	10	15	0	1
Potato Dip Chips	1 oz	160	10	15	0	60
Potato Dip Chips No Salt Added	1 oz	160	10	15	0	1
Herr's						
Potato Chips	1 oz	140	8	16	0	180
Restaurant Style White Corn	10 chips (1 oz)	140	6	18	0	90
Kelly's						
Potato Chips	1 oz	150	9	14	0	160
Potato Chips Bar-B-Q	1 oz	150	9	15	0	230
Potato Chips Crunchy	1 oz	150	9	17	0	140
Potato Chips Rippled	1 oz	150	9	14	0	160
Potato Chips Sour Cream n' Onion	1 oz	150	9	15	0	170
Potato Chips Unsalted	1 oz	150	10	14	0	5
La FAMOUS						
Tortilla	1 oz	140	7	18	0	180
Tortilla No Salt Added	1 oz	140	7	18	0	5

FOOD	PORTION	CALS	FAT	CARB	CHOL	SOD
Lance						
Corn Chips	1 pkg (50 g)	270	17	26	0	350
Corn Chips BBQ	1 pkg (50 g)	260	16	25	0	360
Potato Chips	1 pkg (32 g)	190	15	12	0	220
Potato Chips BBQ	1 pkg (32 g)	190	12	18	0	270
Potato Chips Cajun Style	1 pkg (32 g)	160	11	16	0	250
Potato Chips Ripple	1 pkg (32 g)	190	15	12	0	220
Potato Chips Sour Cream & Onion	1 pkg (32 g)	190	12	18	0	390
Potato Hot Fries	1 pkg (28 g)	160	10	14	0	220
Tortilla Jalapeno Cheese	1 pkg (1⅛ oz)	160	8	—	0	—
Tortilla Nacho	1 pkg (32 g)	160	8	19	0	240
Lay's						
Crunch Tators	16 pieces (1 oz)	150	8	17	0	120
Crunch Tators Amazin' Cajun	16 pieces (1 oz)	150	8	17	0	150
Crunch Tators Hoppin' Jalapeno	16 pieces (1 oz)	140	7	18	0	200
Crunch Tators Mighty Mesquite	16 pieces (1 oz)	150	8	17	0	135
Crunch Tators Supreme Sour Cream	16 pieces (1 oz)	150	8	16	0	180
Potato Chips	17 pieces (1 oz)	150	10	15	0	170
Potato Chips Bar-B-Q	17 pieces (1 oz)	150	9	15	0	270
Potato Chips Cheddar Cheese	17 pieces (1 oz)	150	10	14	tr	300
Potato Chips Flamin' Hot	17 pieces (1 oz)	150	9	15	0	190
Potato Chips Kansas City Style Bar-B-Q	17 pieces (1 oz)	150	9	15	0	270
Potato Chips Salt & Vinegar	17 pieces (1 oz)	150	10	14	0	390
Potato Chips Sour Cream & Onion	17 pieces (1 oz)	160	10	15	tr	220
Potato Chips Tangy Ranch	17 pieces (1 oz)	160	10	15	0	210
Potato Chips Unsalted	17 pieces (1 oz)	150	10	15	0	10
Wow Fat Free Original	1 pkg (0.75 oz)	55	0	13	0	130
Louise's						
Potato Chips "1g" Mesquite BBQ	1 oz	110	1	24	0	180

FOOD	PORTION	CALS	FAT	CARB	CHOL	SOD
Louise's (CONT.)						
Potato Chips "1g" Original	1 oz	110	1	24	0	180
Potato Chips 70% Less Fat Mesquite BBQ	1 oz	110	3	21	0	180
Potato Chips 70% Less Fat Original	1 oz	110	3	21	0	200
Potato Chips Fat-Free Maui Onion	1 oz	110	0	23	0	180
Potato Chips Fat-Free Mesquite BBQ	1 oz	110	0	23	0	180
Potato Chips Fat-Free No Salt	1 oz	110	0	24	0	10
Potato Chips Fat-Free Original	1 oz	110	0	23	0	180
Potato Chips Fat-Free Vinegar & Salt	1 oz	110	0	23	0	300
Tortilla 95% Fat-Free	1 oz	120	2	23	0	170
Mr. Phipps						
Tater Crisps Bar-B-Que	21 (1 oz)	130	4	21	0	270
Tater Crisps Original	23 (1 oz)	120	7	20	0	220
Tater Crisps Sour Cream 'N Onion	22 (1 oz)	130	4	21	0	210
Tortilla Nacho	28 (1 oz)	130	4	20	0	150
Tortilla Original	28 (1 oz)	130	4	21	0	130
New York Deli						
Potato Chips	1 oz	160	11	14	0	120
Old Dutch Foods						
Potato Augratin	1 oz	150	8	15	—	220
Potato Chips	1 oz	150	9	16	—	160
Potato Chips BBQ	1 oz	140	8	16	—	360
Potato Chips Dill Flavored	1 oz	150	8	16	—	340
Potato Chips Onion & Garlic	1 oz	150	9	15	—	420
Potato Chips Ripple	1 oz	150	9	16	—	150
Potato Chips Sour Cream & Onion	1 oz	150	10	15	—	220
Old El Paso						
NACHIPS	9 chips (1 oz)	150	8	17	0	85
Tortilla White Corn	11 chips (1 oz)	140	8	18	0	60
Planters						
Corn Chips	34 chips (1 oz)	170	10	17	0	180

FOOD	PORTION	CALS	FAT	CARB	CHOL	SOD
Planters (CONT.)						
Corn Chips King Size	17 chips (1 oz)	160	10	16	0	180
Corn Chips Snacks To Go	1 pkg (1.5 oz)	240	15	23	0	260
Pringles						
Cheez-ums	14 chips (1 oz)	150	10	—	1	190
Original	14 chips (1 oz)	160	11	—	0	170
Potato Chips BBQ	14 chips (1 oz)	150	6	15	0	200
Ranch	14 chips (1 oz)	150	10	—	0	130
Ridges Cheddar & Sour Cream	12 chips (1 oz)	150	10	—	0	200
Ridges Mesquite BBQ	12 chips (1 oz)	150	10	—	0	220
Ridges Original	12 chips (1 oz)	150	10	—	0	150
Right BBQ	16 chips (1 oz)	140	7	18	0	160
Right Original	16 chips (1 oz)	140	7	—	0	135
Right Ranch	16 chips (1 oz)	140	7	18	0	120
Right Sour Cream 'N Onion	16 chips (1 oz)	140	7	18	0	120
Rippled Original	10 chips (1 oz)	160	11	15	0	150
Sour Cream 'N Onion	14 chips (1 oz)	160	10	15	1	135
Ruffles						
Cheddar Cheese & Sour Cream	18 chips (1 oz)	160	10	15	tr	250
Mesquite Grille B-B-Q	18 chips (1 oz)	160	10	15	0	270
Monterey Jack Cheese Attack	18 chips (1 oz)	160	10	15	tr	200
Potato Chips	18 chips (1 oz)	150	10	15	0	135
Potato Light	18 chips (1 oz)	130	6	19	0	140
Potato Light Sour Cream & Onion	18 chips (1 oz)	130	6	18	tr	190
Ranch	18 chips (1 oz)	160	10	15	0	220
Sour Cream & Onion	18 chips (1 oz)	160	10	15	tr	220
Santitas						
Tortilla Cantina Style	1 oz	140	6	19	0	75
Tortilla Cantina Style Fajita	1 oz	140	7	19	0	95
Tortilla Chips	1 oz	140	7	19	0	50
Tortilla Strips	1 oz	140	7	19	0	65
Snyder's						
Corn Chips	1 oz	160	11	14	0	150
Corn Chips BBQ	1 oz	160	11	14	0	200
Potato Chips	1 oz	150	10	13	0	130
Potato Chips BBQ	1 oz	150	10	13	0	370
Potato Chips Cheddar Bacon	1 oz	150	10	13	0	260

FOOD	PORTION	CALS	FAT	CARB	CHOL	SOD
Snyder's (CONT.)						
Potato Chips Coney Island	1 oz	150	10	13	0	280
Potato Chips Grilled Stead & Onion	1 oz	150	10	13	0	260
Potato Chips Hot Buffalo Wings	1 oz	150	10	13	0	200
Potato Chips Kosher Dill	1 oz	150	10	13	0	400
Potato Chips No Salt	1 oz	150	10	13	0	0
Potato Chips Salt & Vinegar	1 oz	150	10	13	0	200
Potato Chips Sausage Pizza	1 oz	150	10	13	0	230
Potato Chips Sour Cream & Onion	1 oz	150	10	13	0	190
Potato Chips Sour Cream & Onion Unsalted	1 oz	150	10	13	0	10
Tortilla Chips	1 oz	140	7	18	0	130
Tortilla Enchilada	1 oz	140	7	18	0	220
Tortilla Nacho Cheese	1 oz	140	7	18	0	130
Tortilla No Salt	1 oz	140	7	18	0	0
Tortilla Ranch	1 oz	140	7	18	0	150
State Line						
Potato Chips	1 pkg (0.5 oz)	80	5	7	0	70
Sunchips						
Chips	12 pieces (1 oz)	150	8	18	0	100
French Onion	12 pieces (1 oz)	140	7	18	tr	120
Suprimos						
Potato Chips Cheddar & Jack	1 oz	140	6	17	tr	180
Potato Chips Cool Onion	1 oz	140	6	17	tr	170
Terra Chips						
Sweet Potato	1 oz	140	7	18	0	10
Sweet Potato Spiced	1 oz	140	7	16	0	105
Taro Spiced	1 oz	130	5	20	0	170
Vegetable	1 oz	140	7	18	0	70
Top Banana						
Plantain Chips	1 oz	150	8	17	0	85
Tostitos						
Restaurant Style Lime 'N Chili	7 pieces (1 oz)	150	7	18	0	190

FOOD	PORTION	CALS	FAT	CARB	CHOL	SOD
Tostitos (CONT.)						
Restaurant Style White Corn	7 pieces (1 oz)	150	6	20	0	75
Tortilla Baked	1 oz	110	1	24	0	140
Tortilla Baked Cool Ranch	1 oz	130	3	21	0	170
Tortilla Baked Unsalted	1 oz	110	1	24	0	0
Tortilla Bite Size	16 pieces (1 oz)	150	8	18	0	110
Tortilla Chips	11 pieces (1 oz)	140	8	18	0	160
Tyson						
Tortilla Nacho Cheese	1 oz	140	7	17	0	145
Tortilla Ranch Flavor	1 oz	140	2	17	0	—
Tortilla Traditional	1 oz	140	7	17	0	95
Tortilla Unsalted	1 oz	140	7	17	0	7
Weight Watchers						
Potato Chips Barbecue Curls	1 pkg (0.5 oz)	60	3	11	0	110
Wise						
Corn Crunchies	1 oz	160	10	15	0	180
Crispy Corn	1 oz	160	10	15	0	125
Crispy Corn Nacho Cheese	1 oz	160	10	16	0	190
Dipsy Doodles	1 pkg (1.5 oz)	240	15	24	0	270
Potato Chips Natural	1 oz	160	11	14	0	190
Ridgies Barbecue	1 oz	150	10	14	0	240
Tortilla Bravos	1 oz	150	8	18	0	180

CHOCOLATE

FOOD	PORTION	CALS	FAT	CARB	CHOL	SOD
semisweet chips	60 pieces (1 oz)	136	9	18	0	3

CHOCOLATE SYRUP

FOOD	PORTION	CALS	FAT	CARB	CHOL	SOD
chocolate fudge	1 tbsp (0.7 oz)	73	3	12	—	27
syrup as prep w/ whole milk	9 oz	232	9	34	33	156

CLAMS

FOOD	PORTION	CALS	FAT	CARB	CHOL	SOD
raw	9 lg (180 g)	133	2	5	60	100

COCONUT

FOOD	PORTION	CALS	FAT	CARB	CHOL	SOD
fresh	1 piece (1.5 oz)	159	15	7	0	9

COFFEE BEVERAGES

FOOD	PORTION	CALS	FAT	CARB	CHOL	SOD
Starbucks						
Frappuccino	1 bottle (9.5 fl oz)	190	3	39	12	110

FOOD	PORTION	CALS	FAT	CARB	CHOL	SOD
COFFEE WHITENERS						
International Delight						
Amaretto	1 tbsp (0.6 fl oz)	45	2	7	0	5
Cinnamon Hazelnut	1 tbsp (0.6 fl oz)	45	2	7	0	5
Irish Creme	1 tbsp (0.6 fl oz)	45	2	7	0	5
No Fat Amaretto	1 tbsp (0.5 fl oz)	30	0	7	0	5
No Fat French Vanilla Royale	1 tbsp (0.5 fl oz)	30	0	7	0	5
No Fat Hawaiian Macadamia	1 tbsp (0.5 fl oz)	30	0	7	0	5
No Fat Irish Creme	1 tbsp (0.5 fl oz)	30	0	7	0	5
Suisse Chocolate Mocha	1 tbsp (0.6 fl oz)	45	2	7	0	10
Mocha Mix						
Signature Flavors French Vanilla	1 tbsp (0.5 fl oz)	35	0	8	0	5
Signature Flavors Irish Creme	1 tbsp (0.5 fl oz)	35	0	8	0	5
Signature Flavors Kahlua	1 tbsp (0.5 fl oz)	35	0	8	0	5
Signature Flavors Mauna Loa Macadamia Nut	1 tbsp (0.5 fl oz)	35	0	8	0	5
COOKIES						
animal	11 crackers (1 oz)	126	4	21	—	112
animal crackers	1 (2.5 g)	11	tr	2	—	10
animal crackers	1 box (2.4 oz)	299	9	51	11	274
butter	1 (5 g)	23	1	3	—	18
chocolate chip	1 (0.4 oz)	48	2	7	—	32
chocolate chip	1 box (1.9 oz)	233	12	36	12	188
chocolate chip low fat	1 (0.25 oz)	45	2	7	0	38
chocolate chip low sugar low sodium	1 (0.24 oz)	31	1	5	0	1
chocolate chip refrigerated dough	1 (0.42 oz)	59	3	8	3	28
chocolate chip soft-type	1 (0.5 oz)	69	4	9	0	49
chocolate chip unbaked refrigerated dough	1 oz	126	6	17	7	59

FOOD	PORTION	CALS	FAT	CARB	CHOL	SOD
chocolate w/ creme filling	1 (0.35 oz)	47	2	7	—	36
chocolate w/ creme filling chocolate coated	1 (0.60 oz)	82	5	11	—	55
chocolate w/ creme filling sugar free low sodium	1 (0.35 oz)	46	2	7	—	24
chocolate w/ extra creme filling	1 (0.46 oz)	65	3	9	—	64
chocolate wafer	1 (0.2 oz)	26	1	4	0	35
chocolate wafer cookie crumbs	½ cup (5.9 oz)	728	25	120	0	980
digestive biscuits plain	2	141	7	21	—	—
fig bars	1 (0.56 oz)	56	1	11	—	56
fortune	1 (0.28 oz)	30	tr	7	—	22
fudge	1 (0.73 oz)	73	1	17	—	40
gingersnaps	1 (0.24 oz)	29	1	5	0	48
graham	1 square (0.24 oz)	30	1	5	0	42
graham chocolate covered	1 (0.49 oz)	68	3	9	0	41
graham honey	1 (0.24 oz)	30	1	5	0	42
ladyfingers	1 (0.38 oz)	40	1	7	40	16
marshmallow chocolate coated	1 (0.46 oz)	55	2	9	—	22
marshmallow pie chocolate coated	1 (1.4 oz)	165	7	26	—	66
molasses	1 (0.5 oz)	65	2	11	0	69
oatmeal	1 (0.6 oz)	81	3	12	0	69
oatmeal raisin	1 (0.6 oz)	81	3	12	0	69
oatmeal raisin low sugar no sodium	1 (0.24 oz)	31	1	5	0	1
oatmeal raisin refrigerated dough	1 (0.4 oz)	56	3	8	3	39
oatmeal raisin soft-type	1 (0.5 oz)	61	2	10	—	52
oatmeal refrigerated dough	1 (0.4 oz)	56	3	8	3	39
oatmeal soft-type	1 (0.5 oz)	61	2	10	—	52
peanut butter refrigerated dough	1 (0.4 oz)	60	3	7	4	52
peanut butter sandwich	1 (0.5 oz)	67	3	9	0	52
peanut butter sandwich sugar free low sodium	1 (0.35 oz)	54	3	5	—	41

FOOD	PORTION	CALS	FAT	CARB	CHOL	SOD
peanut butter soft-type	1 (0.5 oz)	69	4	9	0	50
peanut butter unbaked refrigerated dough	1 oz	130	7	15	8	112
raisin soft-type	1 (0.5 oz)	60	2	10	0	51
shortbread	1 (0.28 oz)	40	2	5	2	36
shortbread pecan	1 (0.49 oz)	79	5	8	5	39
sugar	1 (0.52 oz)	72	3	10	8	53
sugar low sugar sodium free	1 (0.24 oz)	30	1	5	0	0
sugar refrigerated dough	1 (0.42 oz)	58	3	8	4	56
sugar unbaked refrigerated dough	1 oz	124	6	17	8	120
sugar wafers w/ creme filling	1 (0.12 oz)	18	1	3	0	5
sugar wafers w/ creme filling sugar free sodium free	1 (0.14 oz)	20	1	3	0	0
vanilla sandwich	1 (0.35 oz)	48	2	7	0	35
vanilla wafers	1 (0.21 oz)	28	1	4	—	18
Archway						
Almond Crescents	2 (0.8 oz)	100	4	17	<5	75
Apple N'Raisin	1 (1.1 oz)	130	52	20	<5	105
Apricot Filled	1 (1 oz)	110	4	18	5	90
Bells And Stars	3 (1 oz)	150	7	19	5	100
Blueberry Filled	1 (1 oz)	110	4	19	5	115
Carrot Cake	1 (1 oz)	120	5	18	<5	180
Cherry Nougat	3 (1 oz)	150	9	18	0	40
Chocolate Chip	1 (1 oz)	130	6	19	tr	150
Chocolate Chip & Toffee	1 (1 oz)	140	7	19	<5	120
Chocolate Chip Bag	3 (0.9 oz)	130	7	17	10	70
Chocolate Chip Drop	1 (1 oz)	140	10	11	10	105
Chocolate Chip Ice Box	1 (1 oz)	140	7	19	5	80
Chocolate Chip Mini	12 (1.1 oz)	150	7	20	5	95
Cinnamon Snaps	12 (1.1 oz)	150	7	19	5	115
Coconut Macaroon	1 (0.8 oz)	90	5	14	0	55
Cookie Jar Hermits	1 (1 oz)	110	3	19	<5	160
Dark Chocolate	1 (1 oz)	110	4	20	<5	150
Dutch Chocolate	1 (1 oz)	120	4	19	<5	110
Fig Bars Low Fat	2 (1.1 oz)	100	1	23	0	105
Frosty Lemon	1 (1 oz)	120	5	19	0	110
Frosty Orange	1 (1 oz)	120	4	19	0	140
Fruit And Honey Bar	1 (1 oz)	110	4	18	5	120

FOOD	PORTION	CALS	FAT	CARB	CHOL	SOD
Archway (CONT.)						
Fruit Bar No Fat	1 (1 oz)	90	0	21	0	95
Fruit Cake	1 (1.1 oz)	140	7	20	0	100
Fudge Nut Bar	1 (1 oz)	110	5	17	<5	120
Fun Chip Mini	12 (1.1 oz)	140	6	21	5	100
Gingersnaps	5 (1.1 oz)	130	5	22	0	110
Granola No Fat	1 (0.5 oz)	50	0	11	0	60
Holiday Pak	3 (1.1 oz)	150	8	19	<5	95
Iced Gingerbread	3 (1.1 oz)	140	5	23	5	130
Iced Molasses	1 (1 oz)	110	5	19	0	170
Iced Oatmeal	1 (1 oz)	120	5	19	<5	85
Lemon Snaps	12 (1.1 oz)	150	7	19	5	120
New Orleans Cake	1 (1 oz)	110	4	18	<5	105
Nutty Nougat	3 (1.1 oz)	160	10	18	0	60
Oatmeal	1 (0.9 oz)	110	3	19	<5	95
Oatmeal Apple Filled	1 (1 oz)	110	3	18	<5	105
Oatmeal Date Filled	1 (1 oz)	110	4	18	<5	120
Oatmeal Mini	12 (1.1 oz)	150	8	19	5	130
Oatmeal Pecan	1 (1 oz)	120	5	18	<5	100
Oatmeal Raisin	1 (1 oz)	110	4	19	<5	115
Oatmeal Raisin Bran	1 (1 oz)	110	4	19	<5	100
Old Fashioned Molasses	1 (1 oz)	120	3	20	5	150
Old Fashioned Windmill	1 (0.7 oz)	100	4	15	0	95
Party Treats	3 (1.1 oz)	140	7	20	15	105
Peanut Butter	1 (1 oz)	140	7	16	10	125
Peanut Butter & Chip	3 (0.9 oz)	130	7	16	10	125
Peanut Butter N' Chips	1 (1 oz)	140	7	16	10	115
Peanut Butter Nougat	3 (1.1 oz)	160	9	18	0	**140**
Pecan Crunch	6 (1.1 oz)	150	8	18	10	120
Pecan Ice Box	1 (1 oz)	140	7	18	10	100
Pecan Malted Nougat	3 (1.1 oz)	160	10	17	0	60
Pfeffernusse	2 (1.3 oz)	140	1	32	0	100
Pineapple Filled	1 (0.9 oz)	100	4	16	5	75
Raisin Oatmeal	1 (1 oz)	130	5	19	5	40
Raisin Oatmeal Bag	3 (1 oz)	130	6	19	10	55
Raspberry Filled	1 (1 oz)	110	4	18	5	90
Rocky Road	1 (1 oz)	130	6	18	10	85
Ruth's Golden Oatmeal	1 (1 oz)	120	5	19	<5	135
Select Assortment	3 (0.9 oz)	130	6	18	10	80
Soft Molasses Drop	1 (1 oz)	110	4	18	<5	160
Soft Sugar	1 (1 oz)	110	4	18	5	110

FOOD	PORTION	CALS	FAT	CARB	CHOL	SOD
Archway (CONT.)						
Strawberry Filled	1 (1 oz)	110	4	18	<5	90
Sugar	1 (1 oz)	120	4	20	<5	190
Vanilla Wafer	5 (1.1 oz)	130	4	22	5	130
Wedding Cakes	3 (1.1 oz)	160	8	20	0	45
Bakery Wagon						
Apple Walnut Raisin	1	100	4	16	0	130
Cobbler Apple Cranberry Fat Free	1	70	0	16	0	60
Cobbler Apple Fat Free	1	70	0	17	0	55
Cobbler Mixed Fruit Fat Free	1	70	0	16	0	65
Cobbler Raspberry Fat Free	1	70	0	17	0	60
Ginger Snaps	5	160	7	22	0	140
Honey Fruit Bars	1	100	3	17	5	80
Iced Molasses	1	100	3	18	2	120
Iced Molasses Mini	3	130	3	18	0	170
Oatmeal Apple Filled	1	90	3	14	0	65
Oatmeal Chocolate Chunk	1	100	3	16	0	75
Oatmeal Date Filled	1	90	3	17	0	90
Oatmeal Raspberry Filled	1	100	3	16	0	105
Oatmeal Soft	1	100	4	16	0	90
Oatmeal Walnut Raisin	1	100	4	17	0	125
Vanilla Wafers Cholesterol Free	6	130	6	22	0	140
Baking On The Lite Side						
Oatmeal Crunchy	2 (0.6 oz)	60	0	13	0	20
Raspberry Linzer	1 (0.6 oz)	55	0	12	0	20
Barnum's						
Animal Crackers	12 (1.1 oz)	140	4	23	0	160
Biscos						
Sugar Wafers	8 (1 oz)	140	6	21	0	40
Waffle Cremes	4 (1.2 oz)	180	9	24	0	35
Cadbury						
Fingers	3	85	4	11	2	30
Chip-A-Roos						
Cookies	3 (1.3 oz)	190	10	23	0	150
Chips Ahoy!						
Bit Size Chocolate Chip	14 (1.1 oz)	170	7	21	0	105
Chewy Chocolate Chip	3 (1.3 oz)	170	8	23	<5	125

FOOD	PORTION	CALS	FAT	CARB	CHOL	SOD
Chips Ahoy! (CONT.)						
Chunky Chocolate Chip	1 (0.5 oz)	80	4	11	10	60
Real Chocolate Chip	3 (1.1 oz)	160	8	21	0	105
Reduced Fat	3 (1.1 oz)	150	6	23	0	150
Sprinkled Real Chocolate Chip	3 (1.3 oz)	170	8	24	0	120
Striped Chocolate Chip	1 (0.5 oz)	80	4	10	0	45
Chortles						
Cookies	½ pkg. (1 oz)	125	3	23	0	109
Cookie Lover's						
Blue Ribbon Brownies	1 (0.8 oz)	90	3	14	11	75
Classic Shortbread	1 (0.8 oz)	110	7	12	15	75
Dutch Chocolate Chip	1 (0.8 oz)	90	4	12	14	65
Fancy Peanut Butter	1 (0.8 oz)	100	6	10	7	90
Grahams Cinnamon Honey	2 (1 oz)	110	1	24	0	130
Grahams Honey	2 (1 oz)	100	2	22	0	130
Old-Time Raisin	1 (0.8 oz)	90	3	14	15	60
Delacre						
Cookie Assortment	4 (1.1 oz)	130	<5	18	8	35
Drake's						
Chocolate Chip	2 (1 oz)	140	6	18	0	110
Chocolate- Chocolate Chip	2 (1 oz)	130	5	19	0	85
Coconut	2 (1 oz)	130	5	20	0	95
Coconut Macaroon	1 (1 oz)	135	7	17	0	80
Hermit	1 (2 oz)	230	7	38	10	280
Oatmeal	2 (1 oz)	120	5	19	0	50
Oatmeal Creme	1 (2 oz)	240	9	9	2	250
Peanut Butter Wafers	1 (2.25 oz)	324	16	43	0	135
Dutch Mill						
Chocolate Chip	3 (1.1 oz)	160	10	18	0	85
Coconut Macaroons	3 (1 oz)	120	7	14	0	115
Oatmeal Raisin	3 (1 oz)	130	6	18	0	75
Entenmann's						
Chocolate Chip	3 (0.9 oz)	140	7	19	—	85
Estee						
Chocolate Chip	4 (1.1 oz)	150	7	21	0	30
Coconut	4 (1 oz)	140	6	19	0	25
Creme Wafers Chocolate	7 (1.1 oz)	160	8	21	0	0
Creme Wafers Lemon	5 (1.2 oz)	170	8	23	0	10

FOOD	PORTION	CALS	FAT	CARB	CHOL	SOD
Estee (CONT.)						
Creme Wafers Peanut Butter	5 (1.2 oz)	170	9	21	0	85
Creme Wafers Triple Decker Banana Split	3 (0.9 oz)	140	7	18	0	0
Creme Wafers Triple Decker Chocolate Caramel & Peanut Butter	3 (0.9 oz)	140	7	17	0	45
Creme Wafers Vanilla	7 (1.1 oz)	160	7	22	0	0
Creme Wafers Vanilla & Strawberry	5 (1.2 oz)	170	8	23	0	0
Fig Bars Apple Low Fat	2 (1 oz)	100	1	22	0	25
Fig Bars Cranberry Low Fat	2 (1 oz)	100	1	22	0	20
Fig Bars Low Fat	2 (1 oz)	100	0	23	0	20
Fudge	4 (1 oz)	150	7	19	0	45
Lemon	4 (1 oz)	140	6	19	0	25
Oatmeal Raisin	4 (1 oz)	130	5	19	0	25
Sandwich Chocolate	3 (1.2 oz)	160	6	24	0	60
Sandwich Original	3 (1.2 oz)	160	6	24	0	45
Sandwich Peanut Butter	3 (1.2 oz)	160	7	22	0	55
Sandwich Vanilla	3 (1.2 oz)	160	5	25	0	35
Shortbread Reduced Fat	4 (1 oz)	130	4	22	0	150
Vanilla	4 (1 oz)	140	6	19	0	25
FFV						
Animal Crackers	9	110	3	—	—	—
Caramel Patties	2	150	7	—	—	—
Fig Bars Vanilla	1	60	1	—	—	—
Fig Bars Whole Wheat	1	60	1	—	—	—
Ginger Boys Calcium Enriched	6	120	3	—	—	—
Jelly Tarts	2	110	4	—	—	—
Mint Sandwich	2	160	7	—	—	—
Oatmeal Calcium Enriched	5	130	5	—	—	—
Peanut Butter Sandwich	2	170	8	—	—	—
Regal Grahams	2	140	7	—	—	—
Royal Dainty	2	120	6	—	—	—

FOOD	PORTION	CALS	FAT	CARB	CHOL	SOD
FFV (CONT.)						
T.C. Rounds	2	160	8	—	—	—
Tango	2	160	5	—	—	—
Trolley Cakes Devilsfood	2	120	2	—	—	—
Vanilla Wafers	8	120	5	—	—	—
Famous Amos						
Chocolate Chip	3 (1 oz)	140	6	20	—	100
Chocolate Chip Pecan	3 (1 oz)	150	8	18	—	98
Oatmeal Raisin	3 (1 oz)	134	6	19	—	137
Freihofer's						
Chocolate Chip	2 (0.9 oz)	120	6	16	10	75
Frito Lay						
Peanut Butter Bar	1.75 oz	270	16	30	0	65
Frookie						
7-Grain Oatmeal	1	45	2	7	0	35
Animal Frackers	6	60	2	9	0	25
Apple Cinnamon Oat Bran	1	45	2	7	0	35
Apple Cinnamon Oat Bran	1 lg	120	4	18	0	100
Apple Fruitins	1	60	1	12	0	25
Chocolate Chip	1	45	2	7	0	35
Chocolate Chip	1 lg	120	4	18	0	100
Chocolate Chip Mint	1	45	2	7	0	35
Fig Fruitins	1	60	1	12	0	25
Ginger Spice	1	45	2	7	0	35
Mandarin Chocolate Chip	1	45	2	7	0	35
Oat Bran Muffin	1	45	2	7	0	35
Oat Bran Muffin	1 lg	120	4	18	0	100
Oatmeal Raisin	1	45	2	7	0	35
Oatmeal Raisin	1 lg	120	4	18	0	100
General Mills						
Dunkaroos	1 pkg (1 oz)	130	5	19	0	70
FundaMiddles Vanilla Creme In Chocolate Graham Shells	1 pkg (0.8 oz)	110	4	18	—	120
Girl Scout						
Chalet Cremes Sugar Free	4 (1 oz)	150	6	22	0	55
Do-si-dos	3 (1.2 oz)	170	8	22	0	105
Samoas	2 (1 oz)	160	9	17	0	45
Snaps	7 (1.1 oz)	130	2	26	0	210

FOOD	PORTION	CALS	FAT	CARB	CHOL	SOD
Girl Scout (CONT.)						
Striped Chocolate Chip	3 (1.2 oz)	180	10	20	0	100
Tagalongs	2 (0.9 oz)	150	10	13	0	85
Thin Mints	4 (1 oz)	140	8	18	0	80
Trefoils	5 (1.1 oz)	160	8	20	0	90
Glenny's						
Noah'N Friends Animal Peanut Butter	0.5 oz	65	3	9	—	35
Noah'N Friends Animal Vanilla	0.5 oz	65	2	10	—	35
Noah'N Friends Animal Wheat-Free Oatmeal	0.5 oz	65	2	10	—	20
Nookie Bar	1 (1.15 oz)	138	3	18	—	—
Sesame Nookie	1 (0.5 oz)	60	4	6	—	8
Sesame Nookie	1 pkg (1.5 oz)	180	12	18	—	24
Golden Fruit						
Apple	1 (0.7 oz)	80	2	15	0	55
Cranberry	1 (0.7 oz)	70	1	15	0	55
Cranberry Low Fat	1 (0.7 oz)	70	1	15	0	55
Raisin	1 (0.7 oz)	80	2	15	0	40
Grandma's						
Animal Cookies Candied	5 (1 oz)	140	6	20	0	80
Chocolate Chip	2 (2.75 oz)	370	17	50	5	270
Chocolate Chip Rich'N Chewy	3 (1 oz)	140	6	20	5	80
Fudge Chocolate Chip	2 (2.75 oz)	350	13	54	5	380
Grab Cookie Bits Chocolate	8 (1 oz)	140	6	19	0	180
Grab Cookie Bits Peanut Butter	8 (1 oz)	140	6	19	0	125
Grab Cookie Bits Vanilla	8 (1 oz)	140	6	20	5	75
Oatmeal Apple Spice	2 (2.75 oz)	330	12	51	10	570
Old Time Molasses	2 (2.75 oz)	320	9	58	5	520
Peanut Butter	2 (2.75 oz)	410	30	43	10	410
Raisin Soft	2 (2.75 oz)	320	10	54	10	280
Health Valley						
Amaranth Cookies	1	70	3	12	0	30
Fancy Fruit Chunks Apricot Almond	2	90	4	12	0	45

FOOD	PORTION	CALS	FAT	CARB	CHOL	SOD
Health Valley (CONT.)						
Fancy Fruit Chunks Date Pecan	2	90	4	13	0	45
Fancy Fruit Chunks Raisin Oat Bran	2	70	2	13	0	95
Fancy Fruit Chunks Tropical Fruit	2	90	3	15	0	45
Fancy Peanut Chunks	2	90	3	12	0	55
Fat Free Apple Spice	3	75	tr	17	0	40
Fat Free Apricot Delight	3	75	tr	16	0	40
Fat Free Date Delight	3	75	tr	17	0	40
Fat Free Hawaiian Fruit	3	75	tr	16	0	40
Fat Free Jumbos Apple Raisin	1	70	tr	16	0	35
Fat Free Jumbos Raisin	1	70	tr	16	0	35
Fat Free Jumbos Raspberry	1	70	tr	16	0	35
Fat Free Raisin Oatmeal	3	75	tr	17	0	40
Fiber Jumbos Blueberry Nut	1	100	3	14	0	45
Fiber Jumbos Chunky Pecan	1	100	3	14	0	45
Fiber Jumbos Raisin Nut	1	100	3	14	0	45
Fruit & Fitness	5	200	6	34	0	115
Fruit Jumbos Almond Date	1	70	3	10	0	30
Fruit Jumbos Oat Bran	1	70	2	12	0	35
Fruit Jumbos Raisin Nut	1	70	3	10	0	35
Fruit Jumbos Tropical Fruit	1	70	3	10	0	35
Graham Amaranth	7	110	3	25	0	110
Graham Honey	7	100	4	18	0	125
Graham Oat Bran	7	120	3	20	0	45
Honey Jumbos Crisp Cinnamon	1	70	4	9	0	35
Honey Jumbos Crisp Peanut Butter	1	70	2	11	0	35
Honey Jumbos Fancy Oat Bran	2	130	4	20	0	50

FOOD	PORTION	CALS	FAT	CARB	CHOL	SOD
Health Valley (CONT.)						
Oat Bran Animal Cookies	7	110	4	17	0	50
Oat Bran Fruit & Nut	2	110	4	17	0	70
The Great Tofu	2	90	3	14	0	30
The Great Wheat Free	2	80	3	14	0	35
Heyday						
Caramel & Peanut	1 (0.8 oz)	110	5	13	0	40
Fudge	1 (0.8 oz)	110	5	13	0	40
Honey Maid						
Cinnamon Grahams	10 (1.1 oz)	140	3	26	0	210
Honey Grahams	8 (1 oz)	120	3	22	0	180
Hydrox						
Original	3	150	7	21	0	125
Reduced Fat	3 (1.1 oz)	130	4	24	0	140
Keebler						
Buttercup	3	70	3	11	0	110
Chocolate Fudge Sandwich	1	80	4	12	0	70
Commodore	1	60	2	10	0	65
Cookies Mates	2	50	2	8	0	55
French Vanilla Creme	1	80	4	12	0	80
Graham Honey Fiber Enriched	2	90	2	16	0	110
Graham Kitchen Rich	2	60	2	9	0	55
Homeplate	1	60	2	10	1	130
Keebies	1	80	3	12	0	80
Krisp Kreem Wafers	2	50	3	7	0	20
Old Fashion Chocolate Chip	1	80	4	11	0	75
Old Fashion Double Fudge	1	80	4	11	0	65
Old Fashion Oatmeal	1	80	4	13	0	110
Old Fashion Peanut Butter	1	80	4	10	0	100
Old Fashion Sugar	1	80	3	13	0	70
Pitter Patter	1	90	4	12	0	115
Vanilla Wafers	4	80	4	10	1	60
LU						
Chocolatiers	4 (1.1 oz)	170	8	20	0	35
Chocolatiers Dipped	3 (1 oz)	170	11	17	0	15
Le Petit Ecolier Dark Chocolate	2 (0.9 oz)	130	6	17	5	55
Little Schoolboy Milk Chocolate	2 (0.9 oz)	130	7	15	5	85

FOOD	PORTION	CALS	FAT	CARB	CHOL	SOD
LU (CONT.)						
Marie Lu	3 (1.2 oz)	170	6	25	5	170
Truffle Lu	4 (1.2 oz)	180	11	18	0	410
La Choy						
Fortune	1	15	tr	4	0	1
Lance						
Choc-O-Lunch	1 pkg (37 g)	180	7	26	0	150
Choc-O-Mint	1 pkg (35 g)	180	10	22	0	90
Chocolate Chip Fudge	1 (28 g)	130	5	20	5	130
Chocolate Chip Soft	1 (28 g)	130	5	19	5	100
Coated Graham	1 pkg (50 g)	200	10	24	0	60
Fig Bar	1 pkg (42 g)	150	2	30	0	85
Lem-O-Lunch	1 pkg (48 g)	240	11	32	0	190
Lemon Nekot	1 pkg (42 g)	220	11	28	5	100
Malt	1 pkg (35 g)	190	11	16	0	125
Nut-O-Lunch	1 oz	140	5	—	0	—
Oatmeal	1 (57 G)	130	5	20	0	70
Peanut Butter Creme Filled Wafer	1 pkg (50 g)	240	10	34	0	80
Van-O-Lunch	1 pkg (37 g)	180	7	26	0	150
Little Debbie						
Animal	1 pkg (1.5 oz)	190	5	33	0	110
Caramel Cookie Bars	1 pkg (1.2 oz)	160	8	23	0	90
Chocolate Chip Chewy	1 pkg (2 oz)	370	19	47	10	280
Chocolate Chip Crisp	1 pkg (1.5 oz)	210	12	26	5	150
Cookie Wreaths	1 pkg (0.6 oz)	90	5	11	0	45
Creme Filled Chocolate	1 pkg (1.2 oz)	180	8	24	0	115
Creme Filled Chocolate	1 pkg (1.8 oz)	260	11	36	0	230
Easter Puffs	1 pkg (1.2 oz)	140	5	25	0	65
Figaroos	1 pkg (1.5 oz)	160	4	31	0	115
Figaroos	1 pkg (2 oz)	200	5	40	0	160
Fudge Macaroons	1 pkg (1 oz)	140	8	18	0	65
Ginger	1 pkg (0.7 oz)	90	3	14	5	55
Oatmeal Crisp	1 pkg (1.5 oz)	210	11	27	5	230
Oatmeal Lights	1 pkg (1.3 oz)	140	4	28	0	190
Oatmeal Raisin	1 pkg (2.7 oz)	320	13	50	0	330
Peanut Butter	1 pkg (1.5 oz)	210	10	27	5	230
Peanut Butter & Jelly Sandwich	1 pkg (1.1 oz)	130	5	22	0	100
Peanut Butter Bars	1 pkg (1.9 oz)	270	15	33	0	190
Peanut Clusters	1 pkg (1.4 oz)	190	11	23	0	125
Pecan Shortbread	1 pkg (1.5 oz)	220	13	26	5	170

FOOD	PORTION	CALS	FAT	CARB	CHOL	SOD
Little Debbie (CONT.)						
Pecan Spinwheels	1 pkg (1 oz)	110	4	16	0	100
Lorna Doone						
Cookies	4 (1 oz)	140	7	19	5	130
Mallomars						
Cookies	2 (0.9 oz)	120	5	17	0	35
Mallopuffs						
Cookies	1 (0.6 oz)	70	2	12	0	35
Manischewitz						
Macaroons Chocolate	2 (0.9 oz)	90	4	15	0	80
Mother's						
Almond Shortbread	3	180	11	19	0	115
Butter	5	140	6	21	10	95
Checkerboard Wafers	8	150	8	20	0	40
Chocolate Chip	2	160	8	20	10	105
Chocolate Chip Angel	3	180	9	21	0	70
Chocolate Chip Bag	4	140	5	23	2	85
Chocolate Chip Parade	4	130	5	19	0	100
Circus Animals	6	140	6	20	0	55
Cocadas	5	150	7	20	5	140
Cookie Parade	4	140	7	18	0	95
Dinosaur Grrrahams	2	130	3	24	0	130
Double Fudge	3	170	8	22	0	100
Duplex Creme	3	170	8	23	0	130
English Tea	2	180	7	26	0	100
Fig Bar	2	130	4	24	0	105
Fig Bar Fat Free	1	70	0	16	0	65
Fig Bar Whole Wheat	2	130	5	20	0	140
Fig Bar Whole Wheat Fat Free	1	70	0	17	0	60
Flaky Flix Fudge	2	140	7	17	0	50
Flaky Flix Vanilla	2	140	8	17	0	40
Frosted Holiday	4	130	6	19	0	50
Fudge Bowl Crowns	2	140	6	21	0	55
Fudge Bowl Nuggets	2	140	6	21	0	70
Gaucho Peanut Butter	2	190	10	22	0	200
Gingerbread Man	6	140	6	21	5	160
Iced Oatmeal	2	120	4	20	0	150
Iced Oatmeal Bag	4	120	4	20	0	150
Iced Raisin	2	180	8	24	0	110
MLB Double Header Duplex	3	170	8	23	5	130
Macaroon	2	150	8	18	0	80
Marias	3	170	6	28	5	150

FOOD	PORTION	CALS	FAT	CARB	CHOL	SOD
Mother's (CONT.)						
North Poles	2	140	7	17	0	30
Oatmeal	2	110	5	17	0	150
Oatmeal Chocolate Chip	2	120	5	19	0	140
Oatmeal Raisin	5	150	7	20	5	125
Oatmeal Walnut Chocolate Chip	2	130	6	17	0	135
Pecan Goldens	2	170	11	17	0	110
Rainbow Wafers	8	150	8	20	0	40
Striped Shortbread	3	170	8	22	0	75
Sugar	2	140	6	19	0	75
Taffy	2	180	8	25	0	160
Triplet Assortment	2	140	7	18	0	112
Vanilla Wafers	6	150	6	24	4	85
Walnut Fudge	2	130	7	16	0	90
Zoo Pals	14	140	5	23	0	120
Mystic Mint						
Cookies	1 (0.5 oz)	90	4	11	0	65
Nabisco						
Brown Edge Wafers	5 (1 oz)	140	6	21	<5	80
Bugs Bunny Chocolate Graham	13 (1.1 oz)	140	5	22	0	180
Bugs Bunny Cinnamon Graham	13 (1.1 oz)	140	5	23	0	160
Bugs Bunny Graham	13 (1.1 oz)	140	7	23	0	160
Cameo	2 (1 oz)	130	5	21	0	105
Chocolate Chip Snaps	7 (1.1 oz)	150	5	24	0	115
Chocolate Grahams	3 (1.1 oz)	160	8	21	0	90
Chocolate Snaps	7 (1.1 oz)	140	5	23	0	180
Cookie Break	3 (1.1 oz)	160	6	23	0	115
Danish Imported	5 (1.1 oz)	170	8	22	0	80
Family Favorites Fudge Covered Grahams	3 (1 oz)	140	7	19	0	125
Family Favorites Fudge Striped Shortbread	3 (1.1 oz)	160	8	22	0	140
Family Favorites Oatmeal	1 (0.5 oz)	80	3	12	0	65
Family Favorites Vanilla Sandwich	3 (1.2 oz)	170	8	25	0	120
Famous Chocolate Wafers	5 (1.1 oz)	140	4	24	<5	230

FOOD	PORTION	CALS	FAT	CARB	CHOL	SOD
Nabisco (CONT.)						
Ginger Snaps Old Fashioned	4 (1 oz)	120	3	22	0	170
Grahams	8 (1 oz)	120	3	22	0	180
Marshmallow Puffs	1 (0.75 oz)	90	4	14	0	45
Marshmallow Twirls	1 (1 oz)	130	6	20	0	75
Nilla Wafers	8 (1.1 oz)	140	5	24	5	105
Pecan Passion	1 (0.5 oz)	90	5	9	<5	35
Pinwheels	1 (1 oz)	130	5	21	0	35
National						
Arrowroot	1 (5 g)	20	1	3	0	15
Newtons						
Apple Fat Free	2 (1 oz)	100	0	24	0	60
Cranberry Fat Free	2 (1 oz)	100	0	23	0	95
Fig	2 (1.1 oz)	110	3	20	0	120
Fig Fat Free	1 (1 oz)	100	0	22	0	115
Raspberry Fat Free	2 (1 oz)	100	0	23	0	115
Strawberry Fat Free	2 (1 oz)	100	0	23	0	115
Nutra/Balance						
Chocolate Chip	1 (2 oz)	260	14	34	—	81
Oatmeal Raisin	1 (2 oz)	240	9	36	—	50
Nutter Butter						
Bites Peanut Butter Sandwich	10 (1.1 oz)	150	7	20	<5	125
Peanut Butter Sandwich	2 (1 oz)	130	6	19	<5	110
Peanut Creme Patties	5 (1.1 oz)	160	9	17	0	80
Oreo						
Cookies	3 (1.2 oz)	160	7	23	0	220
Double Stuf	2 (1 oz)	140	7	19	0	150
Fudge Covered	1 (0.75 oz)	110	6	14	0	85
Halloween Treats	2 (1 oz)	140	7	19	0	125
Reduced Fat	3 (1.2 oz)	140	5	24	0	190
White Fudge Covered	1 (0.75 oz)	110	6	14	0	70
Pally						
Butter	4 (0.88 oz)	100	3	17	7	95
Pepperidge Farm						
Beacon Hill Chocolate Chocolate Walnut	1	120	7	14	5	65
Blondie Chocolate Chip Fat Free	1 (1.4 oz)	120	0	29	0	65
Bordeaux	2	70	3	11	0	40
Brownie Chocolate Nut	2	110	7	11	<5	45

FOOD	PORTION	CALS	FAT	CARB	CHOL	SOD
Pepperidge Farm (CONT.)						
Brownie Nut Large	1	140	8	15	5	65
Brussels	2	110	5	13	0	65
Brussels Mint	2	130	7	17	0	40
Butter Chessman	2	90	4	12	10	60
Cappucino	1	50	3	6	<5	20
Capri	1	80	5	10	0	45
Champagne	2	110	6	—	—	—
Chantilly	1	80	2	14	<5	35
Chesapeake Chocolate Chunk Pecan	1	120	7	14	5	60
Cheyenne Peanut Butter Milk Chocolate Chunk	1	110	6	13	5	80
Chocolate Chip	2	100	5	12	5	45
Chocolate Chip Large	1	130	6	16	5	60
Chocolate Chunk Pecan	1	70	4	8	12	25
Dakota Milk Chocolate Oatmeal	1	110	6	15	5	70
Date Pecan	2	110	5	15	10	40
Fruit Filled Apricot-Raspberry	2	100	4	15	10	50
Fruit Filled Strawberry	2	100	5	15	10	50
Geneva	2	130	6	14	0	50
Gingerman	2	70	3	10	5	50
Hazelnut	2	110	6	15	0	75
Irish Oatmeal	2	90	5	13	5	80
Lemon Nut Crunch	2	110	7	13	<5	50
Lido	1	90	5	10	<5	30
Linzer	1	120	4	20	<5	55
Milano	2	120	6	15	15	45
Milk Chocolate Macadamia	2	140	8	—	—	—
Mint Milano	2	150	7	17	5	60
Molasses Crisps	2	70	3	8	0	50
Nantucket Chocolate Chunk	1	120	6	15	5	60
Nassau	1	80	5	9	<5	45
Oatmeal Large	1	120	6	18	5	105
Oatmeal Raisin	2	110	5	15	10	115
Old Fashioned Chocolate Chip	2	100	5	12	5	45

FOOD	PORTION	CALS	FAT	CARB	CHOL	SOD
Pepperidge Farm (CONT.)						
Orange Milano	2	150	7	17	5	60
Orleans	3	90	6	11	0	30
Orleans Sandwich	2	120	8	14	0	40
Paris	2	100	5	—	—	—
Pecan Shortbread	1	70	5	7	0	15
Pirouettes Chocolate Laced	2	70	4	8	<5	20
Pirouettes Original	2	70	4	9	<5	35
Raisin Bran	2	110	5	13	<5	55
Ripple Milk Chocolate Fat Free	1 (0.6 oz)	60	0	13	0	60
Santa Fe Oatmeal Raisin	1	100	4	16	<5	70
Sausalito Milk Chocolate Macadamia	1	120	7	14	5	65
Seville	2	100	5	—	—	—
Shortbread	2	150	8	17	<5	85
Southport	2	170	10	—	—	—
Sugar	2	100	5	13	10	55
Tahiti	1	90	6	9	5	25
Zurich	1	60	2	10	0	30
Pillsbury						
Chocolate Chip	1	70	3	9	5	55
Oatmeal Raisin	1	60	2	10	0	55
Peanut Butter	1	70	3	9	5	75
Sugar	1	70	3	9	5	70
Ritz						
Chocolate Covered	3 (1 oz)	150	9	17	0	95
Sargento						
MooTown Snackers Cookies & Creme Honey Graham Sticks & Vanilla Creme w/Sprinkles	1 pkg (1.1 oz)	140	7	19	0	60
MooTown Snackers Cookies & Creme Vanilla Sticks & Chocolate Fudge Creme	1 pkg (1.1 oz)	140	7	20	0	65
SnackWell's						
Fat Free Cinnamon Grahams	20 (1 oz)	110	0	26	0	90

FOOD	PORTION	CALS	FAT	CARB	CHOL	SOD
SnackWell's (CONT.)						
Fat Free Devil's Food	1 (0.5 oz)	50	0	13	0	25
Fat Free Double Fudge	1 (0.5 oz)	50	0	12	0	70
Golden Devil's Food	1 (0.5 oz)	50	1	12	0	30
Reduced Fat Chocolate Chip	13 (1 oz)	130	4	22	0	170
Reduced Fat Chocolate Sandwich With Chocolate Creme	2 (0.9 oz)	100	3	20	0	190
Reduced Fat Oatmeal Raisin	2 (1 oz)	110	3	20	0	135
Reduced Fat Vanilla Sandwich	2 (0.9 oz)	110	3	21	0	95
Social Tea						
Cookies	6 (1 oz)	120	4	20	5	105
Stella D'Oro						
Almond Toast Mandel	1	60	1	10	tr	43
Angel Bars	1	80	5	7	tr	15
Angel Wings	1	70	5	7	1	40
Angelica Goodies	1	110	4	16	tr	45
Anginetti	1	30	1	5	tr	3
Anisette Sponge	1	50	1	10	tr	40
Anisette Toast	1	50	1	9	tr	50
Anisette Toast Jumbo	1	110	1	23	tr	65
Apple Pastry Low Sodium	1	80	3	14	>5	5
Biscottini Cashews	1	110	6	14	—	50
Breakfast Treats	1	100	4	15	tr	80
Castelets Chocolate	1	60	3	9	tr	33
Chinese Dessert Cookies	1	170	9	19	tr	90
Como Delight	1	150	7	18	1	60
Deep Night Fudge	1	65	4	8	2	33
Dutch Apple Bars	1	110	3	19	1	35
Egg Biscuits Low Sodium	3	120	3	20	40	15
Egg Biscuits Sugared	1	80	1	14	1	45
Egg Jumbo	1	50	1	9	tr	30
Fruit Delight Apple Cinnamon Fat Free	1	70	0	17	0	50
Fruit Delight Peach Apricot Fat Free	1	70	0	17	0	35
Fruit Delight Raspberry Fat Free	1	70	0	17	0	40

FOOD	PORTION	CALS	FAT	CARB	CHOL	SOD
Stella D'Oro (CONT.)						
Fruit Slices	1	60	2	9	tr	45
Fruit Slices Fat Free	1	50	0	12	0	60
Golden Bars	1	110	4	16	tr	65
Holiday Rings & Stars	1	47	1	7	0	12
Holiday Trinkets	1	40	2	5	tr	31
Hostess Assortment	1	40	2	6	tr	20
Indulgente Cashew Biscottini	1 (1.1 oz)	150	8	19	10	70
Kichel Low Sodium	21	150	9	13	80	25
Lady Stella Assortment	1	40	2	6	tr	22
Margherite Chocolate	1	70	3	10	tr	40
Margherite Vanilla	1	70	3	11	tr	45
Peach Apricot Pastry Sodium Free	1	80	3	13	>5	0
Pfeffernusse Spice Drops	1	40	1	7	tr	18
Prune Pastry Dietetic	1	90	3	14	>5	0
Roman Egg Biscuits	1	140	5	20	tr	125
Royal Nuggets	1	2	tr	tr	tr	—
Sesame Regina	1	50	2	6	tr	28
Swiss Fudge	1	70	3	9	tr	33
Sunshine						
Almond Crescents	4 (1.1 oz)	150	6	22	0	105
Animal Crackers	1 box (2 oz)	260	7	43	0	230
Animal Crackers	14 (1.1 oz)	140	4	24	0	125
Classics Chocolate Chip With Pecans	1 (0.7 oz)	110	7	11	3	45
Classics Chocolate Chip With Walnuts	1 (0.7 oz)	100	6	11	5	70
Classics Premier Chocolate Chip	1 (0.7 oz)	100	5	13	5	75
Dixie Vanilla	2 (0.9 oz)	120	5	19	0	105
Fig Bars	2 (1 oz)	110	3	20	0	60
Fudge Family Bears Vanilla	2 (1 oz)	140	6	20	0	115
Fudge Mint Patties	2 (0.8 oz)	130	7	16	0	60
Fudge Striped Shortbread	3 (1.1 oz)	160	8	20	0	85
Ginger Snaps	7 (1 oz)	130	5	22	0	150
Grahams Cinnamon	2 (1.1 oz)	140	6	22	0	150
Grahams Fudge Dipped	4 (1.2 oz)	170	9	21	0	75

FOOD	PORTION	CALS	FAT	CARB	CHOL	SOD
Sunshine (CONT.)						
Grahams Honey	2 (1 oz)	120	4	20	0	130
Grahamy Bears	1 pkg (2 oz)	260	10	41	0	230
Grahamy Bears	10 (1.1 oz)	140	5	22	0	125
Iced Gingerbread	5 (1 oz)	130	6	19	5	135
Iced Oatmeal	2 (0.9 oz)	120	5	18	0	90
Jingles	6 (1.1 oz)	150	5	22	0	115
Lemon Coolers	5 (1 oz)	140	6	21	0	100
Mini Chocolate Chip Cookies	5 (1.1 oz)	160	8	20	0	120
Mini Fudge Royals	15 (1.1 oz)	160	8	20	0	90
Oatmeal Chocolate Chip	3 (1.3 oz)	170	8	23	0	130
Oatmeal Country Style	3 (1.2 oz)	170	7	24	0	160
School House Cookies	20 (1.1 oz)	140	5	23	0	115
Sugar Wafers Chocolate	3 (0.9 oz)	130	7	17	0	30
Sugar Wafers Peanut Butter	4 (1.1 oz)	170	9	19	0	75
Sugar Wafers Vanilla	3 (0.9 oz)	130	6	18	0	20
Tru Blu Chocolate	1 (0.6 oz)	80	3	11	0	64
Tru Blu Lemon	1 (0.6 oz)	80	3	11	0	65
Tru Blu Vanilla	1 (0.5 oz)	80	3	11	0	65
Vanilla Wafers	7 (1.1 oz)	150	7	20	3	110
Vienna Fingers	2 (1 oz)	140	6	21	0	105
Tastykake						
Chocolate Chip Bar	1 (43 g)	190	8	28	5	95
Chocolate Chunk Macadamia Nut	1 pkg (56 g)	310	14	42	40	180
Fudge Bar	1 (50 g)	200	7	35	5	160
Oatmeal Raisin Bar	1 (50 g)	210	8	32	15	250
Soft'N Chewy Chocolate Chip	1 (39 g)	170	7	25	10	170
Soft'n Chewy Chocolate Chocolate Chip	1 (32 g)	170	7	26	5	110
Soft'n Chewy Oatmeal Raisin	1 (39 g)	160	5	27	5	160
Vanilla Sugar Wafer	1 (6 g)	36	2	4	0	10
Teddy Grahams						
Chocolate	24 (1 oz)	140	5	22	0	150
Cinnamon	24 (1 oz)	140	4	23	0	150
Honey	24 (1 oz)	140	4	22	0	150

FOOD	PORTION	CALS	FAT	CARB	CHOL	SOD
Tree Of Life						
Creme Supremes	2 (0.9 oz)	120	5	18	0	90
Creme Supremes Mint	2 (0.9 oz)	120	5	18	0	90
Fat Free Classic Carrot Cake	1 (0.8 oz)	60	0	14	0	50
Fat Free Devil's Food Chocolate	1 (0.8 oz)	70	0	15	0	80
Fat Free Golden Oatmeal Raisin	1 (0.8 oz)	70	0	16	0	40
Fat Free Harvest Fruit & Nut	1 (0.8 oz)	70	0	16	0	45
Fat Free Toasted Almond Butter	1 (0.8 oz)	70	0	16	0	35
Fruit Bars Apple Spice	2 (1.3 oz)	120	3	22	0	120
Fruit Bars Fat Free Fig	1 (0.8 oz)	70	0	16	0	100
Fruit Bars Fat Free Peach Apricot	1 (0.8 oz)	70	0	17	0	110
Fruit Bars Fat Free Wildberry	1 (0.8 oz)	70	0	16	0	170
Fruit Bars Fig	2 (1.3 oz)	120	3	21	0	100
Fruit Bars Peach Apricot	2 (1.3 oz)	120	3	22	0	105
Honey-Sweet Colossal Carrot Cake	1 (0.8 oz)	110	5	16	0	105
Honey-Sweet Lemon Burst	1 (0.8 oz)	110	5	15	0	25
Honey-Sweet Oh-So-Oatmeal	1 (0.8 oz)	110	5	14	0	140
Honey-Sweet Pecans-A-Plenty	1 (0.8 oz)	125	7	14	0	30
Monster Fat Free Carrot Cake	¼ cookie (0.9 oz)	60	0	15	0	30
Monster Fat Free Devil's Food Chocolate	¼ cookie (0.9 oz)	80	0	20	0	45
Monster Fat Free Gingerbread	¼ cookie (0.9 oz)	80	0	19	0	50
Monster Fat Free Maple Pecan	¼ cookie (0.9 oz)	90	0	20	0	50
Royal Vanilla	2 (0.9 oz)	120	5	17	0	115
Small World Animal Grahams	7 (1 oz)	120	3	21	0	60
Small World Chocolate Chip	7 (1 oz)	120	4	20	0	60

FOOD	PORTION	CALS	FAT	CARB	CHOL	SOD
Tree Of Life (CONT.)						
Soft-Bake Chocolate Chip	1 (0.8 oz)	125	7	15	0	15
Soft-Bake Double Fudge	1 (0.8 oz)	110	5	16	0	20
Soft-Bake Maui Macaroon	1 (0.8 oz)	135	10	12	0	0
Soft-Bake Oatmeal	1 (0.8 oz)	115	5	16	0	20
Soft-Bake Peanut Butter	1 (0.8 oz)	125	7	13	0	60
Wheat-Free American Oatmeal	1 (0.8 oz)	90	5	11	0	25
Wheat-Free California Carob	1 (0.8 oz)	105	5	14	0	75
Wheat-Free Georgia Peanut Butter	1 (0.8 oz)	95	6	8	0	110
Wheat-Free Mountain Maple Walnut	1 (0.8 oz)	100	6	9	0	50
Vienna Fingers						
Low Fat	2 (1 oz)	130	4	23	0	95
Weight Watchers						
Apple Raisin Bar	1 (0.75 oz)	70	2	14	0	60
Chocolate Chip	2 (1.06 oz)	140	5	22	0	90
Chocolate Sandwich	2 (1.06)	140	4	23	0	160
Fruit Filled Fig	1 (0.7 oz)	70	0	16	0	50
Fruit Filled Raspberry	1 (0.7 oz)	70	0	16	0	45
Oatmeal Raisin	2 (1.06 oz)	120	2	22	0	90
Vanilla Sandwich	2 (1.06 oz)	140	3	25	0	80

COUGH DROPS

FOOD	PORTION	CALS	FAT	CARB	CHOL	SOD
Halls						
Cough Drops	1 (3.8 g)	15	0	4	0	—
Plus	1 (4.7 g)	18	0	5	0	—
With Vitamin C	1 (3.8 g)	14	0	4	0	—
Lifesavers						
Menthol	2 (0.5 oz)	60	0	14	0	0

CRACKERS

FOOD	PORTION	CALS	FAT	CARB	CHOL	SOD
cheese	14 (½ oz)	71	4	8	2	141
cheese low sodium	14 (½ oz)	71	4	8	2	68
cheese w/ peanut butter filling	1 (0.24 oz)	34	2	4	0	69
crispbread	3	61	2	9	—	—
melba toast	1 (5 g)	19	tr	4	0	41
oyster cracker	1 (1 g)	4	tr	1	0	13

FOOD	PORTION	CALS	FAT	CARB	CHOL	SOD
peanut butter sandwich	1 (7 g)	34	2	4	—	66
saltines	1 (3 g)	13	tr	2	0	38
snack cracker w/ cheese filling	1 (7 g)	33	2	4	0	98
Cheez-It						
Crackers	1 pkg (2 oz)	290	16	31	3	450
Lance						
Bonnie	1 pkg (1.2 oz)	160	7	24	5	170
Captain Wafers w/ Cream Cheese & Chives	1 pkg (1.3 oz)	170	9	23	0	260
Cheese-On-Wheat	1 pkg (1.3 oz)	180	9	22	5	260
Lanchee	1 pkg (1.2 oz)	180	11	19	5	110
Nekot	1 pkg (1.5 oz)	210	10	24	5	95
Nip-Chee	1 pkg (1.3 oz)	180	8	21	5	320
Oyster Crackers	1 pkg (0.5 oz)	70	2	10	0	170
Peanut Butter Wheat	1 pkg (1.3 oz)	190	11	18	0	210
Rye-Chee	1 pkg (1.4 oz)	190	9	22	5	320
Toastchee	1 pkg (1.4 oz)	190	11	19	5	310
Toasty	1 pkg (1.2 oz)	180	10	17	0	160
Little Debbie						
Cheese Crackers With Peanut Butter	1 pkg (0.9 oz)	140	7	16	0	290
Cheese Crackers With Peanut Butter	1 pkg (1.4 oz)	210	10	23	0	430
Toasty Crackers With Peanut Butter	1 pkg (0.9 oz)	140	7	16	0	290
Toasty Crackers With Peanut Butter	1 pkg (1.4 oz)	200	10	20	0	350
Wheat Crackers With Cheddar Cheese	1 pkg (0.9 oz)	140	7	16	5	270
NABS						
Cheese Peanut Butter Sandwich	6 (1.4 oz)	190	10	24	0	390
Peanut Butter Toast Sandwich	6 (1.4 oz)	190	10	24	0	380
Nabisco						
Zings!	1 pkg (1.8 oz)	240	11	34	0	420
Nips						
Cheese	29 (1 oz)	150	6	18	0	310
Pepperidge Farm						
Goldfish Cheddar Cheese	1 pkg (1½ oz)	190	6	28	5	340

FOOD	PORTION	CALS	FAT	CARB	CHOL	SOD
Planters						
Cheese Peanut Butter Sandwiches	1 pkg (1.4 oz)	190	10	24	0	390
Toast Peanut Butter Sandwiches	1 pkg (1.4 oz)	190	10	24	0	380
Ritz						
Sandwiches With Real Cheese	1 pkg (1.4 oz)	210	12	21	5	450
SnackWell's						
Reduced Fat Cheese	38 (1 oz)	130	2	23	0	340

CRANBERRIES
Ocean Spray

FOOD	PORTION	CALS	FAT	CARB	CHOL	SOD
Craisins	⅓ cup (1.4 oz)	130	0	33	0	0

CRANBERRY JUICE
After The Fall

FOOD	PORTION	CALS	FAT	CARB	CHOL	SOD
Cape Cod Cranberry	1 bottle (10 oz)	130	0	30	0	25
Cranberry Ginger Ale	1 can (12 oz)	140	0	35	0	65
Snapple						
Cranberry Royal	10 fl oz	150	0	37	0	25
Tropicana						
Twister Ruby Red	1 bottle (10 fl oz)	150	0	37	0	30

CROISSANT

FOOD	PORTION	CALS	FAT	CARB	CHOL	SOD
cheese	1 (2 oz)	236	12	27	—	316
plain	1 (2 oz)	232	12	26	—	424
plain	1 mini (1 oz)	115	6	13	—	211

DANISH PASTRY
Hostess

FOOD	PORTION	CALS	FAT	CARB	CHOL	SOD
Apple	1 (3.8 oz)	400	22	47	20	340
Apple Fruit Roll	1 (2 oz)	180	4	33	<5	170
Coffee Cake Raspberry	1 (1.2 oz)	110	3	21	<5	110

DATES
Sonoma

FOOD	PORTION	CALS	FAT	CARB	CHOL	SOD
Dried	5-6 (1.4 oz)	110	0	30	0	15

DIP
Breakstone

FOOD	PORTION	CALS	FAT	CARB	CHOL	SOD
Sour Cream Bacon & Onion	2 tbsp (1.1 oz)	60	5	2	20	170
Sour Cream Chesapeake Clam	2 tbsp (1.1 oz)	50	4	2	30	190

FOOD	PORTION	CALS	FAT	CARB	CHOL	SOD
Breakstone (CONT.)						
Sour Cream French Onion	2 tbsp (1.1 oz)	50	4	2	20	160
Sour Cream Jalapeno Cheddar	2 tbsp (1.1 oz)	60	4	2	15	170
Sour Cream Toasted Onion	2 tbsp (1.1 oz)	50	4	2	20	180
Chi-Chi's						
Fiesta Bean	2 tbsp (0.9 oz)	35	2	4	0	140
Fiesta Cheese	2 tbsp (0.9 oz)	40	3	3	10	270
Durkee						
Sour Cream as prep	2 tbsp	25	1	4	0	200
Frito Lay						
Cheddar Cheese	1 oz	45	3	3	6	180
French Onion	1 oz	50	4	3	12	180
Jalapeno Bean	1 oz	30	1	4	0	115
Picante Sauce	1 oz	10	0	3	0	160
Guiltless Gourmet						
Black Bean Mild	1 oz	25	0	5	0	80
Black Bean Spicy	1 oz	25	0	5	0	80
Pinto Bean	1 oz	25	0	5	0	80
Hain						
Hot Bean	4 tbsp	70	1	10	5	250
Mexican Bean	4 tbsp	60	1	9	5	260
Onion Bean	4 tbsp	70	1	10	5	270
Taco Dip & Sauce	4 tbsp	25	1	1	5	350
Heluva Good Cheese						
Bacon Horseradish	2 tbsp (1.1 oz)	60	5	2	20	200
Clam	2 tbsp (1.1 oz)	50	5	2	20	130
French Onion	2 tbsp (1.1 oz)	50	5	2	20	160
Homestyle Onion	2 tbsp (1.1 oz)	60	5	3	20	290
Light French Onion	2 tbsp (1.1 oz)	35	2	3	10	180
Light Jalapeno Cheddar	2 tbsp (1.1 oz)	40	2	3	10	160
Ranch	2 tbsp (1.1 oz)	60	5	2	20	180
Knudsen						
Nacho Cheese	2 tbsp (1.1 oz)	60	4	3	15	200
Sour Cream Bacon & Onion	2 tbsp (1.1 oz)	60	5	2	20	170
Sour Cream French Onion	2 tbsp (1.1 oz)	50	4	2	20	160
Louise's						
Fat Free Honey Mustard	1 oz	40	0	9	0	170

FOOD	PORTION	CALS	FAT	CARB	CHOL	SOD
Louise's (CONT.)						
Fat Free Sour Cream & Onion	1 oz	25	0	4	0	195
Fat Free White Cheese Peppercorn	1 oz	25	0	4	0	195
Marzetti						
Blue Cheese Veggie	2 tbsp	200	21	1	20	230
Lemon Dill Veggie	2 tbsp	140	14	2	25	190
Light Ranch Veggie	2 tbsp	60	7	5	10	290
Ranch Veggie	2 tbsp	140	14	1	25	200
Sour Cream & Onion	2 tbsp	130	14	2	25	200
Southwestern Veggie	2 tbsp	130	14	1	25	170
Spinach Veggie	2 tbsp	130	13	1	20	220
Old El Paso						
Black Bean	2 tbsp (1 oz)	20	0	4	0	150
Cheese 'n Salsa Medium	2 tbsp (1 oz)	40	3	3	<5	300
Cheese 'n Salsa Mild	2 tbsp (1 oz)	40	3	3	<5	300
Chunky Salsa Medium	2 tbsp (1 oz)	15	0	3	0	230
Chunky Salsa Mild	2 tbsp (1 oz)	15	0	3	0	230
Jalapeno	2 tbsp (1 oz)	30	1	4	<5	125
Sealtest						
French Onion	2 tbsp (1.1 oz)	50	4	2	20	160
Snyder's						
Mustard Pretzel	2 tbsp (1.2 oz)	90	4	13	20	20
Wise						
Jalapeno Bean	2 tbsp	25	0	5	0	100
Taco	2 tbsp	12	0	3	0	115

DOUGHNUTS

FOOD	PORTION	CALS	FAT	CARB	CHOL	SOD
cake type unsugared	1 (1.6 oz)	198	11	23	18	257
chocolate coated	1 (1.5 oz)	204	13	21	—	185
chocolate glazed	1 (1.5 oz)	175	8	24	—	143
chocolate sugared	1 (1.5 oz)	175	8	24	—	143
creme filled	1 (3 oz)	307	21	26	20	262
french cruller glazed	1 (1.4 oz)	169	8	24	5	142
frosted	1 (1.5 oz)	204	13	21	—	185
honey bun	1 (2.1 oz)	242	14	27	4	205
jelly	1 (3 oz)	289	16	33	22	249
old fashioned	1 (1.6 oz)	198	11	23	18	257
sugared	1 (1.6 oz)	192	10	23	14	181
wheat glazed	1 (1.6 oz)	162	9	19	9	160
wheat sugared	1 (1.6 oz)	162	9	19	9	160
yeast glazed	1 (2.1 oz)	242	14	27	4	205

FOOD	PORTION	CALS	FAT	CARB	CHOL	SOD
Drake's						
Old Fashion Donuts	1 (1.7 oz)	182	8	25	**10**	238
Powdered Sugar Donut Delites	7 (2.5 oz)	300	15	38	16	316
Dutch Mill						
Cider	1 (2.1 oz)	240	10	35	15	220
Cinnamon	1 (1.8 oz)	210	11	26	15	250
Donut Holes Double-Dipped Chocolate	3 (1.4 oz)	220	16	19	5	140
Donut Holes Shootin' Stars	3 (1.4 oz)	190	10	23	5	110
Double-Dipped Chocolate	1 (2.1 oz)	280	17	31	15	360
Glazed	1 (2.1 oz)	250	12	34	15	220
Glazed Chocolate	1 (2.4 oz)	270	11	40	15	380
Plain	1 (1.8 oz)	210	12	25	15	270
Sugared	1 (1.8 oz)	220	11	27	15	260
Entenmann's						
Crumb Topped	1 (2.1 oz)	260	12	34	—	220
Devil's Food Crumb	1 (2.1 oz)	250	12	34	—	200
Rich Frosted	1 (2 oz)	280	18	27	—	210
Freihofer's						
Assorted	1 (2 oz)	270	17	26	10	170
Hostess						
Assorted Regular	1 (1.6 oz)	200	11	23	10	230
Cinnamon Family Pack	1 (1 oz)	110	5	15	5	140
Cinnamon Swirl	1 (1.6 oz)	180	7	28	<5	220
Crumb Regular	1 (1 oz)	130	8	14	5	115
Frosted Regular	1 (1.4 oz)	180	11	20	5	170
Gem Donettes Cinnamon	6 (3 oz)	320	11	53	10	390
Gem Donettes Frosted	6 (3 oz)	390	23	42	10	360
Gem Donettes Frosted Strawberry Filled	3 (3 oz)	240	13	29	<5	210
Gem Donettes Powdered	6 (3 oz)	350	16	47	10	380
Gem Donettes Powdered Strawberry Filled	3 (3 oz)	210	9	31	<5	210
Glazed Party	1 (2.3 oz)	260	10	39	5	310
Jumbo Frosted	1 (2 oz)	260	16	28	10	240
Jumbo Plain	1 (1.1 oz)	140	7	16	10	190
Jumbo Powdered	1 (1.3 oz)	160	9	19	5	170

FOOD	PORTION	CALS	FAT	CARB	CHOL	SOD
Hostess (CONT.)						
Mini Chocolate	5 (2 oz)	220	9	33	35	220
O's Raspberry Filled Powdered	1 (2.2 oz)	230	10	35	5	230
Old Fashioned Glazed	1 (2.1 oz)	250	12	33	15	230
Old Fashioned Glazed Honey Wheat	1 (2.1 oz)	250	12	33	25	270
Old Fashioned Plain	1 (1.5 oz)	170	9	21	10	230
Plain Regular	1 (1 oz)	120	6	13	5	160
Powdered Family Pack	1 (1 oz)	110	6	15	5	135
Little Debbie						
Donut Sticks	1 pkg (1.6 oz)	210	13	25	5	210
Donut Sticks	1 pkg (2 oz)	250	15	30	5	250
Donut Sticks	1 pkg (2.5 oz)	320	19	37	10	310
Donut Sticks	1 pkg (3 oz)	390	23	45	10	370
Tastykake						
Cinnamon	1 (47 g)	180	8	26	10	210
Frosted Rich	1 (57 g)	260	16	28	10	200
Frosted Rich Mini	1 (14 g)	44	3	8	5	60
Honey Wheat	1 (57 g)	210	8	32	10	200
Honey Wheat Mini	1 (12 g)	40	1	7	5	50
Orange Glazed	1 (57 g)	210	9	32	10	180
Plain	1 (47 g)	190	10	22	10	170
Powdered Sugar	1 (46 g)	180	9	24	24	220
Powdered Sugar Mini	1 (12 g)	40	1	7	5	70

DRINK MIXERS

FOOD	PORTION	CALS	FAT	CARB	CHOL	SOD
whiskey sour mix as prep	3.6 oz	169	0	16	0	48
Bacardi						
Margarita Mix w/ rum	8 fl oz	160	0	24	—	0
Margarita Mix w/o liquor	8 fl oz	100	0	25	0	0
Pina Colada	8 fl oz	140	0	34	0	10
Rum Runner	8 fl oz	140	0	35	0	10
Strawberry Daiquiri w/o liquor	8 fl oz	140	0	35	0	0
Canada Dry						
Collins Mixer	8 fl oz	120	0	25	0	20
Sour Mixer	8 fl oz	90	0	22	0	25
Libby						
Bloody Mary Mix	6 oz	40	0	8	0	1120
McIlhenny						
Tabasco Bloody Mary Mix	8 fl oz	56	tr	11	0	1548

FOOD	PORTION	CALS	FAT	CARB	CHOL	SOD
Schweppes						
Collins Mixer	8 fl oz	100	0	24	0	55
Tabasco						
Bloody Mary Mix Extra Spicy	8 fl oz	58	tr	11	0	1645

EGG ROLLS
Empire

Miniature	6 (4.8 oz)	280	8	43	0	740
La Choy						
Pork Restaurant Style	1 (3 oz)	150	5	20	7	480

EGGNOG

eggnog	1 cup	342	19	34	149	138
eggnog	1 qt	1368	76	138	596	553
Borden						
Light	½ cup	130	2	23	—	80
Hood						
Fat Free	4 fl oz	100	0	21	<5	100
Golden	4 fl oz	180	8	22	65	100

FIGS

fresh	1 med	50	tr	10	0	1
Sonoma						
White Misson Dried	3-4 (1.4 oz)	110	0	26	0	0

FRUIT DRINKS
After The Fall

Amaretto Almond	1 can (12 oz)	170	0	42	0	25
American Pie Cherry	1 can (12 oz)	190	0	35	0	20
Apple Raspberry	1 bottle (10 oz)	110	0	29	0	25
Apple Strawberry	1 bottle (10 oz)	120	0	30	0	23
Banana Casablanca	1 bottle (10 oz)	120	0	24	0	13
Berrymeister	1 can (12 oz)	160	0	40	0	25
Cranberry Meets Raspberry	1 bottle (10 oz)	120	0	29	0	25
Georgia Peach Blend	1 bottle (10 oz)	130	0	33	0	23
Mango Montage	1 bottle (10 oz)	140	0	33	0	15
Maui Grove	1 bottle (10 oz)	120	0	29	0	20
Nantucket Ginger Ale	1 can (12 oz)	140	0	35	0	25
Orange Icicle Cream	1 can (12 oz)	170	0	42	0	25
Oregon Berry	1 bottle (10 oz)	130	0	31	0	30
Passion Of The Islands	1 bottle (10 oz)	125	0	32	0	15
Peach Vanilla	1 can (12 oz)	170	0	42	0	35
Strawberry Vanilla	1 can (12 oz)	160	0	42	0	25

FOOD	PORTION	CALS	FAT	CARB	CHOL	SOD
After The Fall (CONT.)						
Twist O' Strawberry	1 can (12 oz)	190	0	37	0	25
Vanilla Bean Cream	1 can (12 oz)	170	0	42	0	25
Apple & Eve						
Apple Cranberry	6 fl oz	80	0	19	0	5
Apple Grape	6 fl oz	120	0	29	0	0
Cranberry Grape	6 fl oz	100	0	23	0	5
Fruit Punch	6 fl oz	78	0	18	0	0
Raspberry Cranberry	6 fl oz	90	0	21	0	10
BAMA						
Fruit Punch	8.45 fl oz	130	0	32	0	15
Boku						
White Grape Raspberry	16 fl oz	120	0	29	0	75
Crystal Geyser						
Juice Squeeze Citrus Grape	1 bottle (12 fl oz)	145	0	35	0	20
Juice Squeeze Orange & Passion Fruit	1 bottle (12 fl oz)	130	0	31	0	20
Juice Squeeze Passion Fruit & Mango	1 bottle (12 fl oz)	125	0	31	0	20
Juice Squeeze Wild Berry	1 bottle (12 fl oz)	130	0	31	0	20
Dole						
Pineapple Orange	6 fl oz	90	0	22	0	10
Pineapple Orange Banana	6 fl oz	100	0	23	0	10
Pineapple Orange Guava	6 fl oz	100	0	21	0	10
Pineapple Passion Banana	6 fl oz	100	0	21	0	10
Eve Alive						
Citrus	1 bottle (16 fl oz)	120	0	31	0	25
Citrus	1 can (11.5 fl oz)	170	0	43	0	35
Citrus	6 fl oz	90	0	22	0	20
Fresh Samantha						
Banana Strawberry	1 cup (8 oz)	148	1	36	0	—
Beta Yet	1 cup (8 oz)	98	1	24	0	0
Carrot Orange	1 cup (8 oz)	107	1	24	0	—
Colossal C	1 cup (8 oz)	116	0	30	0	—

FOOD	PORTION	CALS	FAT	CARB	CHOL	SOD
Fresh Samantha (CONT.)						
Desperately Seeking C	1 cup (8 oz)	129	1	30	0	0
Protein Blast	1 cup (8 oz)	156	1	30	0	—
Spirulina Fruit Blend	1 cup (8 oz)	129	1	30	0	—
Strawberry Orange	1 cup (8 oz)	120	1	27	0	0
The Big Bang	1 cup (8 oz)	97	1	24	0	0
Hi-C						
Boppin Berry Box	8.45 fl oz	140	0	33	0	30
Double Fruit Box	8.45 fl oz	130	0	32	0	35
Ecto Cooler	1 can (11.5 fl oz)	180	0	45	0	40
Ecto Cooler Box	8.45 fl oz	130	0	32	0	35
Fruit Punch	1 can (11.5 fl oz)	190	0	46	0	40
Fruit Punch Box	8.45 fl oz	140	0	32	0	30
Fruity Bubble Gum Box	8.45 fl oz	130	0	32	0	30
Hula Punch	1 can (11.5 fl oz)	170	0	42	0	40
Hula Punch Box	8.45 fl oz	120	0	30	0	30
Jammin' Apple Box	8.45 fl oz	130	0	33	0	30
Stompin' Banana Berry Box	8.45 fl oz	130	0	32	0	30
Wild Berry Box	8.45 fl oz	130	0	32	0	30
Hood						
Natural Blenders Apple Cranberry Raspberry	1 cup (8 oz)	130	0	32	0	5
Natural Blenders Apple Grape Cherry	1 cup (8 oz)	130	0	32	0	5
Natural Blenders Apple Peach Pear	1 cup (8 oz)	120	0	30	0	5
Natural Blenders Apple Wild Blueberry Strawberry	1 cup (8 oz)	120	0	30	0	5
Natural Blenders Pineapple Orange Kiwi	1 cup (8 oz)	120	0	30	0	5
Juicy Juice						
Apple Grape	1 box (8.45 fl oz)	120	0	29	0	10
Berry	1 bottle (6 fl oz)	90	0	22	0	10
Berry	1 box (8.45 fl oz)	130	0	30	0	15

FOOD	PORTION	CALS	FAT	CARB	CHOL	SOD
Juicy Juice (CONT.)						
Punch	1 bottle (6 fl oz)	100	0	23	0	10
Punch	1 box (8.45 fl oz)	140	0	33	0	10
Tropical	1 bottle (6 fl oz)	110	0	26	0	10
Tropical	1 box (8.45 fl oz)	150	0	36	0	10
Kern's						
Apple Strawberry Nectar	6 fl oz	110	0	26	0	0
Apricot Pineapple Nectar	6 fl oz	110	0	27	0	5
Banana Pineapple Nectar	6 fl oz	110	0	27	0	0
Coconut Pineapple Nectar	6 fl oz	140	0	26	0	25
Orange Banana Nectar	6 fl oz	110	0	25	0	0
Strawberry Banana Nectar	6 fl oz	110	0	28	0	0
Tropical Nectar	6 fl oz	110	0	27	0	5
Kool-Aid						
Koolers Mountainberry Punch	1 box (8.45 fl oz)	142	0	37	0	3
Koolers Rainbow Punch	1 box (8.45 fl oz)	135	0	36	0	3
Koolers Tropical Punch	1 box (8.45 fl oz)	132	0	35	0	3
Libby						
Strawberry Banana Nectar	1 can (11.5 fl oz)	220	0	51	0	10
Mauna La'i						
Island Guava Hawaiian Guava Fruit Juice Drink	8 fl oz	130	0	32	0	35
Mango & Hawaiian Guava Fruit Juice Drink	8 fl oz	130	0	33	0	35
Paradise Guava Hawaiian Guava & Passion Fruit Juice Drink	8 fl oz	130	0	32	0	35
Minute Maid						
Berry Punch Box	8.45 fl oz	130	0	31	0	25

FOOD	PORTION	CALS	FAT	CARB	CHOL	SOD
Minute Maid (CONT.)						
Fruit Punch Box	8.45 fl oz	120	0	31	0	25
Juices To Go Citrus Punch	1 bottle (10 fl oz)	160	0	39	0	35
Juices To Go Citrus Punch	1 can (11.5 fl oz)	180	0	45	0	40
Juices To Go Concord Punch	1 bottle (10 fl oz)	160	0	40	0	35
Juices To Go Concord Punch	1 bottle (16 fl oz)	130	0	32	0	25
Juices To Go Concord Punch	1 can (11.5 fl oz)	180	0	46	0	40
Juices To Go Fruit Punch	1 bottle (10 fl oz)	160	0	39	0	35
Juices To Go Fruit Punch	1 bottle (16 fl oz)	120	0	31	0	25
Juices To Go Fruit Punch	1 can (11.5 fl oz)	180	0	44	0	40
Juices To Go Orange Blend	1 bottle (10 fl oz)	150	0	37	0	35
Juices To Go Orange Blend	1 can (11.5 fl oz)	170	0	43	0	40
Tropical Punch Box	8.45 fl oz	130	0	32	0	25
Odwalla						
Boyzenberry Mango	8 fl oz	140	0	34	0	20
C Monster	16 fl oz	300	0	72	0	110
Fruitshake Blackberry	8 fl oz	160	0	39	0	50
Guanaba Dabba Doo!	8 fl oz	130	0	29	0	35
Lotta Colada	8 fl oz	160	3	33	—	45
Mango Tango	8 fl oz	150	3	37	—	55
Mo Beta	16 fl oz	280	1	69	—	290
Raspberry Smoothie	8 fl oz	140	0	35	0	25
Strawberry Banana Smoothie	8 fl oz	100	0	26	0	10
Strawberry Go Man Go	8 fl oz	100	1	26	—	25
Super Protein	16 fl oz	400	6	40	—	250
Pek						
Mango Guava Ecstasy	1 bottle (20 fl oz)	110	0	27	0	20
Passionate Peach Grapefruit	8 fl oz	110	0	27	0	20
Snapple						
Diet Kiwi Strawberry	8 fl oz	13	0	3	0	10

FOOD	PORTION	CALS	FAT	CARB	CHOL	SOD
Snapple (CONT.)						
Fruit Punch	8 fl oz	120	0	29	0	5
Kiwi Strawberry Cocktail	8 fl oz	130	0	33	0	10
Melonberry Cocktail	8 fl oz	120	0	29	0	10
Vitamin Supreme	10 fl oz	150	0	38	0	20
Squeezit						
Berry B. Wild	1 (6.75 fl oz)	90	0	22	0	0
Chucklin' Cherry	1 (6.75 fl oz)	90	0	23	0	5
Grumpy Grape	1 (6.75 fl oz)	90	0	23	0	0
Mean Green Puncher	1 (6.75 fl oz)	90	0	23	0	0
Silly Billy Strawberry	1 (6.75 fl oz)	90	0	23	0	0
Smarty Arty Orange	1 (6.75 fl oz)	90	0	23	0	50
Tropicana						
Citrus Punch	1 bottle (10 fl oz)	180	0	45	0	15
Cranberry Punch	1 bottle (10 fl oz)	170	0	43	0	10
Cranberry Punch	1 can (11.5 fl oz)	200	0	49	0	15
Fruit Punch	1 bottle (10 fl oz)	150	0	39	0	25
Fruit Punch	1 can (11.5 fl oz)	170	0	42	0	30
Fruit Punch	1 container (10 fl oz)	160	0	39	0	25
Orange Pineapple	1 bottle (10 fl oz)	130	0	32	0	15
Pineapple Punch	1 bottle (10 fl oz)	160	0	39	0	20
Twister Apple Raspberry Blackberry	1 bottle (10 fl oz)	150	0	38	0	25
Twister Apple Raspberry Blackberry	1 can (11.5 fl oz)	180	0	44	0	25
Twister Cranberry Raspberry Strawberry	1 bottle (10 fl oz)	160	0	39	0	5
Twister Light Cranberry Raspberry Strawberry	1 container (10 fl oz)	50	0	13	0	15
Twister Light Orange Cranberry	1 container (10 fl oz)	35	0	9	0	25

FOOD	PORTION	CALS	FAT	CARB	CHOL	SOD
Tropicana (CONT.)						
Twister Light Orange Cranberry	1 container (10 fl oz)	35	0	9	0	25
Twister Light Orange Raspberry	1 container (10 fl oz)	45	0	11	0	25
Twister Light Orange Strawberry Banana	1 container (10 fl oz)	45	0	11	0	25
Twister Light Orange Strawberry Banana	1 container (10 fl oz)	45	0	11	0	25
Twister Orange Cranberry	1 bottle (10 fl oz)	140	0	36	0	20
Twister Orange Cranberry	1 container (10 fl oz)	140	0	35	0	20
Twister Orange Peach	1 bottle (10 fl oz)	140	0	36	0	25
Twister Orange Peach	1 can (11.5 fl oz)	160	0	41	0	20
Twister Orange Raspberry	1 bottle (10 fl oz)	140	0	36	0	20
Twister Orange Strawberry Banana	1 container (10 fl oz)	140	0	35	0	20
Twister Strawberry Banana	1 bottle (10 fl oz)	140	0	35	0	20
Twister Strawberry Banana	1 can (11.5 fl oz)	160	0	41	0	30
Twister Strawberry Guava	1 bottle (10 fl oz)	140	0	35	0	25
FRUIT MIXED						
Big Valley						
Cup A Fruit	1 pkg (4 oz)	50	0	7	0	0
Del Monte						
Snack Cups Mixed Fruit Fruit Naturals	1 serv (4.5 oz)	60	0	16	0	10
Snack Cups Mixed Fruit Fruit Naturals EZ-Open Lid	1 serv (4.5 oz)	60	0	15	0	10
Snack Cups Mixed Fruit In Heavy Syrup	1 serv (4.5 oz)	100	0	24	0	10
Snack Cups Mixed Fruit In Heavy Syrup EZ-Open Lid	1 serv (4.2 oz)	90	0	23	0	10
Snack Cups Mixed Fruit Lite	1 serv (4.5 oz)	60	0	16	0	10

FOOD	PORTION	CALS	FAT	CARB	CHOL	SOD
Del Monte (CONT.)						
Snack Cups Mixed Fruit Lite EZ-Open Lid	1 serv (4.5 oz)	60	0	15	0	10
Planters						
Fruit'n Nut Mix	1 oz	140	9	13	0	105
FRUIT SNACKS						
fruit leather	1 bar (0.8 oz)	81	1	18	0	18
fruit leather pieces	1 pkg (0.9 oz)	92	2	21	0	109
fruit leather rolls	1 lg (0.7 oz)	73	1	18	0	13
fruit leather rolls	1 sm (0.5 oz)	49	tr	12	0	8
Betty Crocker						
String Thing Berry 'N Blue	1 pkg (0.7 oz)	80	1	17	0	40
String Thing Cherry	1 pkg (0.7 oz)	80	1	17	0	40
String Thing Strawberry	1 pkg (0.7 oz)	80	1	17	0	40
Brock						
Beauty & The Beast	1 pkg (0.9 oz)	90	0	21	0	25
Cinderella	1 pkg (0.9 oz)	90	0	21	0	25
Dinosaurs	1 pkg (0.9 oz)	90	0	21	0	25
Ninja Trolls	1 pkg (0.9 oz)	90	0	21	0	25
Sharks	1 pkg (0.9 oz)	90	0	21	0	25
Del Monte						
Sierra Trail Mix	1 pkg (0.9 oz)	110	6	15	0	45
Sierra Trail Mix	1 pkg (1 oz)	120	6	16	0	50
Sierra Trail Mix	¼ cup (1.2 oz)	150	8	20	0	65
Fruit By The Foot						
Cherry	1	80	2	18	—	45
Grape	1	80	2	18	—	45
Strawberry	1	80	2	18	—	45
Fruit Roll-Ups						
Cherry	1 (½ oz)	50	tr	12	—	40
Crazy Colors	1 (½ oz)	50	tr	12	—	40
Fruit Punch	1 (½ oz)	50	tr	12	—	40
Grape	1 (½ oz)	50	tr	12	—	40
Raspberry	1 (½ oz)	50	tr	12	—	40
Strawberry	1 (½ oz)	50	tr	12	—	40
Health Valley						
Bakes Apple	1 bar	100	3	16	0	25
Bakes Date	1 bar	100	3	16	0	25
Bakes Raisin	1 bar	100	3	16	0	20
Fat Free Fruit Bars 100% Organic Apple	1 bar	140	tr	33	0	10

FOOD	PORTION	CALS	FAT	CARB	CHOL	SOD
Health Valley (CONT.)						
Fat Free Fruit Bars 100% Organic Apricot	1 bar	140	tr	33	0	10
Fat Free Fruit Bars 100% Organic Date	1 bar	140	tr	33	0	10
Fat Free Fruit Bars 100% Organic Raisin	1 bar	140	tr	33	0	10
Fruit & Fitness Bars	2 bars	200	5	35	0	75
Oat Bran Bakes Apricot	1 bar	100	3	16	0	15
Oat Bran Bakes Fig & Nut	1 bar	110	3	16	0	10
Oat Bran Jumbo Fruit Bar Almond & Date	1 bar	170	5	28	0	10
Oat Bran Jumbo Fruit Bars Raisin & Cinnamon	1 bar	160	2	32	0	10
Rice Bran Jumbo Fruit Bars Almond & Date	1 bar	160	5	27	0	5
Seneca						
Apple Chips	12 chips (1 oz)	140	7	20	0	15
Sonoma						
Trail Mix	¼ cup (1.4 oz)	160	7	24	0	5
Sovex						
Fruit Bites Jungle Pals	1 pkg (0.9 oz)	90	1	21	0	15
Stretch Island						
Fruit Leather Berry Blackberry	2 pieces (1 oz)	90	0	24	0	0
Fruit Leather Chunky Cherry	2 pieces (1 oz)	90	0	24	0	0
Fruit Leather Great Grape	2 pieces (1 oz)	90	0	24	0	0
Fruit Leather Organic Apple	2 pieces (1 oz)	90	0	24	0	10
Fruit Leather Organic Grape	2 pieces (1 oz)	90	0	24	0	5
Fruit Leather Organic Raspberry	2 pieces (1 oz)	90	0	25	0	10
Fruit Leather Rare Raspberry	2 pieces (1 oz)	90	0	24	0	0
Fruit Leather Snappy Apple	2 pieces (1 oz)	90	0	25	0	0

FOOD	PORTION	CALS	FAT	CARB	CHOL	SOD
Stretch Island (CONT.)						
Fruit Leather Tangy Apricot	2 pieces (1 oz)	90	0	23	0	0
Fruit Leather Truly Tropical	2 pieces (1 oz)	90	0	22	0	0
Sunbelt						
Fruit Boosters Apple	1 (1.3 oz)	130	2	27	0	60
Fruit Boosters Blueberry	1 (1.3 oz)	130	2	27	0	60
Fruit Boosters Strawberry	1 (1.3 oz)	130	2	27	0	65
Fruit Jammers	1 (1 oz)	100	1	23	0	20
Sunkist						
Fruit Roll Apple	1 (0.7 oz)	70	0	17	0	20
Fruit Roll Apricot	1	76	1	18	0	17
Fruit Roll Apricot	1 (0.5 oz)	70	0	17	0	15
Fruit Roll Cherry	1 (0.5 oz)	50	0	11	0	10
Fruit Roll Cherry	1 (0.7 oz)	70	0	17	0	160
Fruit Roll Fruit Punch	1 (0.7 oz)	70	0	17	0	25
Fruit Roll Grape	1	76	tr	19	0	13
Fruit Roll Grape	1 (0.5 oz)	50	0	11	0	25
Fruit Roll Grape	1 (0.7 oz)	80	0	17	0	0
Fruit Roll Raspberry	1 (0.5 oz)	45	0	11	0	15
Fruit Roll Raspberry	1 (0.7 oz)	70	0	17	0	20
Fruit Roll Strawberry	1 (0.5 oz)	45	0	11	0	15
Fruit Roll Strawberry	1 (0.7 oz)	70	0	17	0	20
Weight Watchers						
Apple	1 pkg (0.5 oz)	50	0	13	0	125
Apple Chips	1 pkg (0.75 oz)	70	0	18	0	125
Cinnamon	1 pkg (0.5 oz)	50	0	13	0	125
Peach	1 pkg (0.5 oz)	50	0	13	0	125
Strawberry	1 pkg (0.5 oz)	50	0	13	0	125

GELATIN
Del Monte

FOOD	PORTION	CALS	FAT	CARB	CHOL	SOD
Gel Snack Cups Blue Berry	1 serv (3.5 oz)	70	0	19	0	40
Gel Snack Cups Cherry	1 serv (3.5 oz)	70	0	19	0	40
Gel Snack Cups Orange	1 serv (3.5 oz)	70	0	19	0	40
Gel Snack Cups Strawberry	1 serv (3.5 oz)	70	0	19	0	40

FOOD	PORTION	CALS	FAT	CARB	CHOL	SOD
Hunt's						
Snack Pack Juicy Gels Cherry	1 (4 oz)	100	0	25	0	42
Snack Pack Juicy Gels Lemon Lime	1 (4 oz)	100	0	25	0	42
Snack Pack Juicy Gels Mixed Fruit	1 (4 oz)	100	0	25	0	42
Snack Pack Juicy Gels Orange	1 (4 oz)	100	0	25	0	42
Snack Pack Juicy Gels Strawberry	1 (4 oz)	100	0	25	0	42
Kozy Shack						
Gel Treat Cherry	1 pkg (4 oz)	100	0	25	0	25
Gel Treat Lemon Lime	1 pkg (4 ez)	100	0	25	0	25
Gel Treat Orange	1 pkg (4 oz)	100	0	25	0	25
Gel Treat Strawberry	1 pkg (4 oz)	100	0	25	0	25
Gel Treat Sugar Free Orange	1 pkg (4 oz)	10	0	2	0	25
Gel Treat Sugar Free Strawberry	1 pkg (4 oz)	10	0	2	0	25

GRANOLA BARS

FOOD	PORTION	CALS	FAT	CARB	CHOL	SOD
almond	1 (1 oz)	140	7	18	0	73
chewy chocolate coated chocolate chip	1 (1 oz)	132	7	18	1	57
chewy chocolate coated peanut butter	1 (1 oz)	144	9	15	3	55
chewy raisin	1 (1 oz)	127	5	19	0	80
chocolate chip	1 (1 oz)	124	5	20	0	97
chocolate chip chewy	1 (1 oz)	119	5	10	0	77
chocolate chip graham & marshmallow chewy	1 (1 oz)	121	4	20	0	90
nut & raisin chewy	1 (1 oz)	129	6	18	0	72
peanut	1 (1 oz)	136	6	18	0	79
peanut butter	1 (1 oz)	137	7	18	0	80
peanut butter chewy	1 (1 oz)	121	5	18	0	116
peanut butter & chocolate chip chewy	1 (1 oz)	122	6	18	0	93
plain	1 (1 oz)	134	7	18	0	83
plain chewy	1 (1 oz)	126	5	19	0	79
Carnation						
Chocolate Chunk	1 (1.26 oz)	140	5	23	0	65
Honey & Oats	1 (1.26 oz)	130	4	23	0	60
Fi-Bar						
Coconut	1	120	4	20	0	30

FOOD	PORTION	CALS	FAT	CARB	CHOL	SOD
Fi-Bar (CONT.)						
Peanut Butter	1	130	4	20	0	30
General Mills						
Nature Valley Cinnamon	1	120	5	17	0	70
Nature Valley Oat Bran Honey Graham	1	110	4	16	0	90
Nature Valley Oats N'Honey	1	120	5	17	0	65
Nature Valley Peanut Butter	1	120	6	15	0	70
Nature Valley Rice Bran Cinnamon Graham	1	90	4	13	0	75
Grist Mill						
Chewy Apple Cinnamon	1 (1 oz)	120	4	21	0	35
Chewy Chocolate Chip	1 (1 oz)	130	4	21	0	30
Chewy Chunky Nut & Raisin	1 (1 oz)	130	6	18	0	35
Chewy Peanut Butter	1 (1 oz)	130	5	20	0	45
Chewy Peanut Butter Chocolate	1 (1 oz)	130	4	20	0	40
Chocolate Snack Chocolate Chip	1 (1.2 oz)	180	10	21	5	60
Chocolate Snack Nutty Fudge	1 (1.3 oz)	190	11	19	5	90
Crunchy Cinnamon	1 (0.8 oz)	110	5	16	0	60
Crunchy Oats 'N Honey	1 (0.8 oz)	110	5	15	0	60
Hershey						
Chocolate Covered Chocolate Chip	1 (1.2 oz)	170	8	22	—	50
Chocolate Covered Cocoa Creme	1 (1.2 oz)	180	9	22	5	50
Chocolate Covered Cookies & Creme	1 (1.2 oz)	170	8	22	—	50
Chocolate Covered Peanut Butter	1 (1.2 oz)	180	10	19	5	65
Kellogg's						
Low Fat Crunchy Almond & Brown Sugar	1 (0.7 oz)	80	2	16	0	60
Low Fat Crunchy Apple Spice	1 (0.7 oz)	80	2	16	0	60

FOOD	PORTION	CALS	FAT	CARB	CHOL	SOD
Kellogg's (CONT.)						
Low Fat Crunchy Cinnamon Raisin	1 (0.7 oz)	80	2	16	0	60
Kudos						
Chocolate Chunk	1 (0.7 oz)	90	3	13	0	60
Chocolate Coated Chocolate Chip	1 (1 oz)	120	5	18	5	75
Chocolate Coated Milk & Cookies	1 (1 oz)	130	5	18	5	70
Chocolate Coated Nutty Fudge	1 (1 oz)	130	5	18	5	65
Chocolate Coated Peanut Butter	1 (1 oz)	130	5	18	5	85
Low Fat Blueberry	1 (0.7 oz)	90	2	15	0	90
Low Fat Strawberry	1 (0.7 oz)	80	2	15	0	90
New Country						
Chocolate Covered Cookies & Creme	1	200	11	23	—	85
Quaker						
Chewy Chocolate Chip	1	128	5	19	tr	90
Chewy Chunky Nut & Raisin	1	131	6	17	tr	86
Chewy Cinnamon Raisin	1	128	5	19	tr	92
Chewy Honey & Oats	1	125	4	19	tr	95
Chewy Peanut Butter	1	128	5	18	tr	116
Chewy Peanut Butter Chocolate Chip	1	131	6	17	tr	112
Dipps Caramel Nut	1	148	6	21	2	81
Dipps Chocolate Chip	1	139	6	19	1	78
Dipps Chocolate Fudge	1	160	8	20	—	74
Dipps Peanut Butter	1	170	9	9	2	74
Dipps Peanut Butter Chocolate Chip	1	174	10	10	—	102
Sunbelt						
Chewy Chocolate Chip	1 (1.25 oz)	160	7	23	0	65
Chewy Chocolate Chip	1 (1.8 oz)	220	10	32	0	95
Chewy Oats & Honey	1 (1 oz)	130	5	19	0	65
Chewy Oats & Honey	1 (1.7 oz)	210	9	32	0	105
Chewy With Almonds	1 (1 oz)	130	7	17	0	60
Chewy With Almonds	1 (1.5 oz)	190	10	25	0	95
Chewy With Raisins	1 (1.2 oz)	150	6	25	0	65
Fudge Dipped Chewy Chocolate Chip	1 (1.5 oz)	190	8	28	0	80

FOOD	PORTION	CALS	FAT	CARB	CHOL	SOD
Sunbelt (CONT.)						
Fudge Dipped Chewy Macaroo	1 (1.4 oz)	200	13	22	0	60
Fudge Dipped Chewy Macaroo	1 bar (2 oz)	280	17	32	0	90
Fudge Dipped Chewy With Peanuts	1 (2 oz)	270	15	32	0	95
Fudge Dipped Chewy With Peanuts	1 bar (1.5 oz)	210	12	24	0	65

GRAPE JUICE
Hi-C

Box	8.45 fl oz	130	0	33	0	30
Drink	1 can (11.5 fl oz)	180	0	46	0	45
Juicy Juice						
Drink	1 bottle (6 fl oz)	90	0	22	0	5
Drink	1 box	130	0	31	0	10

GRAPEFRUIT

pink fresh	½	37	tr	9	0	0
pink sections fresh	1 cup	69	tr	18	0	1
red fresh	½	37	tr	9	0	0
white fresh	½	39	tr	10	0	0
white sections fresh	1 cup	76	tr	19	0	0

GRAPEFRUIT JUICE
After The Fall

Pink	1 bottle (10 oz)	100	0	23	0	10
Crystal Geyser						
Juice Squeeze	1 bottle (12 fl oz)	150	0	36	0	20
Fresh Samantha						
Juice	1 cup (8 oz)	101	0	24	0	0
Minute Maid						
Juices To Go	1 bottle (10 fl oz)	120	0	29	0	35
Juices To Go	1 bottle (16 fl oz)	100	0	23	0	25
Juices To Go	1 can (11.5 fl oz)	140	0	33	0	40
Juices To Go Pink Cocktail	1 bottle (10 fl oz)	140	0	34	0	35
Juices To Go Pink Cocktail	1 bottle (16 fl oz)	110	0	27	0	25

FOOD	PORTION	CALS	FAT	CARB	CHOL	SOD
Tropicana						
Juice	1 container (6 fl oz)	80	0	19	0	0
Ruby Red	1 container (10 fl oz)	120	0	30	0	0
Season's Best	1 bottle (10 fl oz)	110	0	27	0	5
Season's Best	1 bottle (7 fl oz)	80	0	19	0	5
Season's Best	1 can (11.5 fl oz)	120	0	31	0	5
Twister Light Pink	1 container (10 fl oz)	50	0	12	0	25
Twister Pink	1 can (11.5 fl oz)	160	0	40	0	30
Twister Pink	1 container (10 fl oz)	140	0	35	0	25
GRAPES						
fresh	10	36	tr	9	0	1
GUANABANA JUICE						
Libby						
Nectar	1 can (11.5 fl oz)	210	0	50	0	25
GUAVA						
fresh	1	45	1	11	0	2
GUAVA JUICE						
Libby						
Nectar	1 can (11.5 fl oz)	220	0	54	0	10
Snapple						
Guava Mania	8 fl oz	110	0	29	0	0
HAM DISHES						
Croissant Pocket						
Stuffed Sandwich Ham & Cheddar	1 piece (4.5 oz)	360	17	39	45	710
Hillshire						
Lunch 'N Munch Cooked Ham/Swiss	1 pkg (4.5 oz)	360	22	19	—	1380
Lunch 'N Munch Cooked Ham/Swiss Oreo	1 pkg (4.125 oz)	370	21	30	—	1160
Lunch 'N Munch Cooked Ham/Swiss Snickers/Hi-C	1 pkg (4.25 oz + 6 fl oz)	470	21	54	—	1180

FOOD	PORTION	CALS	FAT	CARB	CHOL	SOD
Hillshire (CONT.)						
Lunch 'N Munch Honey Ham/ Cheddar/ Snickers/ Hi-C	1 pkg (4.25 oz) + 6 fl oz)	500	23	56	—	1030
Hot Pocket						
Stuffed Sandwich Ham & Cheese	1 (4.5 oz)	340	15	37	45	840
Oscar Mayer						
Lunchables Cookies/ Ham/ Swiss	1 pkg (4.2 oz)	360	19	29	50	1420
Lunchables Dessert Chocolate Pudding/ Ham/ American	1 pkg (6.2 oz)	390	20	34	55	1540
Lunchables Ham/ Cheddar	1 pkg (4.5 oz)	340	20	19	75	1830
Lunchables Ham/ Garden Vegetable Cheese	1 pkg (4.5 oz)	380	21	36	45	1240
Lunchables Honey Ham/Herb & Chive Cheese	1 pkg (4.5 oz)	390	21	37	45	1270
Ovenstuffs						
Ham/Turkey Deli Melt	1 (4.75 oz)	360	15	35	—	1050
Weight Watchers						
Ham & Cheese Pocket Sandwich	1 (5 oz)	240	7	32	10	490
Hickory Smoked Ham & Cheddar Pretzel Sandwich	1 (4 oz)	260	8	33	10	580

HONEYDEW

FOOD	PORTION	CALS	FAT	CARB	CHOL	SOD
fresh cubed	1 cup	60	tr	16	0	17
fresh wedge	1/10	46	tr	12	0	13

ICE CREAM AND FROZEN DESSERTS

FOOD	PORTION	CALS	FAT	CARB	CHOL	SOD
chocolate	1/2 cup (4 fl oz)	143	7	19	22	50
dixie cup chocolate	1 (3.5 fl oz)	125	6	16	20	44
dixie cup strawberry	1 (3.5 fl oz)	112	5	16	17	35
dixie cup vanilla	1 (3.5 fl oz)	116	6	14	25	46
freeze dried ice cream chocolate strawberry & vanilla	1 pkg (0.75 oz)	158	5	24	1	97
french vanilla soft serve	1/2 cup (4 fl oz)	185	11	19	78	52
french vanilla soft serve	1/2 gal	3014	180	306	1226	1228

FOOD	PORTION	CALS	FAT	CARB	CHOL	SOD
strawberry	½ cup (4 fl oz)	127	6	18	19	40
vanilla	½ cup (4 fl oz)	132	7	16	29	53
vanilla light	½ cup (2.3 oz)	92	3	15	9	56
vanilla rich	½ cup (2.6 oz)	178	12	17	45	41
vanilla soft serve	½ cup	111	2	19	10	62
vanilla 10% fat	½ gal	2153	115	254	476	929
vanilla 16% fat	½ gal	2805	190	256	256	868
vanilla light	1 cup	184	6	29	18	105
vanilla light	½ gal	1469	45	232	146	836
vanilla light soft serve	1 cup	223	5	38	13	163
vanilla light soft serve	½ gal	1787	37	307	106	1303
3 Musketeers						
Single Chocolate	1 (2 fl oz)	160	10	16	20	30
Single Vanilla	1 (2 fl oz)	160	10	16	15	30
Snack Chocolate	1 (0.72 fl oz)	60	4	6	5	10
Snack Vanilla	1 (0.72 fl oz)	60	4	6	5	10
Avari						
Creme Glace All Flavors	1 oz	10	0	3	0	35
Ben & Jerry's						
Banana Walnut	½ cup (3.9 oz)	290	21	26	75	50
Butter Pecan	½ cup (3.9 oz)	310	26	20	100	160
Cherry Garcia	½ cup (3.7 oz)	240	16	25	80	60
Cherry Vanilla	½ cup (3.9 oz)	240	15	26	85	60
Chocolate Chip Cookie Dough	½ cup (3.7 oz)	270	17	30	80	95
Chocolate Fudge Brownie	½ cup (3.7 oz)	250	14	31	50	100
Chunky Monkey	½ cup (3.7 oz)	280	19	29	70	50
Coconut Almond	½ cup (3.7 oz)	260	20	19	80	80
Coconut Almond Fudge Chip	½ cup (3.8 oz)	320	25	24	75	85
Coffee Almond Fudge	½ cup (3.7 oz)	290	20	24	75	85
Coffee Toffee Crunch	½ cup (3.7 oz)	280	19	28	80	120
English Toffee Crunch	½ cup (4 oz)	310	21	30	90	130
Mint Chocolate Cookie	½ cup (3.8 oz)	260	17	27	80	120
New York Super Fudge Chunk	½ cup (3.7 oz)	290	20	28	50	55
No Fat Strawberry	½ cup (3.3 oz)	140	0	31	0	60
No Fat Vanilla Fudge Swirl	½ cup (3.1 oz)	150	0	32	0	80
Peanut Butter Cup	½ cup (4.1 oz)	370	26	30	75	140
Pop Chocolate Chip Cookie Dough	1 (4.1 oz)	450	28	48	60	150

FOOD	PORTION	CALS	FAT	CARB	CHOL	SOD
Ben & Jerry's (CONT.)						
Pop English Toffee Crunch	1 (3.7 oz)	340	23	35	75	55
Pop Vanilla	1 (3.9 oz)	360	28	30	75	75
Rain Forest Crunch	½ cup (3.7 oz)	300	23	24	85	140
Smooth Aztec Harvest Coffee	½ cup (3.8 oz)	230	16	22	90	55
Smooth Deep Dark Chocolate	½ cup (3.9 oz)	260	15	32	55	55
Smooth Double Chocolate Fudge	½ cup (4.1 oz)	280	16	35	55	60
Smooth Mocho Fudge	½ cup (4 oz)	270	18	30	85	65
Smooth Vanilla	½ cup (3.8 oz)	230	17	21	95	55
Smooth Vanilla Bean	½ cup (3.8 oz)	230	17	21	95	55
Smooth Vanilla Caramel Fudge	½ cup (4.1 oz)	280	17	33	95	75
Smooth White Russian	½ cup (3.8 oz)	240	16	23	90	55
Vanilla	½ cup (3.7 oz)	230	17	21	95	55
Wavy Gravy	½ cup (4.1 oz)	330	24	29	80	95
Bon Bons						
Vanilla With Milk Chocolate Coating	5 pieces	200	14	17	10	35
Vanilla With Milk Chocolate Coating	8 pieces	330	23	27	20	60
Borden						
Buttered Pecan	½ cup	180	12	16	—	65
Chocolate Swirl	½ cup	130	6	18	—	65
Dutch Chocolate Olde Fashioned Recipe	½ cup	130	6	16	—	65
Fat Free Black Cherry	½ cup	90	tr	21	0	40
Fat Free Chocolate	½ cup	100	tr	21	0	50
Fat Free Peach	½ cup	90	tr	21	0	40
Fat Free Strawberry	½ cup	90	tr	21	0	40
Fat Free Vanilla	½ cup	90	tr	20	0	50
Ice Milk Chocolate	½ cup	100	2	18	—	80
Ice Milk Strawberry	½ cup	90	2	17	—	65
Ice Milk Vanilla	½ cup	90	2	17	—	65
Strawberries 'N Cream Olde Fashioned Recipe	½ cup	130	5	19	—	55
Strawberry	½ cup	130	6	18	—	55
Sundae Cone	1	210	12	23	—	110
Vanilla Olde Fashioned Recipe	½ cup	130	7	15	—	55

FOOD	PORTION	CALS	FAT	CARB	CHOL	SOD
Bounty						
Cherry/Dark	1 (0.84 fl oz)	70	5	8	5	20
Coconut/Dark	1 (0.84 fl oz)	70	5	7	5	20
Coconut/Milk	1 (0.84 fl oz)	70	5	7	5	20
Bresler's						
All Flavors Ice Cream	3.5 oz	230	12	23	36	—
All Flavors Royale Cremes	4 oz	260	16	24	48	—
All Flavors Royale Lites	4 oz	217	0	49	0	—
Breyers						
Bar Vanilla	1 (2.7 oz)	250	17	21	50	45
Bar Vanilla Caramel w/ Chocolate Brittle Coating	1 (2.7 oz)	260	15	26	45	65
Bar Vanilla With Chocolate Coating	1 (2.6 oz)	230	15	20	50	45
Butter Almond	½ cup	170	11	15	35	120
Butter Pecan	½ cup (2.6 oz)	180	12	15	35	125
Cherry Vanilla	½ cup	150	7	17	30	40
Chocolate	½ cup (2.6 oz)	160	8	19	30	30
Chocolate Chip	½ cup (2.5 oz)	170	10	18	35	40
Chocolate Chip Cookie Dough	½ cup (2.5 oz)	190	10	20	40	45
Chocolate Chocolate Chip	½ cup (2.5 oz)	180	10	21	25	30
Chocolate Peanut Butter Twirl	½ cup (2.6 oz)	220	13	20	25	75
Coffee	½ cup (2.6 oz)	150	8	15	35	45
Cookies n'Cream	½ cup (2.6 oz)	170	9	19	30	55
Deluxe Rocky Road	½ cup (2.5 oz)	190	9	24	25	30
French Vanilla	(2.5 oz)	170	10	15	105	45
Light Brownie Marble Fudge	½ cup (2.6 oz)	150	5	23	30	55
Light Chocolate	½ cup (2.4 oz)	130	4	19	30	55
Light Chocolate Fudge Twirl	½ cup (2.6 oz)	140	4	22	25	55
Light Heavenly Hash	½ cup (2.4 oz)	150	5	22	25	55
Light Rocky Road Deluxe	½ cup (2.4 oz)	150	5	22	25	50
Light Strawberry	½ cup (2.4 oz)	120	4	18	30	45
Light Toffee Fudge Parfait	½ cup (2.6 oz)	150	5	23	35	55
Light Vanilla	½ cup (2.4 oz)	130	5	18	35	55

FOOD	PORTION	CALS	FAT	CARB	CHOL	SOD
Breyers (CONT.)						
Light Vanilla Chocolate Strawberry	½ cup (2.4 oz)	120	4	18	30	50
Mint Chocolate Chip	½ cup (2.6 oz)	170	10	18	35	40
Mocha Almond Fudge	½ cup (2.7 oz)	190	10	20	30	45
Peach	½ cup (2.6 oz)	130	6	18	25	30
Reduced Fat Chocolate Chocolate Chip	½ cup (2.4 oz)	150	5	21	25	50
Reduced Fat Heavenly Hash	½ cup (2.4 oz)	150	5	22	25	55
Reduced Fat Mocha Almond Fudge	½ cup (2.5 oz)	160	6	20	30	55
Reduced Fat Praline Almond Crunch	½ cup (2.4 oz)	140	5	20	35	70
Reduced Fat Swiss Almond Fudge Twirl	½ cup (2.5 oz)	160	6	22	30	55
Sandwich Vanilla	1 (2.8 oz)	250	11	32	25	160
Strawberry	½ cup (2.6 oz)	130	6	15	25	35
Toffee Bar Crunch	½ cup (2.5 oz)	180	11	18	40	65
Vanilla	½ cup (2.6 oz)	150	8	15	35	45
Vanilla Caramel Praline	½ cup (2.6 oz)	190	10	23	35	90
Vanilla Chocolate	½ cup (2.5 oz)	160	8	17	35	35
Vanilla Chocolate Strawberry	½ cup (2.5 oz)	150	8	16	30	35
Vanilla Fudge Twirl	½ cup (2.6 oz)	160	8	19	35	50
Vanilla Peanut Butter Fudge Sundae	½ cup (2.5 oz)	170	9	18	35	65
Butterfinger						
Bar	1 (2.5 oz)	170	12	14	15	40
Nuggets	8	340	24	29	20	65
Carnation						
Berry Swirl Bar Raspberry	1 bar	70	3	—	10	—
Berry Swirl Bar Strawberry	1 bar	70	3	—	9	—
Cheesecake Bar Original	1 bar	120	6	—	12	—
Cheesecake Bar Strawberry	1 bar	125	6	—	10	—
Chocolate Malted Bar	1 bar	70	3	—	19	—
Creamy Lites Bar Chocolate	1 bar	50	2	—	8	—

FOOD	PORTION	CALS	FAT	CARB	CHOL	SOD
Carnation (CONT.)						
Creamy Lites Bar Strawberry	1 bar	50	2	—	7	—
Sundae Cup Strawberry	1 (3.3 oz)	200	8	29	30	55
Chiquita						
Cherry & Ice Cream Swirl	1 bar	80	3	—	—	—
Mixed Berry & Ice Cream Swirl	1 bar	80	3	—	—	—
Orange & Ice Cream Swirl	1 bar	80	3	—	—	—
Raspberry & Ice Cream Swirl	1 bar	80	3	—	—	—
Strawberry & Ice Cream Swirl	1 bar	80	3	—	—	—
Cool Creations						
Cookies & Cream Sandwich	1 (3.5 oz)	240	11	34	15	250
Mini Sandwich	1 (2.3 oz)	110	5	16	10	70
DoveBar						
Almond	1 (3.67 fl oz)	335	22	30	35	75
Bite Size Almond Praline	1 (0.75 fl oz)	80	5	8	7	15
Bite Size Cherry Royale	1 (0.75 fl oz)	70	5	8	8	10
Bite Size Classic Vanilla	1 (0.75 fl oz)	70	5	7	8	10
Bite Size French Vanilla	1 (0.75 fl oz)	70	5	7	15	10
Bite Size Mint Supreme	1 (0.75 fl oz)	80	5	8	7	5
Caramel Pecan	1 (3.67 fl oz)	350	35	35	35	85
Chocolate Milk Chocolate	1 (3.8 fl oz)	340	21	35	40	80
Coffee Cashew	1 (3.67 fl oz)	335	22	31	35	55
Crunchy Cookie	1 (3.8 fl oz)	340	21	35	40	65
Peanut	1 (3.8 fl oz)	380	25	35	40	100
Single Vanilla/Dark	1 (2 fl oz)	200	12	24	20	50
Vanilla Dark Chocolate	1 (3.8 fl oz)	340	22	34	45	65
Vanilla Milk Chocolate	1 (3.8 fl oz)	340	21	34	40	60
Drumstick						
Cone Chocolate	1 (4.6 oz)	340	19	37	25	95
Cone Chocolate Dipped	1 (4.6 oz)	340	17	41	25	95

FOOD	PORTION	CALS	FAT	CARB	CHOL	SOD
Drumstick (CONT.)						
Cone Vanilla	1 (4.6 oz)	350	20	36	20	95
Cone Vanilla Caramel	1 (4.6 oz)	360	20	39	25	100
Cone Vanilla Fudge	1 (4.6 oz)	370	21	40	20	105
Eagle Brand						
Vanilla	½ cup	150	9	16	—	55
Edy's						
American Dream Chocolate	3 oz	90	1	20	0	45
American Dream Chocolate Chip	3 oz	100	1	22	0	45
American Dream Cookies'N'Cream	3 oz	100	1	22	0	45
American Dream Mocha Almond Fudge	3 oz	110	1	24	0	45
American Dream Rocky Road	3 oz	110	1	24	0	45
American Dream Strawberry	3 oz	70	tr	16	0	40
American Dream Toasted Almond	3 oz	110	1	24	0	45
American Dream Vanilla	3 oz	80	tr	18	0	45
American Dream Vanilla Chocolate Strawberry	3 oz	80	1	18	0	45
Light Almond Praline	4 oz	140	5	18	15	50
Light Banana-Politan	4 oz	110	4	15	15	50
Light Butter Pecan	4 oz	140	5	18	15	50
Light Cafe Au Lait	4 oz	110	4	13	15	50
Light Candy Bar	4 oz	140	5	20	15	50
Light Chocolate Chip	4 oz	120	4	16	15	50
Light Chocolate Fudge Mousse	4 oz	130	5	18	15	50
Light Cookies'N'Cream	4 oz	120	5	18	15	50
Light Dreamy Caramel Cream	4 oz	140	4	16	15	50
Light Malt Ball 'N' Fudge	4 oz	140	5	20	15	50
Light Marble Fudge	4 oz	120	4	15	15	50
Light Mocha Almond Fudge	4 oz	140	5	19	15	50

FOOD	PORTION	CALS	FAT	CARB	CHOL	SOD
Edy's (cont.)						
Light Peanut Butter & Chocolate	4 oz	130	5	19	15	50
Light Raspberry Truffle	4 oz	110	5	19	15	50
Light Rocky Road	4 oz	130	5	17	15	50
Light Strawberry	4 oz	110	4	15	15	50
Light Vanilla	4 oz	100	4	13	15	50
Vanilla Chocolate Strawberry	4 oz	110	4	14	15	50
Fi-Bar						
Banana Cream	1 bar	93	tr	21	—	—
Cocoa-Fudge 'N Cream	1 bar	93	tr	21	—	—
Raspberries 'N Cream	1 bar	93	tr	21	—	—
Wildberry Cream	1 bar	93	tr	21	—	—
Flintstones						
Cool Cream	1 (2.75 oz)	90	2	18	5	30
Push-Up	1 (2.75 oz)	100	2	20	5	25
Friendly's						
Black Raspberry	½ cup	150	7	17	30	35
Chocolate Almond Chip	½ cup	170	10	18	35	45
Forbidden Chocolate	½ cup	150	9	14	30	40
Fudge Nut Brownie	½ cup	200	11	23	25	60
Heath English Toffee	½ cup (2.7 oz)	190	10	24	30	240
Purely Pistachio	½ cup	160	10	16	35	50
Vanilla	½ cup	150	8	16	35	40
Vanilla Chocolate Strawberry	½ cup	150	8	16	30	35
Vienna Mocha Chunk	½ cup	180	11	19	30	50
Good Humor						
Banana Bob	1 (3 fl oz)	155	7	22	5	55
Bar Classic Almond	1 (3.1 fl oz)	210	12	21	15	50
Bar Classic Toasted Almond	1 (3.1 fl oz)	170	9	22	10	40
Bar Classic Vanilla	1 (3.1 fl oz)	190	10	22	15	35
Bar Sidewalk Sundae	1	280	20	21	15	65
Bubble O'Bill	1 (3.6 fl oz)	170	10	20	15	45
Bubble Play	1	110	1	25	—	5
Chip Burrrger	1 (4.7 oz)	320	15	44	20	190
Chip Sandwich	1 (4.7 fl oz)	320	15	44	20	190
Choco Taco	1 (4.4 fl oz)	320	17	38	20	100
Chocolate Eclair Classic	1 (3.1 fl oz)	170	9	21	10	60

FOOD	PORTION	CALS	FAT	CARB	CHOL	SOD
Good Humor (CONT.)						
Classic Candy Center Crunch Vanilla	1	280	21	21	15	75
Colonel Crunch Chocolate	1 (3.1 oz)	160	7	21	10	60
Colonel Crunch Strawberry	1 (3.1 oz)	170	8	22	10	45
Combo Cup	1 (6.2 fl oz)	200	10	25	35	65
Cone Olde Nut Sundae	1 (3.9 oz)	230	9	32	5	100
Cone Sidewalk Sundae	1 (4.2 oz)	270	14	31	10	125
Creamee Burrrger	1 (4.7 oz)	310	17	40	20	150
Crunch Classic Candy Center	1 (3.1 fl oz)	260	19	21	10	60
Dinosaur Bar	1	110	2	25	—	5
Far Frog	1 (3.6 fl oz)	150	8	19	20	45
Fun Box Ice Cream Sandwich	1 (3.1 fl oz)	160	5	27	10	140
King Cone	1 (5.7 fl oz)	300	14	38	25	110
King Cone Classic Vanilla	1 (4.8 oz)	300	10	48	20	110
King Cone Strawberry	1 (5.7 oz)	250	10	38	25	105
Light Chocolate Chip	½ cup (2.4 oz)	130	4	20	10	45
Light Chocolate Chocolate Chip	½ cup (2.4 oz)	130	4	20	10	40
Light Coffee	½ cup (2.4 oz)	110	3	18	15	45
Light Cookies N'Cream	½ cup (2.4 oz)	130	3	21	10	70
Light Heavenly Hash	½ cup (2.4 oz)	140	4	23	10	45
Light Praline Almond Crunch	½ cup (2.4 oz)	130	3	20	15	65
Light Toffee Bar Crunch	½ cup (2.4 oz)	130	4	20	15	55
Light Vanilla	½ cup (2.4 oz)	110	3	19	15	50
Light Vanilla Chocolate Strawberry	½ cup (2.4 oz)	110	3	19	10	45
Light Vanilla Fudge	½ cup (2.6 oz)	120	3	21	15	50
Magnum Almond	1 (4.2 fl oz)	270	12	35	30	50
Magnum Chocolate	1 (4.2 fl oz)	260	12	38	30	60
Number One Bar	1 (4.1 fl oz)	190	11	22	15	45
Popsicle Ice Cream Bar	1 (3.1 fl oz)	160	11	15	15	35
Popsicle Ice Cream Sandwich	1 (3.6 fl oz)	190	8	28	15	120

FOOD	PORTION	CALS	FAT	CARB	CHOL	SOD
Good Humor (CONT.)						
Sandwich Classic Chip Cookie	1 (4.1 fl oz)	300	13	43	18	215
Sandwich Giant Neapolitan	1 (5.2 fl oz)	260	10	39	20	150
Sandwich Giant Vanilla	1 (5.2 fl oz)	240	10	35	20	160
Sandwich Ice Cream	1	190	8	28	15	120
Sandwich Sidewalk Sundae	1 (3.1 oz)	160	5	27	10	140
Sandwich Sprinkle	1 (3.1 fl oz)	180	6	28	10	65
Strawberry Shortcake Bar Classic	1 (3.1 fl oz)	160	8	20	10	60
Sundae Twist Cup	1	160	3	33	10	100
Toffee Taco	1 (4.4 fl oz)	300	16	35	15	120
Viennetta Chocolate	1 (4.2 fl oz)	160	9	19	10	80
Viennetta Vanilla	1 (4.2 fl oz)	160	10	15	20	80
WWF Bar	1 (3.7 fl oz)	200	10	24	15	100
X-Men Bar	1 (3 fl oz)	150	6	23	15	90
Haagen-Dazs						
Bailey's Original Irish Cream	½ cup (3.6 oz)	280	18	23	110	100
Brownies A La Mode	½ cup (3.7 oz)	280	18	25	100	130
Butter Pecan	½ cup (3.7 oz)	320	24	20	105	140
Cappuccino Commotion	½ cup (3.6 oz)	310	21	25	100	105
Caramel Cone Explosion	½ cup (3.6 oz)	310	20	27	95	130
Chocolate	½ cup (3.7 oz)	270	18	22	115	75
Chocolate Chocolate Chip	½ cup (3.7 oz)	300	20	26	100	70
Coffee	½ cup (3.7 oz)	270	18	21	120	85
Cookie Dough Dynamo	½ cup (3.6 oz)	300	19	29	95	140
Cookies & Cream	½ cup (3.6 oz)	270	17	23	110	115
DiSaronno Amaretto	½ cup (3.6 oz)	260	15	26	95	80
Macadamia Brittle	½ cup (3.7 oz)	300	20	25	110	120
Multi Pack Bars Caramel Cone Explosion	1 (3.1 oz)	330	22	30	60	150
Multi Pack Bars Chocolate & Dark Chocolate	1 (3.2 oz)	320	22	27	70	70
Multi Pack Bars Coffee & Almond Crunch	1 (3 oz)	290	21	22	80	70

FOOD	PORTION	CALS	FAT	CARB	CHOL	SOD
Haagen-Dazs (CONT.)						
Multi Pack Bars Iced Cappuccino Explosion	1 (2.9 oz)	290	21	21	70	60
Multi Pack Bars Triple Brownie Overload	1 (3 oz)	320	23	23	80	95
Multi Pack Bars Vanilla & Almonds	1 (3 oz)	300	22	21	70	65
Multi Pack Bars Vanilla & Dark Chocolate	1 (3.2 oz)	320	22	27	70	50
Multi Pack Bars Vanilla & Milk Chocolate	1 (3 oz)	280	20	20	75	65
Peanut Butter Burst	½ cup (3.6 oz)	330	22	26	95	150
Rum Raisin	½ cup (3.7 oz)	270	17	22	110	75
Single Pack Bars Caramel Cone Explosion	1 (3.3 oz)	350	23	32	65	160
Single Pack Bars Chocolate & Dark Chocolate	1 (3.9 oz)	400	27	33	85	90
Single Pack Bars Coffee & Almond Crunch	1 (3.7 oz)	360	26	27	100	85
Single Pack Bars Cookie Dough Dynamo	1 (3.5 oz)	380	25	34	65	125
Single Pack Bars Iced Cappuccino	1 (3.4 oz)	330	24	24	80	70
Single Pack Bars Triple Brownie Overload	1 (3.5 oz)	380	27	28	95	110
Single Pack Bars Vanilla & Almonds	1 (3.7 oz)	370	27	26	90	80
Single Pack Bars Vanilla & Dark Chocolate	1 (3.9 oz)	400	27	33	85	65
Single Pack Bars Vanilla & Milk Chocolate	1 (3.5 oz)	330	25	24	90	75
Strawberry	½ cup (3.7 oz)	250	16	23	95	80
Strawberry Cheesecake Craze	½ cup (3.7 oz)	290	18	28	100	160

FOOD	PORTION	CALS	FAT	CARB	CHOL	SOD
Haagen-Dazs (CONT.)						
Triple Brownie Overload	½ cup (3.5 oz)	300	20	26	90	100
Vanilla	½ cup (3.7 oz)	270	18	21	120	85
Vanilla Fudge	½ cup (3.7 oz)	280	18	25	105	105
Vanilla Swiss Almond	½ cup (3.7 oz)	310	21	23	105	80
Healthy Choice						
Black Forest	½ cup (2.5 oz)	120	2	23	5	50
Bordeaux Cherry Chocolate Chip	½ cup (2.5 oz)	110	2	19	<5	55
Butter Pecan Crunch	½ cup (2.5 oz)	120	2	22	<5	60
Cappuccino Chocolate Chunk	½ cup (2.5 oz)	120	2	32	10	60
Cookies 'N Cream	½ cup (2.5 oz)	120	2	21	<5	90
Double Fudge Swirl	½ cup (2.5 oz)	120	2	21	<5	50
Fudge Brownie	½ cup (2.5 oz)	120	2	22	5	55
Malt Caramel Cone	½ cup (2.5 oz)	120	2	22	10	60
Mint Chocolate Chip	½ cup (2.5 oz)	120	2	21	<5	50
Peanut Butter Cookie Dough 'N Fudge	½ cup (2.5 oz)	120	2	22	<5	60
Praline & Caramel	½ cup (2.5 oz)	130	2	25	<5	70
Rocky Road	½ cup (2.5 oz)	140	2	28	<5	60
Vanilla	½ cup	100	2	18	5	50
Heath						
Bar	1 (2.5 oz)	160	12	13	15	35
Nuggets	8	180	11	18	25	45
Heaven						
Sundae Bars Chocolate Fudge	1 bar	150	9	—	7	—
Sundae Bars Vanilla Fudge	1 bar	150	9	—	7	—
Vanilla Caramel Nut	1 bar	225	15	—	9	—
Vanilla Nut Fudge	1 bar	222	15	—	9	—
Hood						
Bar Orange Cream	1 bar (1.8 oz)	90	2	18	5	30
Bar Vanilla	1 bar (1.6 oz)	160	12	11	15	45
Caramel Butterscotch Blast	½ cup (2.3 oz)	160	8	20	25	70
Chocolate	½ cup (2.3 oz)	140	7	17	30	40
Chocolate Chip	½ cup (2.3 oz)	160	9	18	30	55
Chocolate Eclair	1 bar (1.6 oz)	150	10	14	5	45
Christmas Tree	½ cup (2.3 oz)	140	7	18	30	45
Coffee	½ cup (2.3 oz)	140	7	16	30	50
Cookie Dough Delight	½ cup (2.3 oz)	160	8	21	30	70

FOOD	PORTION	CALS	FAT	CARB	CHOL	SOD
Hood (CONT.)						
Cookies N Cream	½ cup (2.3 oz)	160	8	19	30	75
Cooler Cups	1 (2.1 oz)	80	1	18	<5	25
Crispy Bar	1 (1.9 oz)	180	13	15	20	40
Egg Nog	½ cup (2.3 oz)	130	6	17	25	45
Fabulous Fudge & Peanut Butter Swirled Fudge Bars	1 bar (2.1 oz)	110	4	17	10	45
Fabulous Fudgies Assorted Bars	1 bar (2.1 oz)	100	3	19	10	50
Fat Free Chocolate Passion	½ cup (2.5 oz)	100	0	23	0	50
Fat Free Classic Harlequin	½ cup (2.5 oz)	100	0	23	0	50
Fat Free Double Brownie Sundae	½ cup (2.5 oz)	120	0	27	0	60
Fat Free Heavenly Hash	½ cup (2.5 oz)	120	0	27	0	75
Fat Free Mississippi Mud Pie	½ cup (2.5 oz)	130	0	29	0	75
Fat Free Praline Pecan Delight	½ cup (2.5 oz)	120	0	27	0	55
Fat Free Raspberry Blush	½ cup (2.5 oz)	120	0	26	0	55
Fat Free Super Strawberry Swirl	½ cup (2.5 oz)	100	0	23	0	40
Fat Free Vanilla Fudge Twist	½ cup (2.5 oz)	120	0	26	0	50
Fat Free Very Vanilla	½ cup (2.5 oz)	100	0	23	0	50
Fudge Bars	1 bar (2.7 oz)	100	1	21	0	80
Grasshopper Pie	½ cup (2.3 oz)	160	7	22	25	70
Heavenly Hash	½ cup (2.3 oz)	140	6	21	20	55
Hendrie's Cherry Chocolate Dips	1 bar (1.3 oz)	120	9	11	15	30
Hoodsie Cup Vanilla & Chocolate	1 (1.7 oz)	100	5	12	20	35
Light Almond Praline Delight	½ cup (2.4 oz)	110	5	23	15	75
Light Brownie Nut Sundae	½ cup (2.4 oz)	140	5	22	10	55
Light Caribbean Coffee Royale	½ cup (2.4 oz)	110	4	18	15	50
Light Chocolate Almond Chip Sundae	½ cup (2.4 oz)	140	5	22	10	60

FOOD	PORTION	CALS	FAT	CARB	CHOL	SOD
Hood (CONT.)						
Light Chocolate Chocolate Chip Cookie Dough	½ cup (2.4 oz)	140	5	21	15	70
Light Cookies N Cream	½ cup (2.4 oz)	130	4	21	15	70
Light Heath Toffee Chunk Swirl	½ cup (2.4 oz)	140	5	23	15	95
Light Heavenly Hash	½ cup (2.4 oz)	130	4	22	10	55
Light Maple Sugar Shack	⅓ cup (2.4 oz)	130	4	23	10	65
Light Massachusetts Mud Pie	½ cup (2.4 oz)	140	5	20	10	60
Light Raspberry Swirl	½ cup (2.4 oz)	120	3	22	10	55
Light Strawberry Supreme	½ cup (2.4 oz)	110	3	19	15	45
Light Triple Nut Cluster Sundae	½ cup (2.4 oz)	140	5	22	10	50
Light Vanilla	½ cup (2.4 oz)	110	4	18	15	50
Light Vanilla Chocolate Strawberry	½ cup (2.4 oz)	110	4	18	15	45
Low Fat No Sugar Added Caramel Swirl	½ cup (2.4 oz)	120	3	18	10	80
Low Fat No Sugar Added Chocolate Supreme	½ cup (2.4 oz)	120	3	19	10	60
Low Fat No Sugar Added Mocha Fudge	½ cup (2.4 oz)	110	3	18	10	45
Low Fat No Sugar Added Raspberry Swirl	½ cup (2.4 oz)	110	3	17	10	45
Low Fat No Sugar Added Vanilla	½ cup (2.4 oz)	100	3	14	10	50
Maple Walnut	½ cup (2.3 oz)	160	9	16	30	45
Rockets	1 (2 oz)	120	5	18	20	50
Sandwich Light	1 (2.2 oz)	160	4	29	10	160
Sandwich Vanilla	1 (2.2 oz)	180	7	27	20	170
Sports Bar	1 (2.9 oz)	250	17	23	25	55
Spumoni	½ cup (2.3 oz)	140	9	17	30	45
Strawberry	½ cup (2.3 oz)	130	7	16	30	45

FOOD	PORTION	CALS	FAT	CARB	CHOL	SOD
Hood (CONT.)						
Super Sortment Chocolate & Banana Fudge Bar	1 bar (2.1 oz)	**100**	3	18	10	30
Super Sortment Root Beer Float & Orange Cream Bar	1 bar (1.5 oz)	70	3	12	10	25
Vanilla	½ cup (2.3 oz)	140	7	16	30	50
Vanilla Chocolate Patchwork	½ cup (2.3 oz)	140	7	17	30	45
Vanilla Chocolate Strawberry	½ cup (2.3 oz)	140	7	16	30	45
Vanilla Fudge	½ cup (2.3 oz)	140	6	20	25	55
Klondike						
Almond Bar	1 (5.2 fl oz)	310	21	26	25	90
Caramel Crunch	1 (5.2 fl oz)	300	18	31	30	95
Chocolate Chocolate Bar	1 (5.2 fl oz)	280	20	22	20	60
Coffee Bar	1 (5.2 fl oz)	290	20	25	15	65
Dark Chocolate Bar	1 (5.2 fl oz)	290	20	24	30	75
Gold Bar	1 (5.2 fl oz)	340	23	30	34	60
Krispy Bar	1 (5.2 fl oz)	300	20	28	25	85
Krunch	1 (3.1 fl oz)	200	13	17	20	160
Lite Bar	1 (2.3 fl oz)	110	6	14	5	55
Lite Bar Caramel	1 (2.4 fl oz)	120	6	18	5	65
Movie Bites Chocolate	8 pieces (4.6 fl oz)	340	26	22	25	50
Movie Bites Vanilla	8 pieces (4.6 fl oz)	320	22	27	25	60
Original Bar	1 (5.2 fl oz)	290	20	24	15	65
Sandwich Chocolate	1 (5.2 fl oz)	270	10	41	20	200
Sandwich Lite	1 (2.9 fl oz)	100	2	18	5	105
Sandwich Vanilla	1 (5.2 fl oz)	250	9	37	20	230
Mars						
Almond Bar	1 (1.85 fl oz)	210	14	20	15	45
Meadow Gold						
Sundae Cone	1	210	12	23	—	110
Milky Way						
Single Chocolate/Milk	1 (2 fl oz)	210	11	24	20	60
Snack Chocolate/Milk	1 (0.72 fl oz)	70	4	9	5	25
Snack Vanilla/Dark	1 (0.72 fl oz)	70	4	9	5	25
Mocha Mix						
Berry Berry Berry	½ cup	140	6	20	0	60
Dutch Chocolate	½ cup (2.3 oz)	140	8	16	0	80

FOOD	PORTION	CALS	FAT	CARB	CHOL	SOD
Mocha Mix (CONT.)						
Mocha Almond Fudge	½ cup (2.3 oz)	150	8	19	0	65
Neapolitan	½ cup (2.3 oz)	140	7	18	0	70
Strawberry Swirl	½ cup (2.3 oz)	140	6	20	0	55
Vanilla	½ cup (2.3 oz)	140	7	18	0	70
Nestle Crunch						
Chocolate	1 bar (3 oz)	200	14	18	15	40
Cones	1 (4.6 oz)	300	16	36	25	95
Crunch King	1 (4 oz)	270	19	21	20	45
Nuggets	8 pieces	140	9	12	10	30
Reduced Fat	1 (2.5 oz)	130	7	14	5	40
Vanilla	1 bar (3 oz)	200	14	17	15	40
Rice Dream						
Bar Chocolate	1	270	16	33	0	115
Bar Chocolate Nutty	1	330	23	29	0	110
Bar Strawberry	1	260	15	31	0	110
Bar Vanilla	1	275	16	33	0	120
Bar Vanilla Nutty	1	330	23	29	0	100
Cappuccino	½ cup	130	5	17	0	80
Carob	½ cup	130	5	20	0	80
Carob Almond	½ cup	140	6	20	0	80
Carob Chip	½ cup	140	6	20	0	80
Carob Chip Mint	½ cup	140	6	20	0	80
Cocoa Marble Fudge	½ cup	140	6	19	0	80
Dream Pie Chocolate	1	380	19	47	0	225
Dream Pie Mint	1	380	19	47	0	225
Dream Pie Mocha	1	380	19	47	0	225
Dream Pie Vanilla	1	380	19	47	0	225
Lemon	½ cup	130	5	17	0	80
Peanut Butter Fudge	½ cup	160	7	19	0	100
Strawberry	½ cup	130	5	17	0	80
Vanilla	½ cup	130	5	17	0	80
Vanilla Fudge	½ cup	140	6	21	0	80
Vanilla Swiss Almond	½ cup	140	6	20	0	80
Wildberry	½ cup	130	5	17	0	80
Sealtest						
American Glory	½ cup (2.4 oz)	130	6	17	25	45
Butter Pecan	½ cup (2.4 oz)	160	9	16	30	115
Candy Cane Crunch	½ cup (2.4 oz)	150	6	21	25	50
Chocolate	½ cup (2.4 oz)	140	7	19	25	50
Chocolate Butter Pecan	½ cup (2.4 oz)	150	8	17	30	85
Chocolate Chip	½ cup (2.4 oz)	150	8	18	30	50
Coconut Chocolate	½ cup (2.4 oz)	160	8	18	25	55

FOOD	PORTION	CALS	FAT	CARB	CHOL	SOD
Sealtest (CONT.)						
Coffee	½ cup (2.4 oz)	140	7	16	30	55
Cupid's Scoops	½ cup (2.5 oz)	140	6	20	25	55
Dessert Bar Free Chocolate Fudge	1	90	0	19	0	30
Dessert Bar Free Vanilla Fudge	1	80	0	18	0	30
Dessert Bar Free Vanilla Strawberry Swirl	1	80	0	17	0	40
Free Black Cherry	½ cup	100	0	25	0	45
Free Chocolate	½ cup	100	0	23	0	50
Free Peach	½ cup	100	0	23	0	45
Free Strawberry	½ cup	100	0	23	0	40
Free Vanilla	½ cup	100	0	24	0	45
Free Vanilla Fudge Royale	½ cup	100	0	24	0	50
Free Vanilla Strawberry Royale	½ cup	100	0	25	0	35
French Vanilla	½ cup (2.4 oz)	140	8	16	60	50
Fudge Royale	½ cup (2.5 oz)	150	7	19	25	55
Heavenly Hash	½ cup (2.4 oz)	150	7	20	25	50
Maple Walnut	½ cup (2.4 oz)	160	9	16	30	50
Strawberry	½ cup (2.4 oz)	130	6	19	25	45
Triple Chocolate Passion	½ cup (2.5 oz)	160	7	21	25	50
Vanilla	½ cup (2.4 oz)	140	7	16	30	55
Vanilla Chocolate Strawberry	½ cup (2.4 oz)	140	6	18	25	50
Vanilla With Orange Sherbet	½ cup (2.7 oz)	130	4	22	20	45
Simple Pleasures						
Chocolate	4 oz	140	tr	25	10	—
Chocolate Caramel Sundae Light	4 oz	90	tr	20	15	—
Chocolate Chip	4 oz	150	3	25	15	—
Chocolate Light	4 oz	80	tr	16	15	—
Coffee	4 oz	120	tr	22	15	—
Cookies n' Cream	4 oz	150	2	25	10	—
Mint Chocolate Chip	4 oz	150	2	26	5	—
Peach	4 oz	120	tr	21	10	—
Pecan Praline	4 oz	140	2	25	5	—
Rum Raisin	4 oz	130	tr	35	15	—
Strawberry	4 oz	120	tr	22	10	—

FOOD	PORTION	CALS	FAT	CARB	CHOL	SOD
Simple Pleasures (CONT.)						
Toffee Crunch	4 oz	130	tr	22	10	—
Vanilla	4 oz	120	tr	22	15	—
Vanilla Fudge Swirl Light	4 oz	90	tr	20	15	—
Vanilla Light	4 oz	80	tr	16	15	—
Snickers						
Single	1 (2 fl oz)	220	13	22	15	65
Snack	1 (1 fl oz)	110	7	11	5	35
Starbucks						
Biscotti Bliss	½ cup	240	12	30	55	70
Caffe Almond Fudge	½ cup	260	13	30	55	80
Caffe Almond Roast	1 bar	280	18	26	3	45
Dark Roast Espresso Swirl	½ cup	220	10	29	55	60
Frappuccino	1 bar (2.8 oz)	110	2	20	10	45
Italian Roast Coffee	½ cup	230	12	26	65	50
Javachip	½ cup	250	13	29	60	55
Low Fat Latte	½ cup	170	3	31	10	65
Low Fat Mocha Mambo	½ cup	170	3	32	10	75
Vanilla Mochachip	½ cup	270	16	27	75	60
Tofu Ice Creme						
Carob	4 fl oz	190	8	28	0	55
Vanilla	4 fl oz	190	8	28	0	55
Tofutti						
Frutti Vanilla Apple Orchard	4 fl oz	100	0	20	0	90
Turkey Hill						
Black Cherry	½ cup (2.3 oz)	140	7	18	25	30
Butter Pecan	½ cup (2.3 oz)	170	11	16	30	50
Choco Mint Chip	½ cup (2.3 oz)	160	10	17	30	45
Cookies 'N Cream	½ cup (2.3 oz)	160	9	19	30	60
Lite Butter Pecan	½ cup (2.3 oz)	130	6	17	15	80
Lite Choco Mint Chip	½ cup (2.3 oz)	140	5	19	15	75
Lite Cookies 'N Cream	½ cup (2.3 oz)	130	5	21	15	90
Lite Vanilla & Chocolate	½ cup (2.3 oz)	110	3	18	15	60
Lite Vanilla Bean	½ cup (2.3 oz)	110	3	18	15	65
Neapolitan	½ cup (2.3 oz)	150	8	18	30	30
Rocky Road	½ cup (2.3 oz)	170	8	23	30	40
Tin Roof Sundae	½ cup (2.3 oz)	160	9	19	30	70
Vanilla	½ cup (2.3 oz)	140	8	16	30	35
Vanilla & Chocolate	½ cup (2.3 oz)	150	8	17	30	35

FOOD	PORTION	CALS	FAT	CARB	CHOL	SOD
Turkey Hill (CONT.)						
Vanilla Bean	½ cup (2.3 oz)	140	8	16	30	35
Ultra Slim-Fast						
Bar Fudge	1	90	tr	17	0	50
Bar Vanilla Cookie Crunch	1	90	4	14	0	70
Chocolate	4 oz	100	tr	19	0	45
Chocolate Fudge	4 oz	120	tr	24	0	65
Peach	4 oz	100	tr	22	0	55
Pralines & Caramel	4 oz	120	tr	25	0	95
Sandwich Vanilla	1	140	2	28	0	220
Sandwich Vanilla Chocolate	1	140	2	28	0	220
Sandwich Vanilla Oatmeal	1	150	3	26	0	160
Vanilla	4 oz	90	tr	19	0	55
Vanilla Fudge Cookie	4 oz	110	tr	24	0	90
Weight Watchers						
Artic D'Lites	1 bar	130	7	4	5	20
Berries 'n Creme Mousse	2 bars	70	2	17	0	75
Caramel Nut Bars	1 bar	130	8	14	5	25
Chocolate Chip Cookie Dough Sundae	1 (5.43 oz)	180	4	34	5	120
Chocolate Dip	1 bar	100	6	11	5	15
Chocolate Mousse Bar	2 bars	70	1	18	5	80
Chocolate Treat	1 bar	100	1	21	10	150
Crispy Pralines 'n Creme Bars	1 bar	130	7	15	5	40
English Toffee Crunch Bars	1 bar	120	7	12	5	25
Light Cookie Dough Craze	½ cup	140	4	24	5	85
Oh! So Very Vanilla!	½ cup	120	3	20	5	65
Orange Vanilla Treat	2 bars	70	1	17	5	80
Positively Praline Crunch	½ cup	140	3	25	5	105
Praline Toffee Crunch Parfait	1 (5.1 oz)	190	3	40	5	140
Reckless Rocky Road	½ cup	140	1	23	5	75
Triple Chocolate Tornado	½ cup	150	1	26	5	80
Vanilla Sandwich	1 bar	160	4	30	5	180

FOOD	PORTION	CALS	FAT	CARB	CHOL	SOD
ICE CREAM CONES						
sugar cone	1	40	tr	8	0	32
wafer cone	1	17	tr	3	0	6
waffle cone	1 (17 g)	70	1	14	0	30
ICE CREAM TOPPINGS						
butterscotch	2 tbsp (1.4 oz)	103	tr	27	—	143
caramel	2 tbsp (1.4 oz)	103	tr	27	—	143
marshmallow cream	1 jar (7 oz)	615	tr	157	0	90
marshmallow cream	1 oz	88	tr	23	0	13
pineapple	1 cup (11.5 oz)	861	—	226	0	214
pineapple	2 tbsp (1.5 oz)	106	0	28	0	26
strawberry	1 cup (11.5 oz)	863	1	225	0	73
strawberry	2 tbsp (1.5 oz)	107	tr	28	0	9
walnuts in syrup	2 tbsp (1.4 oz)	167	9	22	0	—
Ben & Jerry's						
Hot Fudge	(1.3 oz)	140	7	19	10	25
Crumpy						
Chocolate Hazelnut Spread	1 tbsp (0.5 oz)	80	5	8	0	5
Hershey						
Chocolate Fudge	2 tbsp	100	4	14	5	30
Chocolate Shoppe Candy Bar Sprinkles York	2 tbsp (1.1 oz)	170	8	22	<5	0
Kraft						
Butterscotch	2 tbsp (1.4 oz)	130	2	28	<5	150
Caramel	2 tbsp (1.4 oz)	120	0	28	0	90
Chocolate	2 tbsp (1.4 oz)	110	0	26	0	30
Hot Fudge	2 tbsp (1.4 oz)	140	4	24	0	100
Pineapple	2 tbsp (1.4 oz)	110	0	28	0	15
Strawberry	2 tbsp (1.4 oz)	110	0	29	0	15
Marzetti						
Caramel Apple	2 tbsp	60	7	23	5	95
Caramel Apple Reduced Fat	2 tbsp	30	3	26	5	100
Peanut Butter Caramel	2 tbsp	60	6	21	0	135
Planters						
Nut	2 tbsp (0.5 oz)	100	9	3	0	0
Smucker's						
Butterscotch	2 tbsp	140	1	33	—	75
Butterscotch Special Recipe	2 tbsp	160	3	33	—	40
Caramel	2 tbsp	140	1	33	—	110

FOOD	PORTION	CALS	FAT	CARB	CHOL	SOD
Smucker's (CONT.)						
Chocolate	2 tbsp	130	0	27	0	35
Chocolate Fudge	2 tbsp	130	1	31	—	50
Dark Chocolate Special Recipe	2 tbsp	130	1	31	—	45
Hot Caramel	2 tbsp	150	4	28	—	75
Hot Fudge	2 tbsp	110	4	18	—	55
Hot Fudge Light	2 tbsp	70	tr	19	—	35
Hot Fudge Special Recipe	2 tbsp	150	5	23	—	60
Hot Toffee Fudge	2 tbsp	110	4	18	—	55
Magic Shell Chocolate	2 tbsp	190	15	16	—	25
Magic Shell Chocolate Fudge	2 tbsp	190	15	16	0	50
Magic Shell Chocolate Nut	2 tbsp	200	16	25	—	40
Marshmallow	2 tbsp	120	0	29	—	0
Peanut Butter Caramel	2 tbsp	150	2	29	—	120
Pecans in Syrup	2 tbsp	130	1	28	—	0
Pineapple	2 tbsp	130	0	32	0	0
Strawberry	2 tbsp	120	0	30	0	0
Swiss Milk Chocolate Fudge	2 tbsp	140	1	31	—	70
Walnuts in Syrup	2 tbsp	130	1	27	—	0

ICED TEA
Arizona

FOOD	PORTION	CALS	FAT	CARB	CHOL	SOD
Lemon	1 bottle (16 oz)	180	0	50	0	40
Raspberry	8 fl oz	95	0	25	0	20
Clearly Canadian						
Clearly Tea Original	8 fl oz	80	0	19	0	9
Clearly Tea Tangy Lemon	8 fl oz	80	0	19	0	9
Lipton						
Chilled Diet Lemon	8 fl oz	0	0	0	0	10
Chilled Lemon	8 fl oz	80	0	20	0	15
Chilled No Lemon	8 fl oz	90	0	24	0	15
Chilled Peach	8 fl oz	80	0	20	0	15
Chilled Raspberry	8 fl oz	80	0	20	0	15
Nestea						
With Sugar & Lemon	1 bottle (16 fl oz)	176	0	44	0	50
With Sugar & Lemon	1 can (11.5 fl oz)	127	0	32	0	36

FOOD	PORTION	CALS	FAT	CARB	CHOL	SOD
Royal Mistic						
Diet	12 fl oz	8	0	2	0	34
Lemon	12 fl oz	144	0	36	0	26
Orange	12 fl oz	144	0	36	0	26
Wild Berry	12 fl oz	144	0	36	0	34
Schweppes						
Iced Tea	8 fl oz	90	0	22	0	60
Shasta						
Iced Tea	12 oz	124	0	—	0	—
Snapple						
Cranberry	8 fl oz	110	0	27	0	10
Diet	8 fl oz	0	0	1	0	10
Diet Peach	8 fl oz	0	0	1	0	10
Diet Raspberry	8 fl oz	0	0	1	0	10
Lemon	8 fl oz	110	0	27	0	10
Mango	8 fl oz	110	0	27	0	5
Mint	8 fl oz	120	0	29	0	10
Old Fashioned	8 fl oz	80	0	20	0	10
Orange	8 fl oz	110	0	27	0	10
Peach	8 fl oz	110	0	27	0	10
Raspberry	8 fl oz	120	0	29	0	10
Strawberry	8 fl oz	100	0	26	0	10
Tropicana						
Diet Lemon Fruit	8 fl oz	15	0	4	0	25
Lemon Fruit	8 fl oz	100	0	25	0	25
Peach Fruit	1 bottle (10 fl oz)	140	0	35	0	20
Peach Fruit	1 can (11.5 fl oz)	160	0	41	0	20
Peach Fruit	8 fl oz	120	0	28	0	15
Raspberry Fruit	1 bottle (10 fl oz)	140	0	34	0	20
Raspberry Fruit	1 can (11.5 fl oz)	160	0	41	0	15
Raspberry Fruit	8 fl oz	120	0	28	0	15
Tangerine Fruit	1 bottle (10 fl oz)	140	0	34	0	30
Tangerine Fruit	1 can (11.5 fl oz)	170	0	42	0	30
Tangerine Fruit	8 fl oz	110	0	27	0	20
Twister Apple Berry	8 fl oz	100	0	28	0	15
Twister Lemon Citrus	8 fl oz	110	0	28	0	5
Turkey Hill						
Diet Decaffeinated	1 cup (8 oz)	0	0	0	0	0

FOOD	PORTION	CALS	FAT	CARB	CHOL	SOD
Turkey Hill (CONT.)						
Raspberry Cooler	1 cup (8 oz)	110	0	28	0	0
Regular	1 cup (8 oz)	90	0	22	0	0
Veryfine						
With Lemon	8 oz	80	0	16	0	<10
ICES AND ICE POPS						
fruit & juice bar	1 (3 fl oz)	75	tr	19	0	3
gelatin pop	1 (1.5 oz)	31	0	7	0	20
ice coconut pineapple	½ cup (4 fl oz)	109	3	23	0	34
ice fruit w/ Equal	1 bar (1.7 oz)	12	0	3	0	3
ice lime	½ cup (4 fl oz)	75	0	31	0	—
ice pop	1 (2 fl oz)	42	0	11	0	7
Ben & Jerry's						
Cherry Pop	1	330	24	28	55	—
Bresler's						
All Flavors Ice	3.5 oz	120	0	30	0	—
Chiquita						
Fruit & Cream Banana	1 bar	80	2	—	—	—
Fruit & Cream Blueberry	1 bar	80	1	—	—	—
Fruit & Cream Peach	1 bar	80	1	—	—	—
Fruit & Cream Raspberry	1 bar	80	1	—	—	—
Fruit & Cream Strawberry	1 bar	80	1	—	—	—
Fruit & Cream Strawberry Banana	1 bar	80	2	—	—	—
Fruit & Juice Bar Cherry	1 bar (2 oz)	50	0	—	0	—
Fruit & Juice Bar Raspberry	1 bar (2 oz)	50	0	—	0	—
Fruit & Juice Bar Raspberry Banana	1 bar (2 oz)	50	0	—	0	—
Fruit & Juice Bar Strawberry	1 bar (2 oz)	50	0	—	0	—
Fruit & Juice Bar Strawberry Banana	1 bar (2 oz)	50	0	—	0	—
Cool Creations						
10 Pack	1 pop (2 oz)	60	0	14	0	5
Lion King Cone	1 (4 oz)	280	14	36	15	90
Mickey Mouse Bar	1 (2.5 oz)	110	7	12	10	25
Mickey Mouse Bar	1 (4 oz)	170	11	17	15	40
Surprise Pops	1 (2 oz)	60	0	14	0	5

FOOD	PORTION	CALS	FAT	CARB	CHOL	SOD
Dole						
Fruit 'N Juice Coconut	1 bar (4 oz)	210	7	33	10	50
Fruit 'N Juice Lemonade	1 bar (4 oz)	120	0	28	0	55
Fruit 'N Juice Lime	1 bar (4 oz)	110	0	28	0	55
Fruit 'N Juice Peach Passion	1 bar (2.5 oz)	70	0	17	0	5
Fruit 'N Juice Pineapple Coconut	1 bar (4 oz)	140	4	27	0	5
Fruit 'N Juice Pineapple Orange Banana	1 bar (2.5 oz)	70	0	16	0	5
Fruit 'N Juice Pineapple Orange Banana	1 bar (4 oz)	110	0	26	0	5
Fruit 'N Juice Raspberry	1 bar (2.5 oz)	70	0	16	0	5
Fruit 'N Juice Strawberry	1 bar (2.5 oz)	70	0	17	0	5
Fruit 'N Juice Strawberry	1 bar (4 oz)	110	0	26	0	5
Fruit Juice Grape	1 bar (1.75 oz)	45	0	11	0	5
Fruit Juice No Sugar Added Grape	1 bar (1.75 oz)	25	0	6	0	5
Fruit Juice No Sugar Added Strawberry	1 bar (1.75 oz)	25	0	6	0	5
Fruit Juice Raspberry	1 bar (1.75 oz)	25	0	6	0	5
Fruit Juice Raspberry	1 bar (1.75 oz)	45	0	11	0	5
Fruit Juice Strawberry	1 bar (1.75 oz)	45	0	11	0	5
Fi-Bar						
Juice Bar Lemoney-Lime	1 bar	63	tr	15	—	—
Juice Bar Strawberry Nectar	1 bar	63	tr	15	—	—
Juice Bar Tropical Delight	1 bar	63	tr	15	—	—
Flintstones						
Rock Pops	1 (3.5 oz)	80	0	20	0	5
Frozfruit						
Banana Cream	1 bar (4 oz)	150	7	20	25	20
Cantaloupe	1 bar (4 oz)	60	0	35	0	5
Cappuccino Cream	1 bar (3 oz)	140	6	18	25	20
Cherry	1 bar (4 oz)	70	0	18	0	0
Coconut Cream	1 bar (4 oz)	170	11	17	20	25

FOOD	PORTION	CALS	FAT	CARB	CHOL	SOD
Frozfruit (CONT.)						
Kiwi Strawberry	1 bar (4 oz)	90	0	23	0	0
Lemon	1 bar (4 oz)	90	0	22	0	10
Lemon Iced Tea	1 bar (4 oz)	80	0	19	0	10
Lime	1 bar (4 oz)	90	0	21	0	10
Orange	1 bar (4 oz)	90	0	21	0	15
Pina Colada Cream	1 bar (4 oz)	170	8	23	20	20
Pineapple	1 bar (4 oz)	80	0	19	0	0
Raspberry	1 bar (4 oz)	80	0	20	0	5
Strawberry	1 bar (4 oz)	80	0	20	0	20
Strawberry Banana Cream	1 bar (4 oz)	140	6	22	20	20
Strawberry Cream	1 bar (4 oz)	130	5	21	20	20
Tropical	1 bar (4 oz)	90	0	23	0	0
Watermelon	1 bar (4 oz)	50	0	13	0	0
Good Humor						
Big Stick Cherry Pineapple	1 (3.6 fl oz)	50	0	12	0	—
Big Stick Popsicle	1 (3.6 fl oz)	50	0	12	0	5
Calippo Cherry	1 (3.8 fl oz)	100	0	23	0	5
Calippo Grape Lemon	1 (3.9 fl oz)	90	0	22	0	0
Calippo Orange	1 (3.9 fl oz)	90	0	23	0	0
Citrus Bites	1 (1.8 fl oz)	35	0	9	0	0
Creamsicle Orange	1 (1.8 fl oz)	70	2	13	5	15
Creamsicle Orange	1 (2.8 fl oz)	110	3	20	10	30
Creamsicle Orange Raspberry	1 (2.6 fl oz)	100	3	19	10	25
Creamsicle Sugar Free	1 (1.8 fl oz)	25	0	5	0	10
Flintstones Push-Up Yabba Dabba Doo Orange	1 (2.75 fl oz)	90	1	20	—	20
Fudgsicle Bar	1 (2.8 fl oz)	90	1	17	5	55
Fudgsicle Pop	1 (1.8 fl oz)	60	1	12	5	40
Fudgsicle Sugar Free	1 (1.8 fl oz)	40	1	8	<5	35
Fun Box Fudge Bar	1 (2.3 fl oz)	80	1	16	5	65
Fun Box Pops	1 (2 fl oz)	35	0	10	0	5
Fun Box Twin Pop Banana	1 (2.6 fl oz)	50	0	14	0	10
Fun Box Twin Pop Blue Raspberry	1 (2.6 fl oz)	50	0	14	0	10
Fun Box Twin Pop Cherry	1 (2.6 fl oz)	50	0	14	0	10
Fun Box Twin Pop Cherry Lemon	1 (2.6 fl oz)	50	0	14	0	10

FOOD	PORTION	CALS	FAT	CARB	CHOL	SOD
Good Humor (CONT.)						
Fun Box Twin Pop Orange Cherry Grape	1 (2.6 oz)	50	0	14	0	10
Fun Box Twin Pop Root Beer	1 (2.6 fl oz)	50	0	14	0	10
Garfield Bar	1 (3.9 fl oz)	90	0	22	0	0
Great White	1 (3.1 fl oz)	70	1	18	—	0
Hyperstripe	1 (2.8 fl oz)	80	0	21	0	0
Ice Stripe Cherry Orange	1 (1.5 fl oz)	35	0	9	0	0
Jumbo Jet Star	1 (4.7 fl oz)	80	0	20	0	0
Laser Blazer	1 (2.6 oz)	70	0	16	0	5
Popsicle All Natural	1 (1.8 fl oz)	45	0	10	0	5
Popsicle Orange Cherry Grape	1 (1.8 fl oz)	45	0	11	0	0
Popsicle Rainbow Pops	1 (1.8 fl oz)	45	0	11	0	0
Popsicle Rootbeer Banana Lime	1 (1.8 fl oz)	45	0	11	0	0
Popsicle Strawberry Raspberry Wildberry	1 (1.8 fl oz)	45	0	11	0	0
Popsicle Supersicle Traffic Signal	1	80	0	20	0	0
Popsicle Twin Pop Cherry	1 (2.6 fl oz)	70	0	16	0	0
Popsicle Twin Pop Orange Cherry Grape Lime	1 (2.6 fl oz)	70	0	16	0	5
Snow Cone	1	60	0	14	5	5
Snowfruit Coconut Bar	1 (3.75 fl oz)	150	4	27	10	35
Snowfruit Orange Bar	1	140	0	34	0	10
Snowfruit Strawberry Bar	1	120	0	31	0	15
Snowfruit Tropical Fruit Bar	1	110	0	28	0	10
Sugar Free Pop Orange Cherry Grape	1 (1.8 fl oz)	15	0	3	0	0
Super Mario Bar	1	120	1	27	—	10
Supersicle Cherry Banana	1 (4.7 fl oz)	80	0	20	0	0

FOOD	PORTION	CALS	FAT	CARB	CHOL	SOD
Good Humor (CONT.)						
Supersicle Cherry Cola	1 (4.7 fl oz)	80	0	20	0	0
Supersicle Double Fudge	1 (4.7 fl oz)	150	2	29	10	95
Supersicle Firecracker	1 (4.7 fl oz)	90	0	20	0	0
Supersicle Firecracker Jr.	1	72	0	10	0	0
Supersicle Sour Tower	1	80	0	20	0	0
Swirl Bubble Gum	1 (2.7 fl oz)	55	0	13	0	0
Swirl Cherry Banana	1 (2.7 fl oz)	55	0	13	0	0
Torpedo Cherry	1 (1.8 fl oz)	35	0	10	0	5
Twister Blue Raspberry Cherry Cherry Cola Cherry	1 (1.8 fl oz)	45	0	10	0	0
Twister Cherry Lemon Orange Lemon	1 (1.8 fl oz)	45	0	10	0	0
Vampire's Deadly Secret	1 (2.8 fl oz)	100	0	24	0	10
Watermelon Bar	1 (3.6 fl oz)	80	0	20	0	0
Haagen-Dazs						
Sorbet Banana Strawberry	½ cup (4 oz)	140	0	34	0	5
Sorbet Chocolate	½ cup (4 oz)	130	0	30	0	80
Sorbet Mango	½ cup (4 oz)	120	0	30	0	0
Sorbet Orchard Peach	½ cup (4 oz)	140	0	35	0	0
Sorbet Raspberry	½ cup (4 oz)	120	0	29	0	5
Sorbet Strawberry	½ cup (4 oz)	130	0	33	0	0
Sorbet Zesty Lemon	½ cup (4 oz)	130	0	32	0	5
Sorbet & Cream Blueberry	4 oz	190	8	25	—	35
Sorbet & Cream Keylime	4 oz	190	7	29	—	30
Sorbet & Cream Orange	½ cup (3.7 oz)	200	9	27	60	45
Sorbet & Cream Orange	4 oz	190	8	27	—	35
Sorbet & Cream Raspberry	½ cup (3.7 oz)	190	9	23	60	45
Sorbet Bar Chocolate	1 (2.7 oz)	80	0	20	0	50
Sorbet Bar Wild Berry	1 (2.7 oz)	90	0	22	0	5
Hood						
Hendrie's Sizzle'N Sour Stix	1 bar (2 oz)	80	tr	15	5	15

FOOD	PORTION	CALS	FAT	CARB	CHOL	SOD
Hood (cont.)						
Hoodsie Pop	1 (3.3 oz)	60	0	16	0	0
Natural Blenders Pineappple	1 bar (1 oz)	60	0	16	0	0
Natural Blenders Raspberry	1 bar (1 oz)	60	0	16	0	0
Natural Blenders Strawberry	1 bar (1 oz)	60	0	16	0	0
Pop Banana	1 (3.3 oz)	60	0	16	0	0
Pop Blue Raspberry	1 (3.3 oz)	60	0	16	0	0
Pop Cherry	1 (3.3 oz)	60	0	16	0	0
Pop Grape	1 (3.3 oz)	60	0	16	0	0
Pop Orange	1 (3.3 oz)	60	0	16	0	0
Pop Root Beer	1 (3.3 oz)	60	0	16	0	0
Super Sortment Juice Bars	1 bar (1.9 oz)	40	0	10	0	0
Jell-O						
Lemon Lime	1 bar	33	tr	8	—	23
Mixed Berry	1 bar	31	tr	7	0	23
Orange	1 bar	31	tr	7	0	23
Orange Pineapple	1 bar	31	tr	7	0	23
Raspberry	1 bar	29	tr	7	0	24
Raspberry Peach	1 bar	29	tr	7	0	24
Side By Side Apple Cherry	1 bar	36	tr	8	—	7
Side By Side Grape Lemon	1 bar	36	tr	8	—	7
Strawberry	1 bar	31	tr	7	0	23
Strawberry Banana	1 bar	31	tr	7	0	23
Lifesavers						
Ice Pops	1	35	0	9	0	0
Ice Pops	1 (1.75 oz)	35	0	9	0	0
Sunkist						
Orange Juice Bar	1 (3.4 fl oz)	80	1	19	—	5
Wildberry	1 (3.4 fl oz)	120	1	27	—	10
Tofutti						
Frutti Apricot Mango	4 fl oz	100	0	20	0	90
Frutti Three Berry	4 fl oz	100	0	20	0	90
Vitari						
Passion-Fruit	4 oz	80	0	—	0	—
Peach	4 oz	80	0	—	0	—
KIWIS						
fresh	1 med	46	tr	11	0	4

FOOD	PORTION	CALS	FAT	CARB	CHOL	SOD

LEMON JUICE
After The Fall

Spicy Lemon	1 can (12 oz)	150	0	37	0	35

LEMONADE
After The Fall

Apple Raspberry	1 bottle (10 oz)	120	0	29	0	15
Crystal Geyser						
Juice Squeeze Pink	1 bottle (12 fl oz)	140	0	34	0	20
Diet Rite						
Salt/Sodium Free	8 fl oz	2	0	1	0	0
Fruitopia						
Lemonade	8 fl oz	120	0	29	0	25
Kool-Aid						
Koolers	1 pkg (8.45 fl oz)	120	0	32	0	3
Minute Maid						
Chilled	8 fl oz	110	0	28	0	25
Cranberry Chilled	8 fl oz	120	0	31	0	25
Juices To Go	1 bottle (16 fl oz)	110	0	28	0	25
Juices To Go	1 can (11.5 fl oz)	160	0	40	0	40
Juices To Go Cranberry Lemonade	1 bottle (16 fl oz)	110	0	29	0	25
Juices To Go Raspberry Lemonade	1 bottle (16 fl oz)	120	0	29	0	25
Pink Chilled	8 fl oz	110	0	28	0	25
Raspberry Chilled	8 fl oz	120	0	30	0	0
Mott's						
Lemonade	10 fl oz	160	0	41	0	20
Nehi						
Lemonade	8 fl oz	130	0	35	0	35
Newman's Own						
Roadside Virginia	8 fl oz	100	tr	22	0	0
Ocean Spray						
Lemonade	8 fl oz	110	0	29	0	35
With Cranberry Juice	8 fl oz	110	0	26	0	35
With Raspberry Juice	8 fl oz	110	0	27	0	35
Odwalla						
Honey	8 fl oz	70	0	26	0	10
Strawberry	8 fl oz	150	0	40	0	35

FOOD	PORTION	CALS	FAT	CARB	CHOL	SOD
Royal Mistic						
Lemonade Limeade	16 fl oz	230	0	57	0	19
Tropical Pink	16 fl oz	230	0	57	0	11
Santa Cruz						
Organic	8 oz	100	0	24	0	0
Snapple						
Diet Pink	8 fl oz	13	0	3	0	10
Lemonade	8 fl oz	110	0	29	0	10
Pink	8 fl oz	110	0	26	0	15
Strawberry	8 fl oz	110	0	26	0	5
Tropicana						
Lemonade	1 can (11.5 oz)	160	0	39	0	20
Turkey Hill						
Lemonade	8 fl oz	110	0	29	0	0
Veryfine						
Lemonade	8 fl oz	120	0	30	0	<25
LIME JUICE						
After The Fall						
Caribbean Lime	1 can (12 oz)	170	0	42	0	25
Key West	1 cup (8 oz)	100	0	25	0	10
Odwalla						
Summertime Lime	8 fl oz	90	0	23	0	10
LIQUOR/LIQUEUR						
anisette	⅔ oz	74	0	7	0	—
apricot brandy	⅔ oz	64	0	6	0	—
aquavit	3.5 oz	229	0	0	0	—
benedictine	⅔ oz	69	0	7	0	—
bloody mary	5 oz	116	tr	5	0	332
bourbon & soda	4 oz	105	0	0	0	16
coffee liqueur	1½ oz	174	tr	24	0	4
coffee w/ cream liqueur	1½ oz	154	7	10	—	43
cognac	3.5 oz	233	0	1	0	—
creme de menthe	1½ oz	186	tr	21	0	3
curacao liqueur	⅔ oz	54	0	6	0	—
daiquiri	2 oz	111	0	4	0	1
gin	1½ oz	110	0	0	0	1
gin & tonic	7.5 oz	171	0	16	0	10
gin ricky	4 oz	150	0	—	0	—
manhattan	2 oz	128	0	2	0	2
martini	2½ oz	156	0	tr	0	2
mint julep	10 oz	210	0	3	0	—
old-fashioned	2½ oz	127	0	3	0	—
pina colada	4½ oz	262	3	40	0	9

FOOD	PORTION	CALS	FAT	CARB	CHOL	SOD
planter's punch	3½ oz	175	0	—	0	—
rum	1½ oz	97	0	0	0	0
screwdriver	7 oz	174	tr	18	0	2
sloe gin fizz	2½ oz	132	0	4	0	1
tequila sunrise	5½ oz	189	tr	15	0	7
tom collins	7½ oz	121	0	3	0	39
vodka	1½ oz	97	0	0	0	0
whiskey	1½ oz	105	0	tr	0	0
whiskey sour	3 oz	123	tr	5	0	10
whiskey sour mix not prep	1 pkg (0.6 oz)	64	0	16	0	46

MACADAMIA NUTS
Mauna Loa

FOOD	PORTION	CALS	FAT	CARB	CHOL	SOD
Candy Glazed	1 oz	170	14	11	5	80
Chocolate Covered	1 oz	170	13	12	0	21
Honey Roasted	1 oz	200	17	8	0	80
Macadamia Nut Brittle	1 oz	150	8	19	6	140
Roasted & Salted	1 oz	210	21	4	0	75

MALT

FOOD	PORTION	CALS	FAT	CARB	CHOL	SOD
nonalcoholic	12 fl oz	32	0	5	0	—

Bartles & Jaymes

FOOD	PORTION	CALS	FAT	CARB	CHOL	SOD
Malt Cooler Berry	12 fl oz	210	0	32	0	5
Malt Cooler Black Cherry	12 fl oz	190	0	30	0	5
Malt Cooler Light Berry	12 fl oz	140	0	29	0	0
Malt Cooler Mandarin Lemon	12 fl oz	210	0	34	0	5
Malt Cooler Margarita	12 fl oz	250	0	44	0	40
Malt Cooler Original	12 fl oz	180	0	27	0	0
Malt Cooler Peach	12 fl oz	200	0	31	0	5
Malt Cooler Pina Colada	12 fl oz	270	0	48	0	5
Malt Cooler Planter's Punch	12 fl oz	220	0	35	0	5
Malt Cooler Red Sangria	12 fl oz	190	0	29	0	5
Malt Cooler Strawberry	12 fl oz	200	0	31	0	5
Malt Cooler Strawberry Daiquiri	12 fl oz	220	0	35	0	5
Malt Cooler Tropical	12 fl oz	220	0	36	0	5

FOOD	PORTION	CALS	FAT	CARB	CHOL	SOD
Olde English						
Malt	12 oz	163	0	10	0	—
Schaefer						
Malt	12 oz	165	0	12	0	20
Schlitz						
Malt	12 oz	177	0	15	0	21
MALTED MILK						
Kraft						
Instant Chocolate as prep w/ 2% milk	1 serv (9.5 oz)	200	6	29	20	160
Instant Natural as prep w/ 2% milk	1 serv (9.5 oz)	210	7	27	25	205
MANGO						
fresh	1	135	1	35	0	4
Rainforest Farms						
Slices Dried	6 slices (1.3 oz)	140	1	33	0	108
MANGO JUICE						
After The Fall						
Hawaiian Mango	1 can (12 oz)	180	0	45	0	20
Mango Ginger	1 can (12 oz)	150	0	35	0	25
Fresh Samantha						
Mango Mama	1 cup (8 oz)	125	1	33	0	0
Kern's						
Nectar	6 fl oz	100	0	28	0	0
Libby						
Nectar	1 can (11.5 fl oz)	210	0	52	0	10
Snapple						
Diet Mango Madness	8 fl oz	13	0	3	0	10
Mango Madness Cocktail	8 fl oz	110	0	29	0	10
MARSHMALLOW						
marshmallow	1 reg (0.3 oz)	23	0	6	0	3
Campfire						
Large	2	40	0	10	0	10
Miniature	24	40	0	10	0	10
Joyva						
Twists Chocolate Covered	2 (1.5 oz)	190	4	21	0	20
Kraft						
Funmallows	4 (1.1 oz)	110	0	26	0	20
Funmallows Miniature	½ cup (1.1 oz)	100	0	25	0	20

FOOD	PORTION	CALS	FAT	CARB	CHOL	SOD
Kraft (CONT.)						
Jet-Puffed	5 (1.2 oz)	110	0	27	0	40
Marshmallow Creme	2 tbsp (0.4 oz)	40	0	10	0	10
Miniature	½ cup (1.1 oz)	100	0	25	0	30
Teddy Bear Cocoa-Flavored	½ cup (1.1 oz)	100	0	23	0	25

MATZO

FOOD	PORTION	CALS	FAT	CARB	CHOL	SOD
Horowitz Margareten						
Egg Milk Chocolate Coated	1 oz	97	4	16	8	7
Manischewitz						
Egg Dark Chocolate Coated	½ matzo (1 oz)	97	3	17	8	7

MEAT STICKS

FOOD	PORTION	CALS	FAT	CARB	CHOL	SOD
jerky beef	1 lg piece (0.7 oz)	67	3	3	22	569
smoked	1 (0.7 oz)	109	10	1	26	293
Tombstone						
Beef Jerky	1 stick (0.5 oz)	35	0	tr	15	310
Beef Sticks	1 (0.8 oz)	110	10	0	20	270
Snappy Sticks	1 (0.8 oz)	110	10	tr	20	260

MILK DRINKS

FOOD	PORTION	CALS	FAT	CARB	CHOL	SOD
chocolate milk	1 cup	208	8	26	30	149
chocolate milk	1 qt	833	34	103	122	596
chocolate milk 1%	1 cup	158	3	26	7	152
chocolate milk 2%	1 cup	179	5	26	17	150
Body Wise						
Chocolate Nonfat Milk	1 cup (8 fl oz)	180	0	35	5	170
Borden						
Chocolate Lowfat Dutch Brand	8 fl oz	180	5	25	—	180
Bosco						
Chocolate Milk	1 cup (8 fl oz)	230	8	33	—	110
Hershey						
Chocolate Milk 2%	1 cup	190	5	29	20	130
Whole Chocolate Milk	8 oz	210	9	28	—	120
Hood						
Chocolate Lowfat	1 cup (8 oz)	150	2	27	10	240
Lactaid						
Chocolate Milk 1%	8 fl oz	158	3	26	7	152
Meadow Gold						
Chocolate Milk	8 fl oz	210	8	25	—	240

FOOD	PORTION	CALS	FAT	CARB	CHOL	SOD
Parmalat						
Chocolate 2%	1 box (8 oz)	180	5	28	20	115
Quik						
Banana Lowfat Milk	8 oz	190	4	30	—	115
Chocolate Lowfat Milk	8 oz	200	5	29	—	150
Ready To Drink Chocolate	8 oz	230	9	30	—	120
Ready To Drink Lite Chocolate Lowfat	8 oz	130	5	13	—	150
Ready To Drink Strawberry	8 oz	230	8	32	—	140

MILK SUBSTITUTES

FOOD	PORTION	CALS	FAT	CARB	CHOL	SOD
Better Than Milk						
Chocolate	8 fl oz	125	5	17	0	175
Eden						
Original	1 pkg (8.8 oz)	135	4	14	0	110
Edensoy						
Carob	8 fl oz	150	4	23	0	105
Extra Original	1 pkg (8.8 oz)	140	5	13	0	105
Extra Vanilla	1 pkg (8.8 fl oz)	150	3	24	0	95
Vanilla	1 pkg (8.8 fl oz)	150	3	24	0	95

MILKSHAKE

FOOD	PORTION	CALS	FAT	CARB	CHOL	SOD
chocolate	10 oz	360	11	58	37	273
strawberry	10 oz	319	8	53	31	234
thick shake chocolate	10.6 oz	356	8	63	32	333
thick shake vanilla	11 oz	350	10	56	37	299
vanilla	10 oz	314	8	51	32	232
D'Frosta Shake						
Vanilla	1 serv (13.5 oz)	340	9	57	40	200
Freeze Flip						
Fruit Shake No Fat Lactose Free Black Raspberry	1 serv (6 oz)	150	0	37	0	25
Frostee						
Chocolate	8 fl oz	200	8	30	—	160
Strawberry	8 fl oz	180	7	27	—	150
Hood						
Shake Up Chocolate	1 cup (8 oz)	240	6	38	20	290
Shake Up Strawberry	1 cup (8 oz)	220	5	36	20	270
Shake Up Vanilla	1 cup (8 oz)	220	5	36	20	270
Parmalat						
Shake A Shake Chocolate	1 box (6 oz)	180	4	29	15	140

FOOD	PORTION	CALS	FAT	CARB	CHOL	SOD
Parmalat (CONT.)						
Shake A Shake Orange Vanilla	1 box (6 oz)	110	3	14	10	55
Shake A Shake Vanilla	1 box (6 oz)	170	3	28	15	140
Weight Watchers						
Chocolate Fudge Shake Mix as prep	1 pkg	80	1	12	0	140

MINERAL/BOTTLED WATER

FOOD	PORTION	CALS	FAT	CARB	CHOL	SOD
Canada Dry						
Sparkling Water	8 fl oz	0	0	0	0	10
Crystal Geyser						
Sparking Natural Wild Cherry	1 bottle 12 fl oz	0	0	0	0	70
Sparkling Lemon	1 bottle (12 fl oz)	0	0	0	0	70
Sparkling Mineral	1 bottle (12 fl oz)	0	0	0	0	70
Sparkling Natural Cola Berry	1 bottle (12 fl oz)	0	0	0	0	70
Sparkling Orange	1 bottle (12 fl oz)	0	0	0	0	70
Diamond Spring						
Water	1 qt	0	0	0	0	—
Evian						
Water	1 liter	0	0	0	0	5
Glennpatrick						
Irish Spring Pure	8 oz	0	0	0	0	—
LaCroix						
Sparkling Berry	12 fl oz	0	0	0	0	—
Sparkling Lemon	12 fl oz	0	0	0	0	—
Sparkling Lime	12 fl oz	0	0	0	0	—
Sparkling Orange	12 fl oz	0	0	0	0	—
Sparkling Regular	12 fl oz	0	0	0	0	—
Mountain Valley						
Mineral Water	1 qt	0	0	0	0	—
San Pellegrino						
Mineral Water	1 liter (33.8 oz)	0	0	0	0	41
Saratoga						
Sparkling	1 liter	0	0	0	0	19
Water Joe						
Caffeine Enhanced	8 fl oz	0	0	0	0	0

MOUSSE

FOOD	PORTION	CALS	FAT	CARB	CHOL	SOD
chocolate	½ cup (7.1 oz)	447	33	33	299	87

FOOD	PORTION	CALS	FAT	CARB	CHOL	SOD
MUFFIN						
blueberry	1 (2 oz)	158	4	27	17	255
corn	1 (2 oz)	174	5	29	—	297
toaster type blueberry	1	103	3	18	—	158
toaster type corn	1	114	4	19	—	142
toaster type wheat bran w/ raisins	1 (1.3 oz)	106	3	19	—	178
Dutch Mill						
Banana Walnut	1 (2 oz)	220	6	33	5	210
Carrot	1 (2 oz)	190	7	31	30	230
Corn	1 (2 oz)	190	6	31	40	280
Cranberry Orange	1 (2 oz)	170	6	26	55	290
Raisin Bran	1 (2 oz)	230	5	37	30	330
Entenmann's						
Blueberry	1 (2 oz)	200	8	29	—	250
Freihofer's						
Corn Toasters	1 (1.3 oz)	130	6	18	15	210
Hostess						
Mini Apple Cinnamon	5 (2 oz)	260	16	28	45	180
Mini Banana Nut	5 (2 oz)	260	16	28	40	160
Mini Blueberry	5 (2 oz)	240	13	30	40	180
Mini Chocolate Chip	5 (2 oz)	260	15	29	35	170
Muffin Loaf Blueberry	1 (3.8 oz)	440	19	62	80	460
Oat Bran	1 (1.5 oz)	160	8	22	0	150
Oat Bran Banana Nut	1 (1.5 oz)	150	6	22	0	160
MUNCHIES						

MUNCHIES

(FAST FACT: According to the Snack Food Association of America, Americans consume 5.7 billion pounds of salty snack foods a year; an average person eats more than twenty-two pounds.)

FOOD	PORTION	CALS	FAT	CARB	CHOL	SOD
oriental mix	1 oz	155	12	9	0	235
pork skins	1 oz	154	9	0	27	521
pork skins barbecue	1 oz	152	9	1	33	756
trail mix	1 cup (5.3 oz)	693	44	67	0	343
trail mix	1 oz	131	8	13	0	65
trail mix tropical	1 oz	115	5	19	0	3
trail mix w/ chocolate chips	1 cup (5.1 oz)	707	47	66	—	177
trail mix w/ chocolate chips	1 oz	137	9	13	—	34
Bakem-ets						
Hot'N Spicy	21 pieces (1 oz)	150	9	1	25	750
Snacks	21 pieces (1 oz)	160	10	2	25	850

FOOD	PORTION	CALS	FAT	CARB	CHOL	SOD
Big Dipper						
Bagel Chips Lowfat Barbeque	12 (1 oz)	110	2	21	0	190
Bagel Chips Lowfat Garlic	12 (1 oz)	120	2	21	0	295
Bagel Chips Lowfat Original	12 (1 oz)	110	2	21	0	150
Bugles						
Nacho Cheese	1 oz	160	9	17	—	250
Ranch	1 oz	150	9	16	—	290
Snacks	1 oz	150	8	18	—	290
Cheetos						
Cheddar Valley	26 pieces (1 oz)	160	9	16	0	240
Crunchy	26 pieces (1 oz)	150	9	17	0	310
Curls	15 pieces (1 oz)	150	9	17	0	270
Flamin' Hot	26 pieces (1 oz)	150	9	16	0	240
Light	38 pieces (1 oz)	140	6	19	0	280
Paws	16 pieces (1 oz)	160	10	15	0	310
Puffed Ball	38 pieces (1 oz)	160	10	16	0	360
Puffs	33 pieces (1 oz)	160	9	16	0	330
Cheez Doodles						
Crunchy	1 oz	160	10	16	—	230
Puffed	1 oz	150	9	16	—	360
Cheez Waffies						
Snacks	1 oz	140	8	14	—	420
Chex						
Snack Mix Barbeque	½ cup (1.1 oz)	130	5	20	0	330
Snack Mix Cool Sour Cream And Onion	½ cup (1 oz)	130	4	21	0	310
Snack Mix Golden Cheddar	½ cup (1 oz)	130	4	20	0	310
Snack Mix Traditional	⅔ cup (1.2 oz)	150	5	23	0	410
Combos						
Cheddar Cheese Cracker	1 oz	140	8	16	5	300
Cheddar Cheese Cracker	1 pkg (1.7 oz)	250	13	28	5	520
Cheddar Cheese Pretzel	1 oz	130	5	18	0	310
Cheddar Cheese Pretzel	1 pkg (1.8 oz)	240	9	33	5	560
Chili Cheese w/ Corn Shell	1 oz	140	6	17	0	420
Chili Cheese w/ Corn Shell	1 pkg (1.7 oz)	230	11	29	5	710

FOOD	PORTION	CALS	FAT	CARB	CHOL	SOD
Combos (CONT.)						
Mustard Pretzel	1 oz	130	4	19	0	270
Mustard Pretzel	1 pkg (1.8 oz)	230	8	35	0	500
Nacho Cheese Pretzel	1 oz	130	5	19	0	320
Nacho Cheese Pretzel	1 pkg (1.7 oz)	230	8	34	0	580
Nacho Cheese w/ Tortilla Shell	1 oz	140	6	17	0	380
Nacho Cheese w/ Tortilla Shell	1 pkg (1.7 oz)	230	11	30	0	640
Peanut Butter Cracker	1 oz	140	8	15	0	260
Pepperoni & Cheese Pizza	1 oz	140	7	17	5	280
Pepperoni & Cheese Pizza	1 pkg (1.7 oz)	240	11	30	5	480
Pizzeria Pretzel	1 oz	130	5	19	0	290
Pizzeria Pretzel	1 pkg (1.8 oz)	230	8	35	0	520
Tortilla Ranch	1 bag (1.7 oz)	240	12	29	5	610
Tortilla Ranch	1 oz	140	7	17	5	350
Cornnuts						
Barbecue	1 oz	120	4	22	0	270
Nacho Cheese	1 oz	120	4	22	0	180
Original	1 oz	120	4	22	0	170
Original	1 pkg (2 oz)	260	8	40	0	340
Picante	1 oz	120	4	22	0	260
Ranch	1 oz	120	4	20	0	190
Doo Dads						
Snacks	1 oz	130	6	17	0	360
Energy Food Factory						
Poprice Cheddar Cheese	½ oz	60	3	8	0	110
Poprice Herb & Garlic	½ oz	50	2	10	0	70
Poprice Lite	½ oz	50	2	9	0	70
Poprice Original No Salt	½ oz	45	0	11	0	1
Estee						
Snack Crisps Apple Cinnamon	1 pkg (0.66 oz)	90	2	16	0	70
Snack Crisps Apple Cinnamon	27 crisps (1 oz)	130	3	24	0	110
Snack Crisps Chocolate	1 pkg (0.66 oz)	90	2	15	0	70
Snack Crisps Chocolate	30 crisps (1 oz)	130	3	23	0	110
Snack Crisps Lemon	1 pkg (0.66 oz)	90	2	16	0	70

FOOD	PORTION	CALS	FAT	CARB	CHOL	SOD
Estee (CONT.)						
Snack Crisps Lemon	30 (1 oz)	130	3	23	5	110
Snack Crisps Ranch	1 pkg (0.6 oz)	90	2	15	0	135
Snack Crisps Ranch	30 (1 oz)	130	3	22	5	200
Snack Crisps White Cheddar	1 pkg (0.6 oz)	90	2	14	5	135
Snack Crisps With Cheddar	27 crisps (1 oz)	130	3	22	5	200
Frito Lay						
Corn Nuggets Toasted	1.38 oz	170	5	29	0	265
Funyums						
Onion Rings	11 pieces (1 oz)	140	7	18	0	265
Handi-Snacks						
Peanut Butter'n Crackers	1 pkg (1.1 oz)	180	12	12	0	150
Peanut Butter'n Grahamsticks	1 pkg (1.1 oz)	170	10	14	0	130
Hapi						
Chili Bits	½ cup (1 oz)	110	0	25	0	180
Health Valley						
Cheddar Lites	0.75 oz	40	2	4	tr	35
Cheddar Lites With Green Onion	0.75 oz	40	2	4	0	35
Innovative Foods						
Roasted Sweet Corn	1 pkg (0.8 oz)	76	0	17	0	5
Lance						
Cheese Balls	1 pkg (1.1 oz)	190	13	16	5	420
Crunchy Cheese Twists	1 pkg (1.5 oz)	260	16	25	0	290
Gold-N-Chees	1 pkg (1.4 oz)	180	9	23	5	410
Pork Skins	1 pkg (0.5 oz)	80	5	0	20	270
Pork Skins BBQ	1 pkg (0.5 oz)	80	5	0	20	400
Mr. Peanut						
Peanut Butter Crisps Graham	12 pieces (1.1 oz)	150	8	18	0	100
Munchos						
Snack	16 pieces (1 oz)	160	10	15	0	230
Pita Puffs						
Barbeque	35 (1 oz)	120	3	20	0	150
Lowfat Garlic	35 (1 oz)	110	1	22	0	125
Lowfat Original	35 (1 oz)	110	1	22	0	170
Lowfat Salsa	35 (1 oz)	110	1	21	0	290
Pizza	35 (1 oz)	120	2	21	0	230
Ranch	35 (1 oz)	120	2	21	0	195

FOOD	PORTION	CALS	FAT	CARB	CHOL	SOD
Planters						
Cheez Balls	1 oz	150	10	15	2	300
Cheez Balls	1 pkg (1 oz)	150	10	15	2	330
Cheez Curls	1 oz	150	10	15	2	310
Cheez Curls	1 pkg (1.2 oz)	190	12	19	2	380
Heat Snack Mix	1 oz	140	8	13	0	230
Snyder's						
Cheddar Cheese Twists	1 oz	150	8	17	0	200
Kruncheez	1 oz	160	10	15	0	170
Onion Toasters	1 oz	150	8	17	0	280
Snack Mix	1 oz	170	8	11	0	410
Sopaipillas Apple & Cinnamon	1 oz	150	8	18	0	15
Splurge						
Snack Mix Fat Free Original	⅔ cup (1 oz)	100	0	25	0	340
Ultra Slim-Fast						
Lite N' Tasty Cheese Curls	1 oz	110	3	20	0	360
Weight Watchers						
Cheese Curls	1 pkg (0.5 oz)	70	3	10	0	85
Pizza Curls	1 pkg (0.5 oz)	60	2	11	0	125
Ranch Curls	1 pkg (0.5 oz)	60	3	10	0	170
NECTARINE						
fresh	1	67	1	16	0	0
NUTRITIONAL SUPPLEMENTS						
BeneFit						
Chocolate	1 serv	120	2	15	—	200
Nutrition Bar	1 (2 oz)	240	8	33	0	190
Vanilla	1 serv	120	2	15	—	220
Boost						
Chocolate	1 can (8 oz)	240	4	40	5	130
Vanilla	8 oz	240	4	40	5	130
Calorie Shed						
Shake Fat Free No Sugar Caramel Ripple	½ cup (4 fl oz)	70	0	21	5	45
Shake Fat Free No Sugar Chocolate	½ cup (4 fl oz)	70	0	21	5	45
Shake Fat Free No Sugar Marshmallow Nougat	½ cup (4 fl oz)	70	0	21	5	45

FOOD	PORTION	CALS	FAT	CARB	CHOL	SOD
Dynatrim						
Dutch Chocolate as prep w/ 1% milk	8 oz	220	4	33	—	300
Strawberry Royale as prep w/ 1% milk	8 oz	220	4	33	—	300
Vanilla as prep w/ 1% milk	8 oz	220	4	33	—	300
Fi-Bar						
Apple	1 (1 oz)	90	3	15	0	12
Cocoa Almond	1	130	4	21	0	20
Cocoa Peanut	1	130	4	20	0	20
Cranberry & Wild Berries	1 (1 oz)	100	3	13	0	20
Lemon	1 (1 oz)	90	3	15	0	12
Mandarin Orange	1 (1 oz)	99	4	15	0	12
Nuggets Almond Butter Crunch	1 pkg	163	11	12	0	—
Nuggets Almond Cappuccino Crunch	1 pkg	136	6	18	0	—
Nuggets Coconut Almond Crunch	1 pkg	136	6	18	0	—
Nuggets Peanut Butter Crunch	1 pkg	160	10	12	0	—
Raspberry	1 (1 oz)	100	3	13	0	20
Strawberry	1 (1 oz)	100	3	13	0	20
Treat Yourself Right Almond	1	152	6	22	0	38
Treat Yourself Right Peanutty Butter	1	152	5	18	0	56
Vanilla Almond	1	130	4	21	0	20
Vanilla Peanut	1	130	4	20	0	20
Figurines						
Chocolate	1 bar	100	5	11	—	45
Chocolate Caramel	1 bar	100	6	10	—	55
Chocolate Peanut Butter	1 bar	100	6	10	—	45
S'Mores	1 bar	100	5	11	—	54
Vanilla	1 bar	100	5	11	—	45
Gatorade						
GatorBar	1 (1.17 oz)	110	1	13	0	10
GatorLode	1 can (11.6 fl oz)	280	0	71	0	90
GatorPro	1 can (11 fl oz)	360	6	59	0	270
ReLode	1 pkt (0.75 oz)	80	0	17	0	25

FOOD	PORTION	CALS	FAT	CARB	CHOL	SOD
GeniSoy						
Soy Protein Bar Chocolate	1 bar (2.2 oz)	210	0	36	0	190
Soy Protein Bar Chocolate Coated	1 bar (2.2 oz)	220	4	33	0	190
Soy Protein Powder	1 scoop (0.6 oz)	60	0	0	0	180
Soy Protein Shake Chocolate	1 scoop (1.2 oz)	120	0	17	0	170
Soy Protein Shake Vanilla	1 scoop (1.2 oz)	130	0	18	0	180
Gookinaid						
Lemonade	1 cup (8 fl oz)	45	0	12	0	70
Malsovit						
Mealwafers	2	152	8	—	0	—
Meal On The Go						
Apple	1 bar (3 oz)	294	5	50	0	114
Banana w/ Pecans	1 bar (3 oz)	289	10	50	0	109
Original	1 bar (3 oz)	286	9	52	0	119
Nancy Grey's						
Shake Hi-Protein Black Raspberry	1 cup (8 fl oz)	340	16	40	65	160
Shake Hi-Protein Chocolate	1 cup (8 fl oz)	340	15	42	60	140
Shake Hi-Protein Vanilla	1 cup (8 fl oz)	340	16	40	65	160
NiteBite						
Chocolate Fudge	1 bar (0.9 oz)	100	4	15	5	40
Peanut Butter	1 bar (0.9 oz)	100	4	15	5	80
Nutra/Balance						
EggPro	4 oz	200	4	33	18	105
Frozen Pudding Butterscotch	4 oz	225	8	31	0	220
Frozen Pudding Chocolate	4 oz	225	8	31	0	220
Frozen Pudding Tapioca	4 oz	225	8	31	0	220
Frozen Pudding Vanilla	4 oz	225	8	31	0	220
NutraShake						
Chocolate	4 oz	200	6	31	18	55
Strawberry	4 oz	200	6	31	18	55
Vanilla	4 oz	200	6	31	18	55
With Fiber Strawberry	6 oz	300	2	60	0	110

FOOD	PORTION	CALS	FAT	CARB	CHOL	SOD
NutraShake (CONT.)						
With Fiber Vanilla	6 oz	300	2	60	0	110
Power Bar						
Malt-Nut	1 bar (2.3 oz)	230	3	45	0	90
Resource						
Fructose Sweetened	1 pkg (8 oz)	250	11	23	—	230
Fruit Beverage	1 pkg (8 oz)	180	0	36	—	55
Liquid Food	1 pkg (8 oz)	250	9	34	—	210
Plus Liquid Food	1 pkg (8 oz)	355	13	47	—	300
Sego						
Lite Chocolate	10 fl oz	150	3	20	5	480
Lite Dutch Chocolate	10 fl oz	150	3	20	5	480
Lite French Vanilla	10 fl oz	150	4	17	5	390
Lite Strawberry	10 fl oz	150	4	17	5	390
Lite Vanilla	10 fl oz	150	4	17	5	390
Very Chocolate	10 fl oz	225	1	43	5	450
Very Chocolate Malt	10 fl oz	225	1	43	5	450
Very Strawberry	10 fl oz	225	5	34	5	360
Very Vanilla	10 fl oz	225	5	34	5	360
Slim-Fast						
Powder Chocolate as prep w/ skim milk	8 oz	190	1	32	9	210
Powder Chocolate Malt as prep w/ skim milk	8 oz	190	tr	32	9	230
Powder Strawberry as prep w/ skim milk	8 oz	190	1	32	9	220
Powder Vanilla as prep w/ skim milk	8 oz	190	1	32	6	220
Sustacal						
Vanilla	8 oz	240	6	33	<5	220
Sweet Success						
Chewy Bar Chocolate Brownie	1 (1.6 oz)	120	4	28	<5	35
Chewy Bar Chocolate Chip	1 (1.6 oz)	120	4	23	<5	35
Chewy Bar Chocolate Peanut Butter	1 (1.6 oz)	120	4	23	<5	35
Chewy Bar Chocolate Raspberry	1 (1.6 oz)	120	4	23	<5	35
Chewy Bar Oatmeal Raisin	1 (1.6 oz)	120	4	23	<5	30
Chocolate Mocha Supreme	1 can (10 fl oz)	200	3	38	5	220

FOOD	PORTION	CALS	FAT	CARB	CHOL	SOD
Sweet Success (CONT.)						
Chocolate Mocha Supreme as prep w/ skim milk	9 fl oz	180	tr	30	6	356
Chocolate Raspberry Truffle	1 can (10 fl oz)	200	3	38	5	220
Chocolate Raspberry as prep w/ skim milk	9 fl oz	180	1	30	6	360
Classic Chocolate Chip as prep w/ skim milk	9 fl oz	180	1	30	6	288
Creamy Milk Chocolate	1 can (10 fl oz)	200	3	38	5	240
Creamy Milk Chocolate	1 carton (12 fl oz)	220	2	45	<5	300
Creamy Milk Chocolate as prep w/ skim milk	9 fl oz	180	1	30	6	336
Creamy Vanilla Delight as prep w/ skim milk	9 fl oz	180	tr	33	6	312
Dark Chocolate Fudge	1 can (10 fl oz)	200	3	38	5	220
Dark Chocolate Fudge	1 carton (12 fl oz)	220	2	45	<5	310
Dark Chocolate Fudge as prep w/ skim milk	9 fl oz	180	1	30	6	356
Rich Chocolate Almond	1 can (10 fl oz)	200	3	38	5	240
Rich Chocolate Almond	1 carton (12 fl oz)	220	2	45	<5	300
Rich Chocolate Almond as prep w/ skim milk	9 fl oz	180	tr	30	6	356
Smooth Vanilla Creme	1 can (10 fl oz)	200	3	38	5	220
The Pumper						
Body Building Milkshake Chocolate	1 serv (13.5 oz)	390	2	80	5	260
Body Building Milkeshake Banana	1 serv (13.5 oz)	390	2	82	10	230
Ultra Slim-Fast						
Cafe Mocha as prep w/ skim milk	8 oz	200	tr	38	8	280

FOOD	PORTION	CALS	FAT	CARB	CHOL	SOD
Ultra Slim-Fast (CONT.)						
Chocolate Royale as prep w/ skim milk	8 oz	200	1	36	8	230
Crunch Bar Cocoa Almond	1	110	3	19	0	30
Crunch Bar Cocoa Raspberry	1	100	3	21	0	30
Crunch Bar Vanilla Almond	1	110	4	18	0	30
Dutch Chocolate as prep w/ water	8 oz	220	tr	40	8	260
French Vanilla as prep w/ skim milk	8 oz	190	tr	36	8	250
French Vanilla as prep w/ water	8 oz	220	tr	40	8	260
Fruit Juice Mix as prep w/ fruit juice	8 oz	200	tr	43	12	80
Nutrition Bar Dutch Chocolate	1	130	4	17	5	90
Nutrition Bar Peanut Butter	1	140	6	15	5	100
Pina Colada as prep w/ skim milk	8 oz	180	tr	36	8	250
Ready-To-Drink Chocolate Royale	11 oz	230	3	42	5	220
Ready-To-Drink Chocolate Royale	12 oz	250	1	45	5	240
Ready-To-Drink French Vanilla	11 oz	230	5	38	5	190
Ready-To-Drink French Vanilla	12 oz	220	tr	38	5	240
Ready-To-Drink Strawberry Supreme	12 oz	220	1	38	5	240
Strawberry Supreme as prep w/ water	8 oz	220	tr	40	8	260
Strawberry as prep w/ skim milk	8 oz	190	1	36	8	250
Vita-J						
Apple Juice	11.5 fl oz	8	0	2	0	25
Fruit Punch	11.5 fl oz	8	0	2	0	25
Grapefruit Cocktail w/ Raspberry	11.5 fl oz	8	0	2	0	25
Orange Juice	11.5 fl oz	8	0	2	0	25

FOOD	PORTION	CALS	FAT	CARB	CHOL	SOD
NUTS MIXED						
Fisher						
Mixed Deluxe Lightly Salted	1 oz	180	16	5	0	—
Mixed Deluxe Salted	1 oz	180	16	5	0	95
Mixed Oil Roasted 25% More Cashews Lightly Salted	1 oz	180	16	5	0	50
Mixed Oil Roasted 25% More Cashews Salted	1 oz	180	16	5	0	110
Nut & Fruit Pina Colada	1 oz	150	10	13	0	50
Nut & Fruit Raisin Cranberry	1 oz	150	10	12	0	70
Nut & Fruit Tropical Fruit	1 oz	140	8	15	0	90
Peanuts Cashews	1 oz	170	13	8	0	110
Guy's						
Mixed With Peanuts	1 oz	180	16	3	0	140
Tasty Mix	1 oz	130	7	14	0	510
Planters						
Cashews & Peanuts Honey Roasted	1 oz	150	12	10	0	125
Deluxe Oil Roasted	1 oz	170	16	6	0	110
Dry Roasted	1 oz	170	14	7	0	250
Honey Roasted	1 oz	140	13	9	0	85
Lightly Salted Oil Roasted	1 oz	170	15	6	0	55
No Brazils Lightly Salted Oil Roasted	1 oz	170	15	6	0	55
No Brazils Oil Roasted	1 oz	170	15	6	0	110
Oil Roasted	1 oz	170	15	5	0	115
Select Mix Cashews Almonds & Macadamias Oil Roasted	1 oz	170	16	6	0	90
Select Mix Cashews Almonds & Pecans Oil Roasted	1 oz	170	15	7	0	95
Unsalted Oil Roasted	1 oz	170	15	6	0	0
ORANGE						
california navel fresh	1	65	tr	16	0	1

FOOD	PORTION	CALS	FAT	CARB	CHOL	SOD
california valencia fresh	1	59	tr	14	0	0
florida fresh	1	69	tr	17	0	1
sections fresh	1 cup	85	tr	21	0	0

ORANGE JUICE

After The Fall

Juice	1 bottle (10 oz)	110	0	26	0	10

Fresh Samantha

Juice	1 cup (8 oz)	109	1	24	0	0

Hi-C

Box	8.45 fl oz	130	0	33	0	30
Drink	1 can (11.5 fl oz)	180	0	45	0	40

Minute Maid

Box	8.45 fl oz	120	0	28	0	25
Juices To Go	1 bottle (10 fl oz)	140	0	34	0	30
Juices To Go	1 bottle (16 fl oz)	110	0	27	0	25
Juices To Go	1 can (11.5 fl oz)	160	0	39	0	35
Orange Punch Box	8.45 fl oz	130	0	33	0	25

Odwalla

Juice	8 fl oz	110	1	25	—	25

Snapple

Juice	10 fl oz	130	0	29	0	55
Orangeade	8 fl oz	120	0	31	0	10

Tropicana

Juice	1 container (10 fl oz)	130	0	33	0	0
Juice	1 container (6 fl oz)	80	0	20	0	0
Juice	1 container (8 fl oz)	110	0	27	0	0
Season's Best	1 bottle (10 fl oz)	130	0	33	0	5
Season's Best	1 bottle (7 fl oz)	90	0	23	0	0
Season's Best	1 can (11.5 fl oz)	140	0	36	0	5

PAPAYA

cubed fresh	1 cup	54	tr	14	0	4
fresh	1	117	tr	30	0	8

FOOD	PORTION	CALS	FAT	CARB	CHOL	SOD
Sonoma						
Pieces Dried	2 pieces (2 oz)	200	4	41	0	60
PAPAYA JUICE						
Goya						
Nectar	6 oz	110	0	27	0	10
Libby						
Nectar	1 can (11.5 fl oz)	210	0	51	0	10
PASSION FRUIT JUICE						
Snapple						
Passion Supreme	10 fl oz	160	0	39	0	20
PEACH						
fresh	1	37	tr	10	0	0
Del Monte						
Snack Cups Diced Fruit Naturals	1 serv (4.5 oz)	60	0	16	0	10
Snack Cups Diced Fruit Naturals EZ-Open Lid	1 serv (4.2 oz)	60	0	15	0	10
Snack Cups Diced In Heavy Syrup	1 serv (4.5 oz)	100	0	24	0	10
Snack Cups Diced In Heavy Syrup EZ-Open Lid	1 serv (4.2 oz)	90	0	23	0	10
Snack Cups Diced Lite	1 serv (4.5 oz)	60	0	16	0	10
Snack Cups Diced Lite EZ-Open Lid	1 serv (4.2 oz)	60	0	15	0	10
Sonoma						
Pieces Dried	3-5 pieces (1.4 oz)	120	0	31	0	0
PEACH JUICE						
Goya						
Nectar	6 oz	110	0	27	0	30
Libby						
Nectar	1 can (11.5 fl oz)	210	0	52	0	5
Snapple						
Dixie Peach	10 fl oz	140	0	39	0	20
PEANUT BUTTER						
Skippy						
Creamy w/ 2 slices white bread	1 sandwich	340	19	33	0	430

FOOD	PORTION	CALS	FAT	CARB	CHOL	SOD
Skippy (CONT.)						
Super Chunk w/ slices white bread	1 sandwich	340	19	32	0	410

PEANUTS

FOOD	PORTION	CALS	FAT	CARB	CHOL	SOD
chocolate coated	1 cup (5.2 oz)	773	50	74	13	61
chocolate coated	10 (1.4 oz)	208	13	20	4	16
dry roasted	1 oz	164	14	6	0	228
oil roasted	1 oz	163	14	5	0	121
Beer Nuts						
Peanuts	1 pkg (1 oz)	180	14	7	0	60
Lance						
Honey Toasted	1 pkg (1.4 oz)	230	17	11	0	240
Roasted w/ Shell	1 pkg (1.8 oz)	190	15	8	0	0
Salted	1 pkg (1 oz)	190	15	7	0	105
Little Debbie						
Salted	1 pkg (1.2 oz)	230	21	3	0	45
Planters						
Fun Size! Oil Roasted	2 pkg (1 oz)	170	15	6	0	140
Heat Hot Spicy Oil Roasted	1 pkg (1.7 oz)	290	25	9	0	370
Heat Hot Spicy Oil Roasted	1 pkg (2 oz)	330	29	10	0	390
Honey Roasted Dry Roasted	1 pkg (1.7 oz)	260	19	17	0	260
Lightly Salted Dry Roasted	1 pkg (1.75 oz)	290	25	9	0	190
Lightly Salted Oil Roasted	1 pkg (1.8 oz)	300	27	8	0	95
Munch'N Go Singles Heat Hot Spicy Oil Roasted	1 pkg (2.5 oz)	410	36	13	0	480
Reduced Fat Honey Roasted	⅓ cup (1 oz)	130	7	12	0	150
Weight Watchers						
Honey Roasted	1 pkg (0.7 oz)	100	5	7	0	100

PEAR

FOOD	PORTION	CALS	FAT	CARB	CHOL	SOD
asian fresh	1 (4.3 oz)	51	tr	13	0	0
fresh	1	98	1	25	0	1
Del Monte						
Snack Cups Diced In Heavy Syrup	1 serv (4.5 oz)	100	0	24	0	10
Snack Cups Diced In Heavy Syrup EZ-Open Lid	1 serv (4.2 oz)	90	0	23	0	10

FOOD	PORTION	CALS	FAT	CARB	CHOL	SOD
Del Monte (CONT.)						
Snack Cups Diced Lite	1 serv (4.5 oz)	60	0	15	0	10
Snack Cups Diced Lite EZ-Open Lid	1 serv (4.2 oz)	60	0	15	0	10
Sonoma						
Pieces Dried	3-4 pieces (1.4 oz)	120	0	33	0	0
PEAR JUICE						
Kern's						
Nectar	6 fl oz	120	0	28	0	0
Libby						
Nectar	1 can (11.5 fl oz)	220	0	54	0	5
PECANS						
dry roasted salted	1 oz	187	18	6	0	260
oil roasted salted	1 oz	195	20	5	0	252
Planters						
Honey Roasted	1 oz	180	16	9	0	75
PERSIMMONS						
fresh	1	32	tr	8	0	0
Sonoma						
Dried	6-8 pieces (1.4 oz)	140	0	35	0	10
PICKLES						
dill	1 (2.3 oz)	12	tr	3	0	833
dill sliced	1 slice	1	tr	tr	0	77
kosher dill	1 (2.3 oz)	12	tr	3	0	833
quick sour	1 (1.2 oz)	4	tr	1	0	423
sweet gherkin	1 sm (½ oz)	20	tr	5	0	107
PIE						
snack apple blueberry fried	1 (6.4 oz)	404	21	55	—	479
snack pie apple	1 (3 oz)	266	14	33	13	325
snack pie apple fried	1 (6.4 oz)	404	21	55	—	479
snack pie cherry	1 (3 oz)	266	14	33	13	325
snack pie lemon	1 (3 oz)	266	14	33	13	325
snack pie lemon fried	1 (6.4 oz)	404	21	55	—	479
snack pie peach fried	1 (6.4 oz)	404	21	55	—	479
snack pie strawberry fried	1 (6.4 oz)	404	21	55	—	479
Drake's						
Apple	1 (2 oz)	210	10	29	0	135

FOOD	PORTION	CALS	FAT	CARB	CHOL	SOD
Drake's (CONT.)						
Blueberry	1 (2 oz)	210	10	30	0	135
Cherry	1 (2 oz)	220	10	30	0	135
Lemon	1 (2 oz)	210	11	27	0	115
Entenmann's						
Apple Homestyle	1 serv (2.1 oz)	140	7	21	—	150
Coconut Custard	1 serv (1.8 oz)	140	8	16	—	160
Lance						
Pecan	1 (38 g)	350	15	51	40	70
Little Debbie						
Marshmallow Banana	1 pkg (1.4 oz)	160	5	27	0	95
Marshmallow Banana	1 pkg (2 oz)	240	8	40	0	140
Marshmallow Banana	1 pkg (2.7 oz)	320	11	54	0	190
Marshmallow Chocolate	1 pkg (1.4 oz)	160	5	27	0	95
Marshmallow Chocolate	1 pkg (2 oz)	240	9	40	0	135
Marshmallow Chocolate	1 pkg (2.7 oz)	320	11	53	0	190
Oatmeal Creme	1 pkg (1.3 oz)	170	8	25	0	200
Oatmeal Creme	1 pkg (2.5 oz)	300	11	48	0	330
Oatmeal Creme	1 pkg (3 oz)	360	14	58	0	400
Raisin Creme	1 pkg (1.2 oz)	140	5	23	0	120
Raisin Creme	1 pkg (2.5 oz)	290	12	47	0	240
Tastykake						
Apple	1 pkg (4 oz)	300	12	46	0	340
Banana Creme	1 pkg (4.2 oz)	380	16	54	25	430
Blueberry	1 pkg (4 oz)	310	9	55	0	410
Cherry	1 pkg (4 oz)	300	10	49	0	310
Coconut Creme	1 pkg (4 oz)	380	20	46	65	420
French Apple	1 pkg (4 oz)	350	11	63	0	220
Lemon	1 pkg (4 oz)	320	13	48	40	380
Lemon Lime	1 pkg (4 oz)	320	13	49	45	310
Peach	1 pkg (4 oz)	300	12	47	0	360
Pineapple Cheese	1 pkg (4.2 oz)	340	13	54	20	410
Pumpkin	1 pkg (4 oz)	320	14	46	30	520
Strawberry	1 pkg (4 oz)	340	11	57	0	300
Tasty Klair	1 pkg (4 oz)	400	20	51	55	320
PINEAPPLE						
fresh diced	1 cup	77	tr	19	0	1
fresh slice	1 slice	42	tr	10	0	1
Del Monte						
Snack Cups Tidbits In Juice	1 serv (4.5 oz)	70	0	18	0	10

FOOD	PORTION	CALS	FAT	CARB	CHOL	SOD
Del Monte (CONT.)						
Snack Cups Tidbits In Juice EZ-Open Lid	1 serv (4.2 oz)	60	0	17	0	10
Sonoma						
Pieces Dried	2 pieces (1.4 oz)	140	2	30	0	30

PINEAPPLE JUICE
After The Fall						
Mandarin Pineapple	1 can (12 oz)	150	0	37	0	25
Del Monte						
Juice	1 serv (11.5 oz)	190	0	45	0	15
Minute Maid						
Box	8.45 fl oz	130	0	33	0	25

PISTACHIOS
dry roasted salted	1 cup	776	68	35	0	1040
Dole						
Shelled	1 oz	163	14	7	0	—
Shells On	1 oz	90	7	3	0	250
Lance						
Pistachios	1 pkg (1.1 oz)	100	8	4	0	100
Planters						
Munch'N Go Singles Shelled Dry Roasted	1 pkg (2 oz)	330	29	14	0	450
Red Salted Dry Roasted	1 pkg	160	14	7	0	250

PIZZA
Boboli						
Shell + Sauce	⅙ sm shell (2.6 oz)	170	3	29	5	540
Shell + Sauce	⅛ lg shell (2.6 oz)	170	3	28	5	460
Celeste						
Italian Bread Deluxe	1 (5.1 oz)	290	11	36	15	1000
Italian Bread Garlic & Herb Zesty Chicken	1 (5 oz)	260	8	34	20	960
Italian Bread Pepperoni	1 (5 oz)	320	13	37	20	1140
Italian Bread Zesty Four Cheese	1 (4.6 oz)	300	12	32	25	820
Large Cheese	¼ pie (4.4 oz)	320	16	32	25	590
Large Deluxe	¼ pie (5.5 oz)	350	18	35	20	880

FOOD	PORTION	CALS	FAT	CARB	CHOL	SOD
Celeste (CONT.)						
Large Pepperoni	¼ pie (4.7 oz)	350	20	33	20	990
Large Suprema With Meat	⅕ pie (4.6 oz)	290	16	27	15	770
Large Zesty Four Cheese	¼ pie (4.4 oz)	330	16	34	30	610
Small Cheese	1 (7.5 oz)	540	25	60	45	1090
Small Deluxe	1 (8.2 oz)	540	29	53	25	1320
Small Hot & Zesty Four Cheese	1 (7 oz)	530	27	50	50	1090
Small Original Four Cheese	1 (7 oz)	540	30	47	50	1040
Small Pepperoni	1 (6.7 oz)	520	27	53	25	1280
Small Sausage	1 (7.5 oz)	530	27	52	25	1400
Small Suprema Vegetable	1 (7.5 oz)	480	23	52	5	1270
Small Suprema With Meat	1 (9 oz)	580	31	56	30	1480
Small Zesty Four Cheese	1 (7 oz)	530	27	50	50	1090
Croissant Pocket						
Stuffed Sandwich Pepperoni Pizza	1 piece (4.5 oz)	350	15	39	30	870
Empire						
3 Pack	1 (3 oz)	210	9	23	20	630
Bagel	1 (2 oz)	150	5	15	15	390
English Muffin	1 (2 oz)	130	5	15	15	390
Pizza	½ pie (5 oz)	340	13	38	30	970
Fox						
Deluxe Golden Topping	½ pizza	240	11	25	—	600
Deluxe Hamburger	½ pizza	260	12	26	—	700
Deluxe Pepperoni	½ pizza	250	13	26	—	640
Deluxe Sausage	½ pizza	260	13	26	—	630
Deluxe Sausage & Pepperoni	½ pizza	260	13	26	—	640
Healthy Choice						
French Bread Cheese	1 (5.6 oz)	310	4	49	10	470
French Bread Pepperoni	1 (6 oz)	360	9	48	25	580
French Bread Sausage	1 (6 oz)	330	4	52	20	470
French Bread Supreme	1 (6.35 oz)	340	6	49	25	510

FOOD	PORTION	CALS	FAT	CARB	CHOL	SOD
Hot Pocket						
Stuffed Sandwich Pepperoni & Sausage Pizza	1 (4.5 oz)	340	16	38	30	630
Stuffed Sandwich Pepperoni Pizza	1 (4.5 oz)	350	17	38	30	780
Jeno's						
4-Pack Cheese	1 pizza	160	8	17	—	460
4-Pack Combination	1 pizza	180	9	17	—	470
4-Pack Hamburger	1 pizza	180	9	17	—	500
4-Pack Pepperoni	1 pizza	170	9	17	—	460
4-Pack Sausage	1 pizza	180	9	17	—	460
Crisp 'n Tasty Canadian Bacon	½ pizza	250	11	27	—	880
Crisp 'n Tasty Cheese	½ pizza	270	14	28	—	770
Crisp 'n Tasty Hamburger	½ pizza	290	15	28	—	810
Crisp 'n Tasty Pepperoni	½ pizza	280	15	27	—	760
Crisp 'n Tasty Sausage	½ pizza	300	16	28	—	850
Crisp 'n Tasty Sausage & Pepperoni	½ pizza	300	16	27	—	840
Microwave Pizza Rolls Pepperoni & Cheese	6	240	13	23	—	440
Microwave Pizza Rolls Sausage & Cheese	6	250	13	24	—	440
Pizza Rolls Cheese	6	240	12	23	—	350
Pizza Rolls Hamburger	6	240	13	21	—	280
Pizza Rolls Pepperoni & Cheese	6	230	13	22	—	390
Pizza Rolls Sausage & Pepperoni	6	230	13	22	—	380
Kid Cuisine						
Cheese	1 (8 oz)	430	11	71	20	440
Hamburger	1 (8.30 oz)	400	11	61	25	530
Kineret						
Bagel Pizza	2 (4 oz)	300	10	39	30	700
Slice	1 (4.9 oz)	490	9	93	20	510
Lean Cuisine						
French Bread Cheese	1 pkg (6 oz)	350	8	48	20	400

FOOD	PORTION	CALS	FAT	CARB	CHOL	SOD
Lean Cuisine (CONT.)						
French Bread Deluxe	1 pkg (6.1 oz)	350	6	45	30	560
French Bread Pepperoni	1 pkg (5.25 oz)	330	7	46	25	590
Lean Pockets						
Stuffed Sandwich Pizza Deluxe	1 (4.5 oz)	270	8	37	25	680
MicroMagic						
Deep Dish Combination	1 (6.5 oz)	605	34	60	28	1280
Deep Dish Pepperoni	1 (6.5 oz)	615	32	65	42	1300
Deep Dish Sausage	1 (6.5 oz)	590	31	62	18	1250
Mrs. P's						
Combination	½ pizza	260	13	26	—	640
Golden Topping	½ pizza	240	11	25	—	600
Hamburger	½ pizza	260	12	26	—	700
Pepperoni	½ pizza	250	13	26	—	640
Sausage	½ pizza	260	13	26	—	630
Old El Paso						
Pizza Burrito Cheese	1 (3.5 oz)	320	9	27	20	430
Pizza Burrito Pepperoni	1 (3.5 oz)	260	10	31	20	510
Pizza Burrito Sausage	1 (3.5 oz)	260	9	32	15	420
Pappalo's						
French Bread Cheese	1 pizza	360	15	40	—	830
French Bread Combination	1 pizza	430	21	41	—	1120
French Bread Pepperoni	1 pizza	410	20	41	—	1130
French Bread Sausage	1 pizza	410	18	41	—	1000
Pan Combination	⅙ pizza	340	15	34	—	700
Pan Hamburger	⅙ pizza	310	12	34	—	580
Pan Pepperoni	⅙ pizza	330	14	34	—	710
Pan Sausage	⅙ pizza	360	18	34	—	550
Thin Crust Combination	⅙ pizza	260	10	29	—	590
Thin Crust Hamburger	⅙ pizza	240	8	28	—	470
Thin Crust Pepperoni	⅙ pizza	270	11	28	—	600
Thin Crust Sausage	⅙ pizza	250	9	28	—	490
Pepperidge Farm						
Croissant Pastry Cheese	1	430	23	41	—	640
Croissant Pastry Deluxe	1	440	23	43	—	790

FOOD	PORTION	CALS	FAT	CARB	CHOL	SOD
Pepperidge Farm (CONT.)						
Croissant Pastry Pepperoni	1	420	22	43	—	690
Pillsbury						
Microwave Cheese	½ pizza	240	10	28	—	540
Microwave Combination	½ pizza	310	15	29	—	780
Microwave French Bread	1 pizza	370	15	41	—	680
Microwave French Bread Pepperoni	1 pizza	430	19	46	—	940
Microwave French Bread Sausage	1 pizza	410	16	48	—	860
Microwave French Bread Sausage & Pepperoni	1 pizza	450	21	47	—	950
Microwave Pepperoni	½ pizza	300	15	29	—	790
Microwave Sausage	½ pizza	280	13	29	—	680
Small World						
Four Cheese	1 (4 oz)	240	6	38	13	350
Special Delivery						
Organic	⅓ pizza (5.3 oz)	320	9	46	20	500
Organic Soy Kaas	⅓ pizza (5.3 oz)	320	7	47	0	600
Stouffer's						
French Bread Bacon Cheddar	1 piece (5.8 oz)	440	22	44	30	940
French Bread Cheese	1 piece (5.2 oz)	350	14	42	15	660
French Bread Cheeseburger	1 piece (6 oz)	440	26	31	55	1110
French Bread Deluxe	1 piece (6.2 oz)	440	22	42	35	980
French Bread Double Cheese	1 piece (5.9 oz)	420	19	44	30	790
French Bread Garden Vegetable	1 piece (5.8 oz)	340	12	45	15	540
French Bread Pepperoni	1 piece (5.6 oz)	420	20	42	35	930
French Bread Pepperoni & Mushroom	1 piece (6.1 oz)	430	21	43	30	1000
French Bread Sausage	1 piece (6 oz)	420	20	41	35	900
French Bread Sausage & Pepperoni	1 piece (6.25 oz)	460	25	45	40	1130
French Bread Vegetable Deluxe	1 piece (6.4 oz)	380	17	43	25	830

FOOD	PORTION	CALS	FAT	CARB	CHOL	SOD
Stouffer's (CONT.)						
French Bread White Pizza	1 piece (5.1 oz)	460	28	43	25	760
Lunch Express Deluxe	1 pkg (6.6 oz)	460	25	40	45	1000
Lunch Express Double Cheese	1 pkg (5.9 oz)	420	19	41	35	710
Lunch Express Pepperoni	1 pkg (5.75 oz)	440	23	39	40	960
Lunch Express Sausage	1 pkg (6.5 oz)	460	25	40	40	1090
Lunch Express Sausage & Pepperoni	1 pkg (6.4 oz)	500	27	41	60	1140
Tombstone						
12 in Canadian Bacon	⅕ pie (5.5 oz)	360	15	36	40	920
12 in Cheese & Hamburger	⅕ pie (4.4 oz)	320	16	29	30	660
12 in Cheese & Pepperoni	⅕ pie (4.4 oz)	340	18	29	35	750
12 in Cheese & Sausage	⅕ pie (4.4 oz)	320	16	29	30	650
12 in Cheese Sausage & Mushroom	⅕ pie (4.5 oz)	320	16	29	30	630
12 in Deluxe	⅕ pie (4.7 oz)	320	16	29	30	640
12 in Extra Cheese	⅕ pie (5.1 oz)	370	17	36	30	680
12 in Sausage & Pepperoni	⅕ pie (4.4 oz)	340	18	29	35	740
12 in Special Order Four Cheese	⅕ pie (5.2 oz)	400	19	37	40	760
12 in Special Order Four Meat	⅙ pie (4.7 oz)	350	18	31	40	810
12 in Special Order Pepperoni	⅙ pie (4.5 oz)	360	19	31	40	790
12 in Special Order Super Supreme	⅙ pie (4.8 oz)	350	18	31	40	800
12 in Special Order Three Sausage	⅙ pie (4.6 oz)	340	17	31	35	740
12 in Supreme	⅕ pie (4.6 oz)	330	17	29	35	720
12 in ThinCrust Italian Style Three Cheese	¼ pie (4.8 oz)	380	22	25	45	730
9 in Cheese & Hamburger	⅓ pie (4.1 oz)	310	16	28	30	620
9 in Cheese & Pepperoni	⅓ pie (4.1 oz)	340	19	28	30	740

FOOD	PORTION	CALS	FAT	CARB	CHOL	SOD
Tombstone (CONT.)						
9 in Cheese & Sausage	⅓ pie (4.1 oz)	310	16	28	30	610
9 in Deluxe	⅓ pie (4.5 oz)	320	16	28	30	620
9 in Extra Cheese	⅓ pie (5.6 oz)	420	19	42	30	730
9 in Pepperoni & Sausage	⅓ pie (4.4 oz)	360	21	28	35	820
9 in Special Order Four Meat	⅓ pie (5.3 oz)	400	20	35	45	910
9 in Special Order Pepperoni	⅓ pie (5.1 oz)	400	21	35	45	880
9 in Special Order Super Supreme	⅓ pie (5.5 oz)	400	21	36	45	900
9 in Special Order Three Sausage	⅓ pie (5.2 oz)	390	19	35	40	830
Double Top Pepperoni With Double Cheese	⅙ pie (4.5 oz)	350	20	25	45	850
Double Top Sausage & Pepperoni With Double Cheese	⅙ pie (4.7 oz)	360	20	25	45	800
Double Top Sausage With Double Cheese	⅙ pie (4.7 oz)	350	19	25	40	740
For One ½ Less Fat Cheese	1 pie (6.5 oz)	360	10	45	15	920
For One ½ Less Fat Pepperoni	1 pie (6.7 oz)	400	13	45	35	1040
For One ½ Less Fat Supreme	1 pie (7.7 oz)	400	13	45	35	1090
For One ½ Less Fat Vegetable	1 pie (7.2 oz)	360	10	46	15	730
For One Cheese & Pepperoni	1 pie (7 oz)	580	35	41	50	1170
For One Extra Cheese	1 pie (7 oz)	540	30	41	45	910
For One Italian Sausage	1 pie (7 oz)	560	33	40	55	1130
For One Sausage & Pepperoni	1 pie (7 oz)	590	37	40	55	1200
For One Supreme	1 pie (7.5 oz)	570	34	41	50	1130
Light Supreme	⅕ pie (4.8 oz)	270	9	30	20	710
Light Vegetable	⅕ pie (4.6 oz)	240	7	31	10	500
ThinCrust Italian Style Four Meat Combo	¼ pie (5.1 oz)	410	25	25	50	940

FOOD	PORTION	CALS	FAT	CARB	CHOL	SOD
Tombstone (CONT.)						
ThinCrust Italian Style Pepperoni	¼ pie (5 oz)	420	27	25	55	950
ThinCrust Italian Style Sausage	¼ pie (5.1 oz)	400	24	25	50	880
ThinCrust Italian Style Supreme	¼ pie (5.3 oz)	400	24	26	45	880
ThinCrust Mexican Style Supreme Taco	¼ pie (5.1 oz)	380	23	26	50	850
Totino's						
Microwave Cheese	1 pizza	250	8	34	—	760
Microwave Pepperoni	1 pizza	280	12	34	—	880
Microwave Sausage	1 pizza	320	16	33	—	870
Microwave Sausage Pepperoni Combination	1 pizza	310	15	31	—	970
My Classic Deluxe Cheese	⅙ pizza	210	9	23	—	420
My Classic Deluxe Combination	⅙ pizza	270	14	23	—	630
My Classic Deluxe Pepperoni	⅙ pizza	260	13	23	—	630
Pan Pepperoni	⅙ pizza	330	14	34	—	730
Pan Sausage	⅙ pizza	320	13	34	—	630
Pan Sausage & Pepperoni Combination	⅙ pizza	340	15	34	—	720
Pan Three Cheese	⅙ pizza	290	10	33	—	510
Party Bacon	½ pizza	370	20	35	—	1030
Party Canadian Bacon	½ pizza	310	14	35	—	1150
Party Cheese	½ pizza	340	17	34	—	1000
Party Combination	½ pizza	380	21	35	—	1230
Party Hamburger	½ pizza	370	19	35	—	1060
Party Mexican Style	½ pizza	380	21	35	—	970
Party Pepperoni	½ pizza	370	20	35	—	1310
Party Sausage	½ pizza	390	21	35	—	1180
Party Vegetable	½ pizza	300	13	36	—	910
Slices Cheese	1	170	7	20	—	350
Slices Combination	1	200	10	20	—	630
Slices Pepperoni	1	190	9	20	—	530
Slices Sausage	1	200	10	20	—	540
Weight Watchers						
Deluxe Combo	1 (6.57 oz)	380	11	47	40	550
Deluxe Pocket Pizza Sandwich	1 (5 oz)	300	7	46	15	490

FOOD	PORTION	CALS	FAT	CARB	CHOL	SOD
Weight Watchers (CONT.)						
Extra Cheese	1 (5.74 oz)	390	12	49	35	590
Pepperoni	1 (5.56 oz)	390	12	46	45	650

PLANTAINS
Chifles

FOOD	PORTION	CALS	FAT	CARB	CHOL	SOD
Plantain Chips	1 pkg (2 oz)	170	11	17	0	14

PLUMS

FOOD	PORTION	CALS	FAT	CARB	CHOL	SOD
fresh	1	36	tr	9	0	0

POMEGRANATES

FOOD	PORTION	CALS	FAT	CARB	CHOL	SOD
pomegranate	1	104	tr	26	0	5

POPCORN

(FAST FACT: The Popcorn Institute reports that Americans eat 18 billion quarts of popcorn a year. That's 71 quarts for each person. A healthy snack of popcorn will have about 200 calories, no more than 5 to 6 grams of fat and less than 300 milligrams of sodium.)

FOOD	PORTION	CALS	FAT	CARB	CHOL	SOD
air-popped	1 cup (0.3 oz)	31	tr	6	0	0
air-popped	1 oz	108	1	22	0	1
caramel coated	1 cup (1.2 oz)	152	5	28	—	72
caramel coated	1 oz	122	4	22	—	58
caramel coated w/ peanuts	⅔ cup (1 oz)	114	2	23	0	84
cheese	1 cup (0.4 oz)	58	4	6	1	98
cheese	1 oz	149	9	15	3	252
oil popped	1 cup (0.4 oz)	55	3	6	0	97
oil popped	1 oz	142	8	16	0	251
Barrel O' Fun						
Baked Curl	1 oz	150	9	17	0	260
Caramel Corn	1 oz	115	1	25	0	170
Corn Pop	1 oz	190	16	10	0	230
Popcorn	1 oz	160	12	13	0	240
White Cheddar Pops	1 oz	170	13	11	0	370
Cheetos						
Cheddar Cheese	0.5 oz	80	6	6	0	160
Chesters						
Cheddar Cheese	0.5 oz	80	5	7	0	200
Microwave	3 cups	110	7	13	0	170
Microwave Butter	3 cups	120	7	13	0	180
Microwave Cheese	3 cups	110	8	11	0	230
Popcorn	0.5 oz	70	3	9	0	200
Cracker Jack						
Original	1 oz	120	3	22	—	85

FOOD	PORTION	CALS	FAT	CARB	CHOL	SOD
Estee						
No Sugar Added Caramel	1 cup (1 oz)	120	2	26	0	90
Greenfield						
Caramel	1 cup (1 oz)	120	2	22	0	100
Herr's						
Regular	3 cups (1 oz)	140	11	11	0	250
Jiffy Pop						
Bag Butter	3 cups	90	5	11	0	140
Bag Lite	3 cups	70	3	11	0	110
Bag Regular	3 cups	100	6	11	0	140
Glazed Popcorn Clusters	1 oz	120	2	25	5	120
Microwave Butter	4 cup	140	7	17	0	270
Microwave Regular	4 cup	140	7	17	0	270
Pan Butter	4 cup	130	6	16	0	270
Pan Regular	4 cup	130	6	16	0	270
Lance						
Cheese	1 pkg (25 g)	130	8	13	5	280
Plain	1 pkg (25 g)	140	9	13	0	210
White Cheddar Cheese	1 pkg (25 g)	140	9	12	5	170
Louise's						
Fat-Free Apple Cinnamon	1 oz	100	0	24	0	80
Fat-Free Buttery Toffee	1 oz	100	0	24	0	80
Fat-Free Caramel	1 oz	100	0	24	0	80
Newman's Own						
Oldstyle Picture Show	3⅓ cups	80	1	16	0	0
Oldstyle Picture Show Microwave Natural Butter	3 cups	150	8	18	0	200
Oldstyle Picture Show Microwave No Salt	3 cups	150	8	18	0	0
Oldstyle Picture Show Microwave Light Butter	3 cups	90	3	18	0	100
Oldstyle Picture Show Microwave Light Natural	3 cups	90	3	18	0	100
Orville Redenbacher's						
Gourmet Hot Air	3 cups	40	tr	10	0	0
Gourmet Original	3 cups	80	4	10	0	0
Gourmet White	3 cups	80	4	10	0	0
Microwave Gourmet	3 cups	100	6	11	0	200

FOOD	PORTION	CALS	FAT	CARB	CHOL	SOD
Orville Redenbacher's (CONT.)						
Microwave Gourmet Butter	3 cups	100	6	11	0	240
Microwave Gourmet Butter Toffee	2½ cups	210	12	26	tr	85
Microwave Gourmet Caramel	2½ cups	240	14	29	tr	90
Microwave Gourmet Cheddar Cheese	3 cups	130	8	14	2	280
Microwave Gourmet Frozen	3 cups	100	6	11	0	200
Microwave Gourmet Frozen Butter	3 cups	100	6	11	0	240
Microwave Gourmet Light	3 cups	70	3	8	0	115
Microwave Gourmet Light Butter	3 cups	70	3	8	0	110
Microwave Gourmet Salt Free	3 cups	100	6	11	0	0
Microwave Gourmet Salt Free Butter	3 cups	100	6	11	0	0
Microwave Gourmet Sour Cream 'n Onion	3 cups	160	12	12	0	270
Pillsbury						
Microwave Butter	3 cups	210	13	20	—	410
Microwave Original	3 cups	210	13	20	—	410
Microwave Salt Free	3 cups	170	7	23	—	0
Pop Secret						
Butter Flavor	3 cups	100	6	11	1	170
Butter Flavor Singles	6 cups	250	16	23	0	310
Light Butter Flavor	3 cups	70	3	12	0	115
Light Butter Flavor Singles	6 cups	140	6	23	0	190
Light Natural Flavor	3 cups	70	3	12	0	160
Light Natural Flavor Singles	6 cups	150	6	23	0	320
Natural Flavor	3 cups	100	6	11	0	170
Natural Flavor Salt Free	3 cups	100	6	11	0	<5
Pop Chips	1½ cups (1 oz)	130	4	23	0	400
Pop Qwiz Butter Flavor	3 cups	100	6	11	0	170
Pop Qwiz Natural Flavor	3 cups	100	6	11	0	170

FOOD	PORTION	CALS	FAT	CARB	CHOL	SOD
Smartfood						
Cheddar Cheese	0.5 oz	80	5	7	6	130
Light Butter	0.5 oz	70	3	9	8	105
Snyder's						
Butter	1 oz	140	9	13	0	140
Ultra Slim-Fast						
Lite N' Tasty	½ oz	60	2	10	0	150
Weight Watchers						
Butter	1 pkg (0.66 oz)	90	3	14	0	100
Butter Toffee	1 pkg (0.9 oz)	110	3	21	0	90
Caramel	1 pkg (0.9 oz)	100	1	22	0	45
Microwave	1 pkg (1 oz)	90	1	22	0	0
White Cheddar Cheese	1 pkg (0.66 oz)	90	4	12	0	125
Wise						
Tender Eating	0.5 oz	70	6	4	—	120
With Real Premium White Cheddar Cheese	0.5 oz	70	5	4	—	170

POPCORN CAKES

FOOD	PORTION	CALS	FAT	CARB	CHOL	SOD
popcorn cake	1 (0.3 oz)	38	tr	8	0	29
General Mills						
Popcorn Bars Caramel	1 (0.6 oz)	70	1	16	0	55
Lundberg						
Organic Lightly Salted	1	60	1	12	—	140
Organic Unsalted	1	60	1	12	—	3
Rye With Caraway Lightly Salted	1	59	0	14	—	5
Mother's						
Butter Flavor	1 (0.3 oz)	35	0	7	0	0
Unsalted	1 (0.3 oz)	35	0	7	0	0
Orville Redenbacher's						
Chocolate Peanut Crunch Mini	6 pieces (0.5 oz)	60	1	12	0	20
Quaker						
Blueberry Crunch	1 (0.5 oz)	50	0	11	0	0
Butter Mini	6 (0.5 oz)	50	1	11	0	140
Butter Popped	1 (0.3 oz)	35	0	7	0	45
Caramel	1 (0.5 oz)	50	0	12	0	30
Caramel Mini	5 (0.5 oz)	50	1	12	0	70
Cheddar Cheese Mini	6 (0.5 oz)	50	1	11	0	200
Lightly Salted Mini	7 (0.5 oz)	50	1	12	0	120
Monterey Jack	1 (0.4 oz)	40	0	8	0	80
Strawberry Crunch	1 (0.5 oz)	50	0	11	0	0

FOOD	PORTION	CALS	FAT	CARB	CHOL	SOD

Quaker (CONT.)

FOOD	PORTION	CALS	FAT	CARB	CHOL	SOD
White Cheddar	1 (0.4 oz)	40	0	8	0	90

PRETZELS

(FAST FACT: Pretzels are the oldest snack in the world. In A.D. 610, monks in southern France gave them to children as rewards for learning their prayers. Pretzels are the fastest growing snack food in the United States.)

FOOD	PORTION	CALS	FAT	CARB	CHOL	SOD
chocolate covered	1 (0.4 oz)	50	2	8	—	—
chocolate covered	1 oz	130	5	20	—	—
dutch twist	4 (2.1 oz)	229	2	48	0	1029
pretzels	1 oz	108	1	23	0	486
rods	4 (2 oz)	229	2	48	0	1029
sticks	10	10	tr	2	tr	48
sticks	120 (2 oz)	229	2	48	0	1029
twist	1 (½ oz)	65	1	13	tr	258
twists	10 (2.1 oz)	229	2	48	0	1029
whole wheat	2 med (2 oz)	205	2	46	0	115
whole wheat	2 sm (1 oz)	103	1	23	0	58
Barrel O' Fun						
Mini	1 oz	110	1	23	0	100
Sticks	1 oz	110	1	23	0	100
Twists	1 oz	110	1	23	0	100
Estee						
Dutch Unsalted	2 (1.1 oz)	130	1	26	0	40
Nuggets Ranch Reduced Sodium	23 (1 oz)	130	2	24	0	240
Nuggets Reduced Sodium	30 (1 oz)	120	2	24	0	180
Unsalted	23 (1 oz)	120	1	25	0	30
Formagg						
Pretzel Nuts	1 oz	120	4	21	0	390
Herr's						
Hard Sourdough	1 (1 oz)	100	0	23	0	450
J&J						
Soft	1 (2.25 oz)	170	0	37	0	140
Soft Bites	5 bites	110	0	23	0	95
Lance						
Twist	1 pkg (42 g)	150	1	30	0	700
Manischewitz						
Bagel Pretzels Original	4 (1 oz)	110	0	22	0	260
Mister Salty						
Chips	16 (1 oz)	110	3	21	0	620
Dutch	2 (1.1 oz)	120	1	25	0	580

FOOD	PORTION	CALS	FAT	CARB	CHOL	SOD
Mister Salty (CONT.)						
Fat Free Chips	16 (1 oz)	100	0	22	0	620
Mini	22 (1 oz)	110	1	22	0	440
Sticks Fat Free	47 (1 oz)	110	0	23	0	370
Twist Fat Free	9 (1 oz)	110	0	23	0	380
Mr. Phipps						
Chips Lower Sodium	16 (1 oz)	120	3	21	0	410
Chips Original	16 (1 oz)	120	3	21	0	630
Chips Original Fat Free	16 (1 oz)	100	0	22	0	630
Planters						
Twists	1 oz	100	1	23	0	420
Twists	1 pkg (1.5 oz)	160	1	35	0	640
Quinlan						
Beers	1 oz	110	2	22	0	550
Hard Sourdough	1 oz	110	2	22	0	550
Logs	1 oz	110	2	22	0	550
Nuggets	1 oz	110	2	22	0	550
Rods	1 oz	110	2	22	0	550
Sticks	1 oz	110	2	22	0	550
Thins	1 oz	110	2	22	0	550
Rold Gold						
Bavarian	3 pieces (1 oz)	120	2	22	0	430
Pretzel Chips	1 oz	110	1	22	0	310
Pretzel Chips Cheese	1 oz	120	3	22	0	240
Rods	3 pieces (1 oz)	110	2	23	0	410
Snack Mix	½ cup (1 oz)	140	6	18	0	330
Sour Dough	1½ pieces (1 oz)	110	2	22	0	230
Sticks	50 pieces (1 oz)	110	2	23	0	490
Thin Twist	10 pieces (1 oz)	110	1	23	0	510
Tiny Twist	15 pieces (1 oz)	110	1	23	0	420
Seyfart's						
Butter Rods	1 oz	110	1	21	—	530
Snyder's						
Logs	1 oz	310	0	22	0	360
Minis	1 oz	310	0	22	0	460
Minis Unsalted	1 oz	310	0	22	0	70
Nibblers	1 oz	310	0	22	0	460
Oat Bran	1 oz	120	1	14	0	300
Old Fashioned Hard	1 oz	111	0	23	0	655
Old Fashioned Hard Unsalted	1 oz	100	0	23	0	89
Old Tyme	1 oz	310	0	22	0	310
Old Tyme Unsalted	1 oz	110	0	22	0	70

FOOD	PORTION	CALS	FAT	CARB	CHOL	SOD
Snyder's (CONT.)						
Rods	1 oz	310	0	22	0	320
Sourdough Hard Buttermilk Ranch	1 oz	130	5	19	0	250
Sourdough Hard Cheddar Cheese	1 oz	160	7	13	0	320
Sourdough Hard Honey Mustard & Onion	1 oz	130	5	19	0	250
Stix	1 oz	310	0	22	0	900
Very Thins	1 oz	310	0	22	0	720
Sunshine						
California Pretzels	1 oz	110	2	22	0	350
Ultra Slim-Fast						
Lite N' Tasty	1 oz	100	tr	21	0	460
Wege						
Sourdough	1 oz	102	tr	23	0	548
Unsalted	1 oz	102	tr	23	0	60
Whole Wheat	1 oz	109	1	21	0	25
Weight Watchers						
Oat Bran Nuggets	1 pkg (1.5 oz)	170	3	33	0	250
PRUNES						
Del Monte						
Pitted	¼ cup (1.4 oz)	120	0	29	0	5
Unpitted	⅓ cup (1.4 oz)	110	0	12	0	5
Sunsweet						
Orange Essence Pitted Prunes	6 (1.4 oz)	100	0	26	0	5
PUDDING						
banana	1 pkg (5 oz)	180	5	30	—	278
chocolate	1 pkg (5 oz)	189	6	32	5	183
lemon	1 pkg (5 oz)	177	4	36	0	199
rice	1 pkg (5 oz)	231	11	31	—	121
tapioca	1 pkg (5 oz)	169	5	28	—	168
vanilla	1 pkg (4 oz)	146	4	25	8	153
Del Monte						
Snack Cups Banana	1 serv (4 oz)	140	4	25	0	190
Snack Cups Butterscotch	1 serv (4 oz)	140	4	25	0	170
Snack Cups Chocolate	1 serv (4 oz)	160	4	27	0	130
Snack Cups Chocolate Fudge	1 serv (4 oz)	150	4	25	0	190
Snack Cups Chocolate Peanut Butter	1 serv (4 oz)	160	4	28	0	270

FOOD	PORTION	CALS	FAT	CARB	CHOL	SOD
Del Monte (CONT.)						
Snack Cups Lite Chocolate	1 serv (4 oz)	100	1	19	0	140
Snack Cups Lite Vanilla	1 serv (4 oz)	90	1	18	0	190
Snack Cups Tapioca	1 serv (4 oz)	140	4	23	0	110
Snack Cups Vanilla	1 serv (4 oz)	150	4	26	0	150
Hunt's						
Snack Pack Banana	1 (4 oz)	158	6	25	tr	163
Snack Pack Butterscotch	1 (4 oz)	153	6	24	1	211
Snack Pack Chocolate	1 (4 oz)	167	6	25	1	173
Snack Pack Chocolate Fudge	1 (4 oz)	167	6	26	1	191
Snack Pack Chocolate Marshmallow	1 (4 oz)	155	6	23	tr	124
Snack Pack Fat Free Chocolate	1 (4 oz)	96	tr	21	tr	212
Snack Pack Fat Free Tapioca	1 (4 oz)	95	tr	21	tr	185
Snack Pack Fat Free Vanilla	1 (4 oz)	93	tr	21	1	167
Snack Pack Lemon	1 (4 oz)	162	3	33	0	100
Snack Pack Swirl Chocolate Caramel	1 (4 oz)	168	6	26	1	176
Snack Pack Swirl Chocolate Peanut Butter	1 (4 oz)	166	6	25	1	165
Snack Pack Swirl Milk Chocolate	1 (4 oz)	164	6	26	1	175
Snack Pack Swirl Smores	1 (4 oz)	154	6	25	1	129
Snack Pack Tapioca	1 (4 oz)	151	6	23	1	134
Snack Pack Vanilla	1 (4 oz)	163	6	25	1	176
Imagine Foods						
Lemon Dream	1 (4 oz)	120	0	30	0	5
Jell-O						
Chocolate	1 (4 oz)	171	6	28	1	121
Chocolate Caramel Swirl	1 (4 oz)	175	6	28	2	122
Chocolate Fudge	1 (4 oz)	171	6	28	1	121
Chocolate Fudge Milk Chocolate Swirl	1 (4 oz)	171	6	29	2	123
Chocolate Vanilla Swirl	1 (4 oz)	175	6	28	2	125

FOOD	PORTION	CALS	FAT	CARB	CHOL	SOD
Jell-O (CONT.)						
Chocolate Vanilla Swirl	1 (5.5 oz)	240	8	39	2	173
Light Chocolate	1 (4 oz)	104	2	21	5	113
Light Chocolate Fudge	1 (4 oz)	101	1	22	3	113
Light Chocolate Vanilla	1 (4 oz)	104	2	21	5	116
Light Vanilla	1 (4 oz)	104	2	20	6	118
Milk Chocolate	1 (4 oz)	173	6	29	2	126
Tapioca	1 (4 oz)	167	4	29	2	135
Tapioca	1 (5.5 oz)	229	6	40	2	186
Vanilla	1 (4 oz)	182	7	28	2	133
Vanilla	1 (5.5 oz)	250	9	38	2	183
Vanilla Chocolate Swirl	1 (4 oz)	178	6	28	2	129
Kozy Shack						
Banana	1 pkg (4 oz)	130	3	22	10	150
Chocolate	1 pkg (4 oz)	140	4	24	5	150
Light Chocolate	1 pkg (4 oz)	110	1	22	5	150
Light Vanilla	1 pkg (4 oz)	110	1	22	10	160
Rice	1 pkg (4 oz)	130	3	23	17	140
Tapioca	1 pkg (4 oz)	140	3	25	5	160
Vanilla	1 pkg (4 oz)	130	3	22	10	150
Matthew Walker						
Plum	1 serv (3.5 oz)	290	7	60	—	100
Snack Pack						
Banana	1 serv (4.25 oz)	145	6	22	1	180
Butterscotch	1 serv (4.25 oz)	170	6	27	1	210
Chocolate	1 serv (4.25 oz)	170	6	26	1	120
Chocolate Fudge	1 serv (4.25 oz)	165	6	27	1	125
Chocolate Marshmallow	1 serv (4.25 oz)	165	6	26	1	125
Lemon	1 serv (4.25 oz)	150	4	30	0	75
Light Chocolate	1 serv (4.25 oz)	100	2	20	1	120
Light Tapioca	1 serv (4.25 oz)	100	2	18	1	105
Tapioca	1 serv (4.25 oz)	150	5	23	1	125
Vanilla	1 serv (4.25 oz)	170	6	27	1	150
Swiss Miss						
Butterscotch	1 pkg (4 oz)	180	6	29	5	135
Chocolate	1 pkg (4 oz)	180	6	29	5	160
Chocolate Fudge	1 pkg (4 oz)	220	6	38	5	180
Chocolate Sundae	1 pkg (4 oz)	220	7	36	5	140
Light Chocolate	1 pkg (4 oz)	100	1	20	0	120
Light Chocolate Fudge	1 pkg (4 oz)	100	1	20	0	120

FOOD	PORTION	CALS	FAT	CARB	CHOL	SOD
Swiss Miss (CONT.)						
Light Vanilla	1 pkg (4 oz)	100	1	20	0	105
Light Vanilla Chocolate Parfait	1 pkg (4 oz)	100	1	20	0	110
Tapioca	1 pkg (4 oz)	160	5	27	5	170
Vanilla	1 pkg (4 oz)	190	7	30	5	140
Vanilla Parfait	1 pkg (4 oz)	180	6	29	1	150
Vanilla Sundae	1 pkg (4 oz)	200	7	36	5	180
Ultra Slim-Fast						
Butterscotch	1 pkg (4 oz)	100	tr	21	0	230
Chocolate	1 pkg (4 oz)	100	tr	21	0	240
Vanilla	1 pkg (4 oz)	100	tr	21	0	230

PUDDING POPS

FOOD	PORTION	CALS	FAT	CARB	CHOL	SOD
chocolate	1 (1.6 oz)	72	2	12	1	77
vanilla	1 (1.6 oz)	75	2	13	1	50

PUMPKIN SEEDS

FOOD	PORTION	CALS	FAT	CARB	CHOL	SOD
roasted	1 oz	148	12	4	0	5
salted & roasted	1 oz	148	12	4	0	144

QUINCE

FOOD	PORTION	CALS	FAT	CARB	CHOL	SOD
fresh	1	53	tr	14	0	4

RAISINS

FOOD	PORTION	CALS	FAT	CARB	CHOL	SOD
chocolate coated	10 (0.4 oz)	39	2	7	0	4
Del Monte						
Golden	¼ cup (1.4 oz)	130	0	31	0	10
Raisins	1 box (0.5 oz)	45	0	11	0	0
Raisins	1 box (1 oz)	90	0	22	0	5
Raisins	1 box (1.5 oz)	140	0	33	0	10
Raisins	¼ cup (1.4 oz)	130	0	31	0	10
Yogurt Raisins Strawberry	1 pkg (0.9 oz)	110	3	20	0	25
Yogurt Raisins Vanilla	1 pkg (0.9 oz)	110	3	20	0	25
Yogurt Raisins Vanilla	1 pkg (1 oz)	120	3	22	0	25
Tree Of Life						
Organic	¼ cup (1.4 oz)	130	0	31	0	10

RASPBERRIES

FOOD	PORTION	CALS	FAT	CARB	CHOL	SOD
fresh	1 cup	61	1	14	0	0

RASPBERRY JUICE

FOOD	PORTION	CALS	FAT	CARB	CHOL	SOD
Crystal Geyser						
Juice Squeeze Mountain Raspberry	1 bottle (12 fl oz)	135	0	32	0	20

FOOD	PORTION	CALS	FAT	CARB	CHOL	SOD
Fresh Samantha						
Raspberry Dream	1 cup (8 oz)	120	1	30	0	0
RICE CAKES						
brown rice	1 (0.3 oz)	35	tr	7	0	29
brown rice & buckwheat	1 (0.3 oz)	34	tr	7	0	10
brown rice & buckwheat unsalted	1 (0.3 oz)	34	tr	7	0	tr
brown rice & corn	1 (0.3 oz)	35	tr	7	0	26
brown rice & rye	1 (0.3 oz)	35	tr	7	0	10
brown rice & sesame seed	1 (0.3 oz)	35	tr	7	0	20
brown rice multigrain	1 (0.3 oz)	35	tr	7	0	23
brown rice multigrain unsalted	1 (0.3 oz)	35	tr	7	0	tr
brown rice unsalted	1 (0.3 oz)	35	tr	7	0	3
Hain						
5-Grain	1	40	tr	8	—	10
Mini Apple Cinnamon	½ oz	60	tr	12	0	10
Mini Barbeque	½ oz	70	3	10	0	50
Mini Cheese	½ oz	60	2	10	<5	100
Mini Honey Nut	½ oz	60	tr	11	0	30
Mini Nacho Cheese	½ oz	70	2	10	<5	90
Mini Plain	½ oz	60	tr	12	0	20
Mini Plain No Salt Added	½ oz	60	tr	12	0	5
Mini Ranch	½ oz	70	3	9	0	90
Mini Teriyaki	½ oz	50	tr	12	0	75
Plain	1	40	tr	8	—	10
Plain No Salt Added	1	40	tr	8	—	<5
Sesame	1	40	tr	8	—	10
Sesame No Salt	1	40	tr	8	—	<5
Ka-Me						
Cheese	16 pieces (1 oz)	120	2	24	0	180
Onion	16 pieces (1 oz)	120	1	25	0	75
Plain	16 pieces (1 oz)	120	2	25	0	15
Seaweed	16 pieces (1 oz)	120	2	25	0	100
Sesame	16 pieces (1 oz)	120	2	24	0	85
Unsalted	16 pieces (1 oz)	120	1	26	0	0
Lundberg						
Organic Lightly Salted	1	60	1	14	—	120
Organic Unsalted	1	60	1	14	—	3
Premium Lightly Salted	1	60	1	14	—	120

FOOD	PORTION	CALS	FAT	CARB	CHOL	SOD
Lundberg (CONT.)						
Premium Unsalted	1	60	1	14	—	3
Sesame Lightly Salted	1	59	0	16	—	6
Mother's						
Mini Apple	5 (0.5 oz)	50	0	12	0	40
Mini Caramel	5 (0.5 oz)	50	0	12	0	40
Mini Cinnamon	5 (0.5 oz)	50	0	12	0	40
Mini Plain Unsalted	7 (0.5 oz)	60	0	12	0	0
Multigrain Lightly Salted	1 (0.3 oz)	35	0	7	0	30
Rye Unsalted	1 (0.3 oz)	35	0	7	0	0
Wheat Unsalted	1 (0.3 oz)	35	0	7	0	0
Pritikin						
Mini Apple Crisp	5 (0.5 oz)	50	0	12	0	20
Multigrain	1 (0.3 oz)	35	0	7	0	20
Multigrain Unsalted	1 (0.3 oz)	35	0	7	0	0
Plain	1 (0.3 oz)	35	0	7	0	20
Plain Unsalted	1 (0.3 oz)	35	0	7	0	0
Sesame Low Sodium	1 (0.3 oz)	35	0	7	0	20
Sesame Unsalted	1 (0.3 oz)	35	0	7	0	0
Quaker						
Apple Cinnamon	1 (0.5 oz)	50	0	11	0	0
Banana Crunch	1 (0.5 oz)	50	0	11	0	45
Cinnamon Crunch	1 (0.5 oz)	50	0	11	0	25
Mini Apple Cinnamon	5 (0.5 oz)	50	0	12	0	0
Mini Banana Nut	5 (0.5 oz)	50	0	12	0	40
Mini Butter Popped Corn	6 (0.5 oz)	50	0	12	0	120
Mini Caramel Corn	5 (0.5 oz)	50	0	12	0	25
Mini Chocolate Crunch	5 (0.5 oz)	50	0	12	0	10
Mini Cinnamon Crunch	5 (0.5 oz)	50	0	12	0	25
Mini Honey Nut	5 (0.5 oz)	50	0	12	0	25
Mini Monterey Jack	6 (0.5 oz)	50	0	11	0	100
Mini White Cheddar	6 (0.5 oz)	50	0	11	0	120
Salt-Free	1 (0.3 oz)	35	0	7	0	0
Salted	1 (0.3 oz)	35	0	7	0	15
Tree Of Life						
Fat Free Mini Apple Cinnamon	15	60	0	13	0	5
Fat Free Mini Caramel	15	60	0	13	0	10
Fat Free Mini Honey Nut	15	60	0	13	0	0

FOOD	PORTION	CALS	FAT	CARB	CHOL	SOD
Tree Of Life (CONT.)						
Fat Free Mini Jalapeno	15	60	0	13	0	25
Fat Free Mini Plain	15	50	0	12	0	45

ROLL

cinnamon w/ frosting	1	109	4	17	—	250
crescent	1 (1 oz)	98	4	14	0	341
dinner	1 (1 oz)	85	2	14	0	148
hard	1 (3½ in)	167	2	30	0	310
hot cross bun	1	202	4	38	—	—
kaiser	1 (3½ in)	167	2	30	0	310
raisin & nut	1 (2 oz)	196	7	30	13	185
rye	1 (1 oz)	81	1	15	0	253
whole wheat	1 (1 oz)	75	1	15	0	135

SALAD
Dole

Caesar Salad Mix	⅓ pkg (3.5 oz)	170	14	9	5	480
Classic Blend Mix	3.5 oz	25	1	4	0	20
French Blend Mix	3.5 oz	25	1	4	0	15
Italian Blend Mix	3.5 oz	25	1	3	0	45
Salad-In-A-Minute Oriental	3.5 oz	110	7	12	0	290
Salad-In-A-Minute Spinach	3.5 oz	180	9	19	0	660
Fresh Express						
American Salad Mix	1½ cups (3 oz)	20	0	3	0	10
Caesar Salad Mix	1½ cups (3 oz)	140	11	8	10	320
European Salad Mix	1½ cups (3 oz)	20	0	3	0	10
Garden Salad Mix	1½ cups (3 oz)	20	0	3	0	10
Italian Salad Mix	1½ cups (3 oz)	20	0	3	0	0
Oriental Salad Mix	1½ cups (3 oz)	120	8	11	0	330
Spinach Salad Mix	1½ cups (3 oz)	130	3	23	0	430

SARDINES
Empress

Skinless & Boneless Olive Oil	1 can (3.8 oz)	420	38	2	—	530
Port Clyde						
In Louisiana Hot Sauce	1 can (3.75 oz)	170	9	1	105	760
In Mustard Sauce	1 can (3.75 oz)	150	9	1	110	450
In Soybean Oil With Hot Chilies	1 can (3.3 oz)	155	9	0	80	310
In Spring Water	1 can (3.3 oz)	170	10	0	140	240

FOOD	PORTION	CALS	FAT	CARB	CHOL	SOD
Port Clyde (CONT.)						
In Tomato Sauce	1 can (3.75 oz)	150	9	0	100	480
Viking's Delight						
Brisling In Olive Oil drained	1 can (3.75 oz)	260	20	1	—	450

SAUSAGE DISHES

FOOD	PORTION	CALS	FAT	CARB	CHOL	SOD
Jimmy Dean						
Italian Sausage & Mozzarella Sandwich	1 (4.5 oz)	380	22	28	40	1030
Ovenstuffs						
French Roll Pepperoni	1 (4.75 oz)	370	20	30	—	870

SHERBET

FOOD	PORTION	CALS	FAT	CARB	CHOL	SOD
orange	1 bar (2.75 fl oz)	91	1	20	3	30
orange	½ cup (4 fl oz)	132	2	29	5	44
orange	½ gal	2158	31	469	113	706
orange home recipe	½ cup	120	2	24	9	30
Borden						
Orange	½ cup	110	1	25	—	40
Bresler's						
All Flavors	3.5 oz	140	2	30	6	—
Hood						
Lime Orange Lemon	½ cup (3.1 oz)	120	1	26	<5	35
Orange	½ cup (3.1 oz)	120	1	26	<5	35
Rainbow Swirl	½ cup (3.1 oz)	120	1	26	<5	30
Raspberry Orange Lime	½ cup (3.1 oz)	120	1	26	<5	30
Sealtest						
Lime	½ cup (3 oz)	130	1	28	5	30
Orange	½ cup (3 oz)	130	1	28	5	30
Rainbow Orange Red Raspberry Lime	½ cup (3 oz)	130	1	28	5	25
Red Raspberry	½ cup (3 oz)	130	1	28	5	25

SODA

(FAST FACT: Americans drink over 50 gallons of soft drinks per person each year.)

FOOD	PORTION	CALS	FAT	CARB	CHOL	SOD
club	12 oz	0	0	0	0	75
cola	12 oz	151	tr	39	0	14
cream	12 oz	191	0	49	0	43
diet cola	12 oz	2	0	tr	0	21
diet cola w/ equal	12 oz	2	0	tr	0	21

FOOD	PORTION	CALS	FAT	CARB	CHOL	SOD
diet cola w/ saccharin	12 oz	2	0	tr	0	57
ginger ale	12 oz can	124	0	32	0	25
grape	12 oz	161	0	42	0	57
lemon lime	12 oz	149	0	38	0	41
orange	12 oz	177	0	46	0	49
pepper type	12 oz	151	tr	38	0	38
quinine	12 oz	125	0	32	0	15
root beer	12 oz	152	0	39	0	49
tonic water	12 oz	125	0	32	0	15
7UP						
Cherry	1 oz	13	0	—	0	—
Cherry Diet	1 oz	tr	0	—	0	—
Diet	1 oz	tr	0	—	0	—
Gold	1 oz	13	0	—	0	—
Gold Diet	1 oz	tr	0	—	0	—
Original	1 oz	12	0	—	0	—
After The Fall						
Raspberry Ginger Ale	1 can (12 oz)	150	0	36	0	25
Barrelhead						
Root Beer	8 fl oz	110	0	27	0	25
Burst						
Cola Strawberry	8 fl oz	117	0	31	0	0
Canada Dry						
Birch Beer Brown	8 fl oz	110	0	27	0	40
Birch Beer Clear	8 fl oz	110	0	27	0	40
Black Cherry Wishniak	8 fl oz	130	0	32	0	40
Cactus Cooler	8 fl oz	110	0	27	0	40
California Strawberry	8 fl oz	110	0	27	0	45
Club	8 fl oz	0	0	0	0	60
Club Sodium Free	8 fl oz	0	0	0	0	0
Concord Grape	8 fl oz	120	0	29	0	45
Diet Ginger Ale	8 fl oz	0	0	0	0	60
Diet Ginger Ale Cherry	8 fl oz	0	0	0	0	60
Diet Ginger Ale Cranberry	8 fl oz	0	0	tr	0	50
Diet Ginger Ale Lemon	8 fl oz	5	0	0	0	60
Diet Tonic Water	8 fl oz	0	0	0	0	35
Diet Tonic Water Twist Of Lime	8 fl oz	0	0	0	0	45
Ginger Ale	8 fl oz	100	0	25	0	20
Ginger Ale Cherry	8 fl oz	110	0	27	0	25
Ginger Ale Cranberry	8 fl oz	100	0	25	0	15
Ginger Ale Golden	8 fl oz	100	0	24	0	10
Ginger Ale Lemon	8 fl oz	100	0	25	0	20

FOOD	PORTION	CALS	FAT	CARB	CHOL	SOD
Canada Dry (CONT.)						
Half & Half	8 fl oz	110	0	27	0	25
Hi-Spot	8 fl oz	110	0	28	0	50
Island Lime	8 fl oz	140	0	33	0	15
Jamaica Cola	8 fl oz	110	0	27	0	10
Lemon Sour	8 fl oz	100	0	21	0	15
Peach	8 fl oz	120	0	30	0	40
Pina Pineapple	8 fl oz	110	0	26	0	40
Seltzer	8 fl oz	0	0	0	0	10
Seltzer Cherry	8 fl oz	0	0	0	0	10
Seltzer Cranberry Lime	8 fl oz	0	0	0	0	10
Seltzer Grapefruit	8 fl oz	0	0	0	0	10
Seltzer Lemon Lime	8 fl oz	0	0	0	0	10
Seltzer Mandarin Orange	8 fl oz	0	0	0	0	10
Seltzer Peach	8 fl oz	0	0	0	0	10
Seltzer Raspberry	8 fl oz	0	0	0	0	10
Seltzer Strawberry	8 fl oz	0	0	0	0	10
Seltzer Tropical	8 fl oz	0	0	0	0	10
Sunripe Orange	8 fl oz	140	0	35	0	45
Tahitian Treat	8 fl oz	150	0	36	0	45
Tonic Water	8 fl oz	100	0	24	0	15
Tonic Water Twist Of Lime	8 fl oz	100	0	24	0	20
Vanilla Cream	8 fl oz	120	0	30	0	40
Vichy Water	8 fl oz	0	0	0	0	490
Wild Cherry	8 fl oz	110	0	28	0	40
Clearly 2						
Black Cherry	8 fl oz	2	0	0	—	9
Key Lime	8 fl oz	2	0	0	—	9
Clearly Canadian						
Alpine Fruit & Berries	8 fl oz	90	0	23	—	9
Boysenberry Mist	8 fl oz	2	0	0	—	9
Coastal Cranberry	8 fl oz	90	0	22	—	9
Country Raspberry	8 fl oz	80	0	19	—	9
Green Apple	8 fl oz	80	0	19	—	9
Mountain Blackberry	8 fl oz	100	0	24	—	9
Orchard Peach Strawberry	8 fl oz	90	0	22	—	9
Soda	8 fl oz	0	0	0	0	5
Summer Strawberry	8 fl oz	80	0	19	—	9
Western Longanberry	8 fl oz	80	0	19	—	9
Wild Cherry	8 fl oz	90	0	23	—	9

FOOD	PORTION	CALS	FAT	CARB	CHOL	SOD
Coca-Cola						
Cherry	8 fl oz	104	0	28	0	4
Classic	8 fl oz	97	0	27	0	9
Classic Caffeine-Free	8 fl oz	97	0	27	0	9
Coke II	8 fl oz	105	0	29	0	4
Diet	8 fl oz	1	0	tr	0	4
Diet Cherry	8 fl oz	1	0	tr	0	4
Diet Coke Caffeine-free	8 fl oz	1	0	tr	0	4
Cott						
Cola	8 fl oz	110	0	27	0	10
Ginger Ale	8 fl oz	90	0	20	0	20
Grape	8 fl oz	130	0	30	0	25
Orange	8 fl oz	140	0	33	0	25
Pineapple	8 fl oz	130	0	32	0	25
Punch	8 fl oz	130	0	32	0	25
Seltzer	8 fl oz	0	0	0	0	0
Crush						
Cherry	8 fl oz	140	0	35	0	30
Grape	8 fl oz	110	0	—	0	—
Orange	8 fl oz	140	0	—	0	—
Orange Diet	8 fl oz	0	0	0	0	—
Pineapple	8 fl oz	140	0	35	0	30
Strawberry	8 fl oz	130	0	—	0	—
Tropical Fruit Punch	1 bottle (10 fl oz)	180	0	44	0	20
Tropical Fruit Punch	1 can (11.5 fl oz)	200	0	—	0	—
Diet Rite						
Black Cherry Salt/ Sodium Free	8 fl oz	2	0	1	0	0
Cola	8 fl oz	1	0	tr	0	0
Cola Caffeine/Sugar Free	8 fl oz	1	0	tr	0	7
Cola Salt/Sodium Free	8 fl oz	1	0	tr	0	tr
Fruit Punch Salt/ Sodium Free	8 fl oz	2	0	tr	0	0
Golden Peach Salt/ Sodium Free	8 fl oz	2	0	tr	0	0
Key Lime Salt/Sodium Free	8 fl oz	7	0	2	0	0
Pink Grapefruit Salt/ Sodium Free	8 fl oz	2	0	1	0	0
Red Raspberry Salt/ Sodium Free	8 fl oz	3	0	1	0	tr

FOOD	PORTION	CALS	FAT	CARB	CHOL	SOD
Diet Rite (CONT.)						
Tangerine Salt/Sodium Free	8 fl oz	2	0	tr	0	0
White Grape Salt/ Sodium Free	8 fl oz	1	0	tr	0	0
Dr Pepper						
Diet	1 oz	tr	0	—	0	—
Free	1 oz	12	0	—	0	—
Free Diet	1 oz	tr	0	—	0	—
Original	1 oz	13	0	—	0	—
Fanta						
Ginger Ale	8 fl oz	86	0	23	0	4
Grape	8 fl oz	117	0	31	0	9
Orange	8 fl oz	118	0	32	0	9
Root Beer	8 fl oz	111	0	29	0	4
Fresca						
Soda	8 fl oz	3	0	tr	0	1
Health Valley						
Ginger Ale	12 oz	153	1	35	0	30
Rootbeer Old Fashioned	12 oz	120	1	26	0	12
Sarsaparilla Rootbeer	12 oz	153	1	35	0	27
Wild Berry	12 oz	142	1	33	0	27
Hires						
Cream	8 fl oz	130	0	0	0	30
Cream Soda Diet	8 fl oz	0	0	0	0	35
Original Mocha	8 fl oz	100	0	24	0	45
Original Mocha Diet	8 fl oz	5	0	0	0	45
Root Beer	8 fl oz	130	0	31	0	45
Root Beer Diet	8 fl oz	0	0	0	0	70
Kick						
Soda	8 fl oz	120	0	32	0	35
Like						
Cola	1 oz	13	0	—	0	—
Cola Sugar Free	1 oz	tr	0	—	0	—
Lucozade						
Soda	7 oz	136	0	36	0	—
Manischewitz						
Seltzer No Salt Added No Calories	8 fl oz	0	0	0	0	9
Mello Yellow						
Diet	8 fl oz	4	0	tr	0	tr
Soda	8 fl oz	119	0	32	0	9

FOOD	PORTION	CALS	FAT	CARB	CHOL	SOD
Minute Maid						
Berry	8 fl oz	111	0	30	0	9
Diet Orange	8 fl oz	2	0	0	0	0
Fruit Punch	8 fl oz	117	0	32	0	10
Grape	8 fl oz	121	0	32	0	9
Grapefruit	8 fl oz	108	0	29	0	9
Orange	8 fl oz	118	0	32	0	0
Peach	8 fl oz	110	0	29	0	9
Pineapple	8 fl oz	109	0	30	0	9
Raspberry	8 fl oz	111	0	30	0	9
Soda	8 fl oz	110	0	29	0	11
Strawberry	8 fl oz	122	0	33	0	9
Mountain Dew						
Diet	8 fl oz	2	0	tr	0	0
Soda	8 fl oz	118	0	30	0	21
Mr. PiBB						
Diet	8 fl oz	1	0	tr	0	2
Soda	6 oz	97	0	26	0	7
Mug						
Cream	8 fl oz	122	0	32	0	21
Diet Cream	8 fl oz	2	0	0	0	29
Diet Root Beer	8 fl oz	1	0	tr	0	26
Root Beer	8 fl oz	141	0	29	0	26
Nehi						
Cream	8 fl oz	120	0	32	0	0
Fruit Punch	8 fl oz	120	0	34	0	35
Ginger Ale	8 fl oz	90	0	24	0	35
Grape	8 fl oz	120	0	32	0	35
Orange	8 fl oz	130	0	35	0	35
Peach	8 fl oz	130	0	34	0	35
Pineapple	8 fl oz	130	0	36	0	0
Quinine Water	8 fl oz	90	0	23	0	35
Root Beer	8 fl oz	120	0	32	0	35
Strawberry	8 fl oz	120	0	32	0	35
Wild Red	8 fl oz	120	0	32	0	33
Old Colony						
Grape	8 fl oz	140	0	32	0	40
Orangina						
Sparkling Citrus	6 fl oz	80	0	19	0	0
Pepsi						
Caffeine Free	8 fl oz	105	0	27	0	0

FOOD	PORTION	CALS	FAT	CARB	CHOL	SOD
Pepsi (CONT.)						
Diet	8 fl oz	1	0	tr	0	tr
Diet Caffeine Free	8 fl oz	1	0	tr	0	tr
Regular	8 fl oz	105	0	27	0	0
Ramblin' Root Beer						
Ramblin'Root Beer	8 fl oz	120	0	33	0	4
Razing Razberry						
Cola	8 fl oz	117	0	31	0	0
Royal Crown						
Caffeine Free Cola	8 fl oz	110	0	29	0	35
Cherry	8 fl oz	110	0	29	0	35
Cola	8 fl oz	100	0	28	0	35
Diet	8 fl oz	1	0	tr	0	tr
Diet Caffeine Free	8 fl oz	1	0	tr	0	tr
Diet Cranberry Apple Salt/Sodium Free	8 fl oz	2	0	tr	0	1
Diet Cranberry Salt/ Sodium Free	8 fl oz	2	0	tr	0	1
Royal Mistic						
'N Juice Black Cherry	12 fl oz	146	0	36	0	26
'N Juice Peach Vanilla	12 fl oz	146	0	36	0	18
'N Juice Tangerine Orange	12 fl oz	146	0	36	0	30
'N Juice Tropical Supreme	12 fl oz	152	0	38	0	14
'N Juice Wild Berry	12 fl oz	156	0	38	0	30
Caribbean Fruit Punch	16 fl oz	230	0	57	0	5
Grape Strawberry	16 fl oz	230	0	57	0	5
Sparkling Diet With Lime Kiwi	11.1 fl oz	0	0	0	0	<90
Sparkling Diet With Raspberry Boysenberry	11.1 fl oz	0	0	0	0	<90
Sparkling Diet With Royal Peach	11.1 fl oz	0	0	0	0	<90
Sparkling Diet With Wild Cherry	11.1 fl oz	0	0	0	0	<90
Sparkling With Lime Kiwi	11.1 fl oz	112	0	28	0	38
Sparkling With Mandarin Orange Pineapple	11.1 fl oz	120	0	30	0	18
Sparkling With Mango Passion	11.1 fl oz	112	0	28	0	34

FOOD	PORTION	CALS	FAT	CARB	CHOL	SOD
Royal Mistic (CONT.)						
Sparkling With Raspberry Boysenberry	11.1 fl oz	112	0	28	0	24
Sparkling With Royal Peach	11.1 fl oz	112	0	28	0	30
Sparkling With Wild Cherry	11.1 fl oz	112	0	28	0	28
Schweppes						
Bitter Lemon	8 fl oz	110	0	28	0	45
Club	8 fl oz	0	0	0	0	70
Club Sodium Free	8 fl oz	0	0	0	0	0
Diet Ginger Ale	8 fl oz	0	0	0	0	75
Diet Ginger Ale Dry Grape	8 fl oz	2	0	0	0	90
Diet Ginger Ale Raspberry	8 fl oz	0	0	0	0	75
Ginger Ale	8 fl oz	90	0	22	0	50
Ginger Ale Dry Grape	8 fl oz	100	0	26	0	50
Ginger Ale Raspberry	8 fl oz	100	0	26	0	50
Ginger Beer	8 fl oz	100	0	25	0	90
Grape	8 fl oz	130	0	33	0	55
Grapefruit	8 fl oz	110	0	27	0	75
Lemon Sour	8 fl oz	110	0	26	0	25
Lemon-Lime	8 fl oz	100	0	25	0	75
Seltzer Black Berry	8 fl oz	0	0	0	0	10
Seltzer Lemon	8 fl oz	0	0	0	0	10
Seltzer Lemon Lime	8 fl oz	0	0	0	0	10
Seltzer Lime	8 fl oz	0	0	0	0	10
Seltzer Orange	8 fl oz	0	0	0	0	10
Seltzer Peaches & Cream	8 fl oz	0	0	0	0	10
Seltzer Raspberry	8 fl oz	0	0	0	0	0
Tonic Citrus	8 fl oz	90	0	20	0	25
Tonic Cranberry	8 fl oz	90	0	20	0	25
Tonic Raspberry	8 fl oz	90	0	20	0	25
Tonic Water Diet	8 fl oz	0	0	0	0	85
Shasta						
Black Cherry	12 oz	162	0	—	0	—
Cherry Cola	12 oz	140	0	—	0	—
Citrus Mist	12 oz	170	0	—	0	—
Club	12 oz	0	0	—	0	—
Cola	12 oz	147	0	—	0	—
Cola	8 oz	98	0	—	0	—

FOOD	PORTION	CALS	FAT	CARB	CHOL	SOD
Shasta (CONT.)						
Collins	12 oz	118	0	—	0	—
Creme	12 oz	154	0	—	0	—
Diet Birch Beer	12 oz	4	0	—	0	—
Diet Cola	8 oz	0	0	—	0	—
Diet Ginger Ale	8 oz	0	0	—	0	—
Diet Lemon Lime	8 oz	0	0	—	0	—
Dr. Diablo	12 oz	140	0	—	0	—
Free Cola	12 oz	151	0	—	0	—
Fruit Punch	12 oz	173	0	—	0	—
Ginger Ale	12 oz	120	0	—	0	—
Ginger Ale	8 oz	80	0	—	0	—
Grape	12 oz	177	0	—	0	—
Lemon Lime	12 oz	146	0	—	0	—
Lemon Lime	8 oz	97	0	—	0	—
Orange	12 oz	177	0	—	0	—
Red Berry	12 oz	158	0	—	0	—
Red Pop	12 oz	158	0	—	0	—
Root Beer	12 oz	154	0	—	0	—
Strawberry	12 oz	147	0	—	0	—
Tonic Water	12 oz	0	0	—	0	—
Slice						
Diet Lemon Lime	8 fl oz	5	0	tr	0	1
Diet Mandarin	8 fl oz	5	0	tr	0	10
Lemon Lime	8 fl oz	100	0	26	0	10
Mandarin Orange	8 fl oz	128	0	33	0	10
Red	8 fl oz	128	0	33	0	10
Snapple						
Amazin' Grape	8 fl oz	120	0	28	0	5
Cherry Lime Ricky	8 fl oz	110	0	27	0	0
Creme D'Vanilla	8 fl oz	130	0	33	0	0
French Cherry	8 fl oz	120	0	29	0	0
Kiwi Peach	8 fl oz	120	0	29	0	0
Kiwi Strawberry	8 fl oz	130	0	33	0	5
Mango Madness	8 fl oz	130	0	33	0	5
Passion Supreme	8 fl oz	120	0	29	0	0
Peach Melba	8 fl oz	120	0	31	0	0
Raspberry	8 fl oz	120	0	31	0	0
Seltzer Black Cherry	8 fl oz	0	0	0	0	0
Seltzer Lemon Lime	8 fl oz	0	0	0	0	0
Seltzer Original	8 fl oz	0	0	0	0	0
Seltzer Tangerine	8 fl oz	0	0	0	0	0
Tru Root Beer	8 fl oz	110	0	29	0	0

FOOD	PORTION	CALS	FAT	CARB	CHOL	SOD
Sprite						
Diet	8 fl oz	3	0	0	0	0
Soda	8 fl oz	100	0	26	0	31
Sundrop						
Cherry	8 fl oz	130	0	21	0	15
Diet	8 fl oz	5	0	0	0	65
Soda	8 fl oz	140	0	34	0	20
Sunkist						
Cactus Cooler	8 fl oz	110	0	27	0	40
Cherry	8 fl oz	140	0	35	0	35
Diet Citrus	8 fl oz	0	0	0	0	90
Diet Orange	8 fl oz	5	0	0	0	75
Fruit Punch	8 fl oz	130	0	33	0	35
Orange	8 fl oz	140	0	35	0	40
Peach	8 fl oz	120	0	30	0	40
Pineapple	8 fl oz	140	0	35	0	35
Strawberry	8 fl oz	140	0	34	0	35
TAB						
Soda	8 fl oz	1	0	tr	0	4
Tropical Chill						
Cola	8 fl oz	117	0	31	0	0
Diet	8 fl oz	1	0	tr	0	0
Upper 10						
Diet	8 fl oz	3	0	1	0	0
Diet Salt/Sodium Free	8 fl oz	3	0	1	0	0
Salt Free	8 fl oz	100	0	29	0	0
Soda	8 fl oz	100	0	28	0	35
Welch's						
Sparkling Apple	12 oz	180	0	—	0	—
Sparkling Grape	12 oz	180	0	—	0	—
Sparkling Orange	12 oz	180	0	—	0	—
Sparkling Strawberry	12 oz	180	0	—	0	—
Wink						
Diet	8 fl oz	5	0	1	0	95
Soda	8 fl oz	130	0	31	0	35
Yoo-Hoo						
Original	9 fl oz	150	tr	31	0	200
SOYBEANS						
honey toasted	¼ cup (1 oz)	130	4	19	0	45
roasted & toasted	1 oz	129	7	9	0	1
roasted & toasted salted	1 oz	129	7	9	0	54
SPORTS DRINKS						
Gatorade						
Citrus Cooler	1 cup (8 oz)	50	0	14	0	110

FOOD	PORTION	CALS	FAT	CARB	CHOL	SOD
Gatorade (CONT.)						
Fruit Punch	1 cup (8 oz)	50	0	14	0	110
Grape	1 cup (8 oz)	50	0	14	0	110
Iced Tea Cooler	1 cup (8 oz)	50	0	14	0	110
Lemon-Lime	1 cup (8 oz)	50	0	14	0	110
Lemonade	1 cup (8 oz)	50	0	14	0	110
Orange	1 cup (8 fl oz)	50	0	14	0	110
Tropical Fruit	1 cup (8 oz)	50	0	14	0	110
PowerAde						
Fruit Punch	8 fl oz	72	0	19	0	28
Grape	8 fl oz	73	0	19	0	28
Lemon-Lime	8 fl oz	72	0	19	0	28
Orange	8 fl oz	72	0	19	0	28
Slice						
All Sport Diet Lemon Lime	8 fl oz	1	0	0	0	40
All Sport Lemon Lime	8 fl oz	72	0	19	0	55
All Sport Orange	8 fl oz	74	0	19	0	55
All Sport Punch	8 fl oz	81	0	22	0	55
Snapple						
Sport Fruit	1 bottle	80	0	20	0	60
Sport Lemon	1 bottle	80	0	20	0	60
Sport Lemon Lime	1 bottle	80	0	20	0	60
Sport Orange	1 bottle	80	0	20	0	60
Ultra Fuel						
Lemon Lime	16 fl oz	400	0	100	0	55

SQUASH SEEDS

roasted	1 oz	148	12	4	0	5
salted & roasted	1 oz	148	12	4	0	5

STAR FRUIT

Sonoma						
Dried	7-9 pieces (1.4 oz)	140	0	34	0	0

STRAWBERRIES

fresh	1 cup	45	1	10	0	2
Dole						
Fresh	8	50	0	13	0	0

STRAWBERRY JUICE

Kern's						
Nectar	6 fl oz	110	0	28	0	0
Kool-Aid						
Koolers	1 (8.45 oz)	136	0	36	—	3

FOOD	PORTION	CALS	FAT	CARB	CHOL	SOD
Libby						
Nectar	1 can (11.5 fl oz)	210	0	52	0	10

SUNFLOWER SEEDS

FOOD	PORTION	CALS	FAT	CARB	CHOL	SOD
dried	1 cup	821	71	27	0	4
dried	1 oz	162	14	5	0	1
dry roasted	1 cup	745	64	31	0	4
dry roasted	1 oz	165	14	7	0	1
dry roasted salted	1 cup	745	64	31	0	975
dry roasted salted	1 oz	165	14	7	0	195
oil roasted	1 cup	830	78	20	0	4
oil roasted salted	1 cup	830	78	20	0	804
oil roasted salted	1 oz	175	16	4	0	201
toasted	1 cup	826	76	28	0	4
toasted	1 oz	176	16	6	0	1
toasted & salted	1 cup	826	76	28	0	817
toasted & salted	1 oz	176	16	6	0	204
Fisher						
Oil Roasted	1 oz	170	15	6	0	170
Salted In Shell Shelled	1 oz	160	14	6	0	100
Salted In Shell Unshelled	1 oz	170	15	6	0	110
Frito Lay						
Seeds	1 oz	160	14	6	0	265
Planters						
Kernels	1 pkg (1.7 oz)	290	25	9	0	260
Kernels	1 pkg (2 oz)	340	29	11	0	310
Kernels Barbecue	1 pkg (1.7 oz)	290	25	10	0	180
Kernels Honey Roasted	1 pkg (1.7 oz)	280	22	15	0	105
Kernels Salted	1 oz	170	14	4	0	140
Munch'N Go Singles Dry Roasted	1 pkg	120	11	4	0	70
Nuts Dry Roasted	¼ cup (1.1 oz)	190	17	6	0	230
Original With Shell Dry Roasted	¾ cup	160	15	5	0	35
Stone-Buhr						
Seeds Raw	4 tsp (1 oz)	170	14	6	0	10

TANGERINE

FOOD	PORTION	CALS	FAT	CARB	CHOL	SOD
fresh	1	37	tr	9	0	1

TANGERINE JUICE

FOOD	PORTION	CALS	FAT	CARB	CHOL	SOD
After The Fall						
Juice	1 can (12 oz)	170	0	40	0	35

FOOD	PORTION	CALS	FAT	CARB	CHOL	SOD
Fresh Samantha						
Fresh Juice	1 cup (8 oz)	106	1	24	0	0
TEA/HERBAL TEA						
brewed tea	6 oz	2	0	tr	0	5
instant unsweetened as prep w/ water	8 oz	2	0	tr	0	8
Bigelow						
Almond Orange	5 fl oz	tr	tr	tr	0	tr
Apple Orchard	5 fl oz	5	tr	1	0	tr
Apple Spice	5 fl oz	tr	tr	tr	0	1
Chamomile	5 fl oz	tr	tr	—	0	2
Chamomile Mint	5 fl oz	tr	tr	tr	0	1
Chinese Fortune	5 fl oz	1	tr	tr	0	tr
Cinnamon Orange	5 fl oz	tr	tr	tr	0	tr
Cinnamon Stick	5 fl oz	1	tr	tr	0	tr
Constant Comment	5 fl oz	1	tr	tr	0	tr
Darjeeling Blend	5 fl oz	1	tr	tr	0	tr
Earl Gray	5 fl oz	1	tr	tr	0	tr
Early Riser	5 fl oz	3	tr	1	0	tr
English Teatime	5 fl oz	1	tr	tr	0	tr
Feeling Free	5 fl oz	1	tr	tr	0	1
Fruit & Almond	5 fl oz	1	tr	tr	0	tr
Hibiscus & Rose Hips	5 fl oz	1	tr	tr	0	1
I Love Lemon	5 fl oz	1	tr	tr	0	tr
Lemon & C	5 fl oz	tr	tr	tr	0	tr
Lemon Lift	5 fl oz	1	tr	tr	0	tr
Looking Good	5 fl oz	1	tr	1	0	1
Mint Blend	5 fl oz	tr	tr	tr	0	3
Mint Medley	5 fl oz	1	tr	tr	0	3
Orange & C	5 fl oz	tr	tr	tr	0	tr
Orange & Spice	5 fl oz	1	tr	tr	0	1
Orange Pekoe	5 fl oz	1	tr	tr	0	tr
Peppermint	5 fl oz	tr	tr	tr	0	2
Peppermint Stick	5 fl oz	1	tr	tr	0	1
Plantation Mint	5 fl oz	1	tr	tr	0	1
Raspberry Royale	5 fl oz	1	tr	tr	0	tr
Roasted Grains & Carob	5 fl oz	3	tr	1	0	1
Spearmint	5 fl oz	tr	tr	tr	0	tr
Sweet Dreams	5 fl oz	1	tr	tr	0	1
Take-A-Break	5 fl oz	3	tr	1	0	1
Celestial Seasonings						
Almond Sunset	8 fl oz	3	tr	1	0	2

FOOD	PORTION	CALS	FAT	CARB	CHOL	SOD
Celestial Seasonings (CONT.)						
Bengal Spice	8 fl oz	5	tr	tr	0	3
Caffeine Free	8 fl oz	2	tr	1	0	5
Chamomile	8 fl oz	2	tr	1	0	1
Cinnamon Apple Spice	8 fl oz	<3	tr	tr	0	1
Cinnamon Rose	8 fl oz	<4	tr	1	0	1
Cinnamon Vienna	8 fl oz	2	tr	1	0	1
Country Peach Spice	8 fl oz	3	tr	1	0	1
Cranberry Cove	8 fl oz	2	tr	1	0	1
Earl Grey Extraordinary	8 fl oz	3	tr	1	0	tr
Emperor's Choice	8 fl oz	4	tr	1	0	2
English Breakfast Classic	8 fl oz	3	tr	tr	0	tr
Ginseng Plus	8 fl oz	3	tr	1	0	4
Grandma's Tummy Mint	8 fl oz	2	tr	tr	0	7
Lemon	8 fl oz	7	tr	1	0	1
Lemon Mist	8 fl oz	3	tr	tr	0	3
Lemon Zinger	8 fl oz	4	tr	1	0	1
Mama Bear's Cold Care	8 fl oz	6	tr	tr	0	2
Mandarin Orange Spice	8 fl oz	5	tr	1	0	2
Mellow Mint	8 fl oz	2	tr	tr	0	5
Mint	8 fl oz	4	tr	tr	0	1
Mint Magic	8 fl oz	1	tr	tr	0	13
Morning Thunder	8 fl oz	3	tr	tr	0	1
Naturally Decaffeinated	8 fl oz	10	1	tr	0	1
Orange Spice	8 fl oz	7	tr	1	0	1
Orange Spice Decaf	8 fl oz	7	tr	1	0	1
Orange Zinger	8 fl oz	6	tr	1	0	1
Organically Grown	8 fl oz	12	tr	1	0	1
Peppermint	8 fl oz	2	tr	1	0	9
Raspberry	8 fl oz	7	tr	1	0	1
Raspberry Patch	8 fl oz	4	tr	1	0	1
Red Zinger	8 fl oz	4	tr	1	0	2
Roastaroma	8 fl oz	10	tr	2	0	3
Sleepytime	8 fl oz	4	tr	1	0	2
Spearmint	8 fl oz	5	1	tr	0	6
Strawberry Fields	8 fl oz	4	tr	1	0	1
Sunburst C	8 fl oz	3	tr	1	0	6
Tropical Escape	8 fl oz	1	tr	tr	0	7

FOOD	PORTION	CALS	FAT	CARB	CHOL	SOD
Celestial Seasonings (CONT.)						
Wild Forest Blackberry	8 fl oz	2	tr	1	0	1
Lipton						
English Blend as prep	1 cup	0	0	0	0	0
Family Size Bags Decaf as prep	1 qt	0	0	0	0	0
Family Size Bags as prep	1 qt	0	0	0	0	0
Instant as prep	1 serv	0	0	0	0	0
Instant Decaf as prep	1 serv	0	0	0	0	0
Instant Lemon as prep	1 serv	0	0	0	0	0
Special Blends Amaretto as prep	1 cup	0	0	0	0	0
Special Blends Blackberry as prep	1 cup	0	0	0	0	0
Special Blends Cinnamon as prep	1 cup	0	0	0	0	0
Special Blends Earl Grey as prep	1 cup	0	0	0	0	0
Special Blends English Breakfast as prep	1 cup	0	0	0	0	0
Special Blends Honey & Cinnamon as prep	1 cup	0	0	0	0	0
Special Blends Honey & Lemon as ep	1 cup	0	0	0	0	0
Special Blends Honey & Orange as prep	1 cup	0	0	0	0	0
Special Blends Mint as prep	1 cup	0	0	0	0	0
Special Blends Orange & Spice as prep	1 cup	0	0	0	0	0
Special Blends Peach as prep	1 cup	0	0	0	0	0
Special Blends Raspberry	1 cup	0	0	0	0	0
Tea Bag Almond Pleasure as prep	1 cup	0	0	tr	0	0
Tea Bag Cinnamon Apple as prep	1 cup	0	0	0	0	0

FOOD	PORTION	CALS	FAT	CARB	CHOL	SOD
Lipton (CONT.)						
Tea Bag Cinnamon Spice as prep	1 cup	0	0	tr	0	0
Tea Bag Country Cranberry as prep	1 cup	0	0	0	0	0
Tea Bag Decaf as prep	1 cup	0	0	0	0	0
Tea Bag Gentle Orange as prep	1 cup	0	0	tr	0	0
Tea Bag Ginger Twist as prep	1 cup	0	0	0	0	0
Tea Bag Golden Honey & Lemon as prep	1 cup	0	0	tr	0	0
Tea Bag Green Tea as prep	1 cup	0	0	0	0	0
Tea Bag Lemon Mint Refresher as prep	1 cup	0	0	0	0	0
Tea Bag Lemon Smoother as prep	1 cup	0	0	0	0	0
Tea Bag Moonlight Mint as prep	1 cup	0	0	0	0	0
Tea Bag Mountain Berry	1 cup	0	0	tr	0	0
Tea Bag Orange Refresher as prep	1 cup	0	0	tr	0	0
Tea Bag Peppermint as prep	1 cup	0	0	0	0	0
Tea Bag Quietly Chamomile as prep	1 cup	0	0	tr	0	0
Tea Bag Wildflower & Honey as prep	1 cup	0	0	tr	0	0
Tea Bag as prep	1 cup	0	0	0	0	0
Natural Touch						
Kaffree	8 fl oz	0	0	0	0	<1
Nestea						
Tea Bag as prep	6 oz	0	0	0	0	0
TOFU YOGURT						
Stir Fruity						
Black Cherry	6 oz	141	2	25	—	51
Blueberry	6 oz	140	1	26	—	43
Lemon Chiffon	6 oz	152	3	26	—	43
Mixed Berry	6 oz	149	2	26	—	34
Orange	6 oz	143	2	26	—	51

FOOD	PORTION	CALS	FAT	CARB	CHOL	SOD
Stir Fruity (CONT.)						
Peach	6 oz	160	3	27	—	34
Pina Colada	6 oz	162	3	28	—	43
Raspberry	6 oz	155	2	29	—	34
Spiced Apple	6 oz	167	2	31	—	43
Strawberry	6 oz	140	2	25	—	51
Tropical Fruit	6 oz	170	2	32	—	43

TOMATO
fresh red	1 (4.5 oz)	26	tr	6	0	11

TOMATO JUICE
Campbell						
Juice	6 oz	40	0	8	0	540
Mott's						
Beefamato	8 fl oz	80	0	20	0	780
Clamato	8 fl oz	100	0	24	0	720
Muir Glen						
Organic	8 oz	40	0	7	0	550

VEGETABLE JUICE
Odwalla						
Vegetable Cocktail	8 fl oz	70	0	18	0	290
V8						
No Salt Added	6 fl oz	35	0	8	0	45
Original	6 fl oz	35	0	8	0	560
Spicy Hot	6 fl oz	35	0	8	0	650

WATERMELON
fresh cut up	1 cup	50	1	11	0	3
seeds dried	1 oz	158	13	4	0	28
wedge	1/16	152	2	35	0	10

WHIPPED TOPPINGS
cream pressurized	1 tbsp (3 g)	8	tr	tr	2	4
nondairy pressurized	1 tbsp (4 g)	11	1	1	0	2
Cool Whip						
Extra Creamy	1 tbsp	13	1	1	tr	3
Lite	1 tbsp	9	1	1	tr	3
Non Dairy	1 tbsp	11	1	1	tr	1
Kraft						
Real Cream	2 tbsp (0.4 oz)	20	2	1	5	0
Whipped Topping	2 tbsp (0.4 oz)	20	2	1	0	0
La Creme						
Topping	1 tbsp	16	1	1	tr	5
Reddiwip						
Lite	2 tbsp (8 g)	15	1	2	0	5

FOOD	PORTION	CALS	FAT	CARB	CHOL	SOD
Reddiwip (CONT.)						
Non-Dairy	2 tbsp (8 g)	20	2	2	0	5
Real Whipped Heavy Cream	2 tbsp (8 g)	30	3	tr	10	0
Real Whipped Light Cream	2 tbsp (8 g)	20	2	tr	<5	0
WINE						
madeira	3.5 oz	169	0	10	—	—
port	3.5 oz	156	0	11	—	4
red	3½ oz	74	0	2	0	6
rosé	3½ oz	73	0	2	0	5
sherry	2 oz	84	0	5	0	—
sweet dessert	2 oz	90	0	7	0	5
vermouth dry	3½ oz	105	0	1	0	—
vermouth sweet	3½ oz	167	0	12	0	—
white	3½ oz	70	0	1	0	5
Boone's						
Country Kwencher	1 fl oz	24	0	3	0	1
Delicious Apple	1 fl oz	21	0	3	0	1
Sangria	1 fl oz	22	0	3	0	1
Snow Creek Berry	1 fl oz	18	0	3	0	tr
Strawberry Hill	1 fl oz	22	0	3	0	1
Sun Peak Peach	1 fl oz	18	0	3	0	1
Wild Island	1 fl oz	18	0	3	0	tr
Carlo Rossi						
Blush	1 fl oz	21	0	1	0	1
Burgundy	1 fl oz	22	0	tr	0	1
Chablis	1 fl oz	21	0	tr	0	1
Paisano	1 fl oz	23	0	tr	0	3
Red Sangria	1 fl oz	24	0	2	0	1
Rhine	1 fl oz	21	0	1	0	1
Vin Rosé	1 fl oz	21	0	1	0	1
White Grenache	1 fl oz	20	0	1	0	tr
Fairbanks						
Cream Sherry	1 fl oz	42	0	4	0	1
Port	1 fl oz	44	0	4	0	1
Sherry	1 fl oz	34	0	2	0	2
White Port	1 fl oz	44	0	4	0	1
Gallo						
Blush Chablis	1 fl oz	22	0	1	0	2
Burgundy	1 fl oz	22	0	tr	0	1
Cabernet Sauvignon	1 fl oz	22	0	0	0	tr
Chablis Blanc	1 fl oz	20	0	tr	0	1

FOOD	PORTION	CALS	FAT	CARB	CHOL	SOD
Gallo (CONT.)						
Chardonnay	1 fl oz	23	0	tr	0	1
Classic Burgundy	1 fl oz	21	0	0	0	tr
French Colombard	1 fl oz	21	0	1	0	1
Hearty Burgundy	1 fl oz	22	0	tr	0	1
Johannisbery Riesling '88	1 fl oz	20	0	1	0	1
Pink Chablis	1 fl oz	20	0	1	0	1
Red Rosé	1 fl oz	23	0	1	0	2
Rhine	1 fl oz	22	0	1	0	1
Sauvignon Blanc '90	1 fl oz	20	0	tr	0	1
White Grenache '92	1 fl oz	20	0	1	0	1
White Grenache New Vintage	1 fl oz	20	0	1	0	tr
White Zinfandel '91	1 fl oz	18	0	tr	0	1
White Zinfandel New Vintage	1 fl oz	18	0	tr	0	1
Zinfandel '87	1 fl oz	23	0	0	0	tr
Ka-Me						
Chinese Cooking	2 tbsp (1 fl oz)	20	0	5	0	170
Sheffield Cellars						
Sherry	1 fl oz	44	0	4	0	1
Tawny Port	1 fl oz	45	0	4	0	2
Vermouth Extra Dry	1 fl oz	28	0	1	0	1
Vermouth Sweet	1 fl oz	43	0	4	0	2
Very Dry Sherry	1 fl oz	32	0	1	0	2

WINE COOLERS

FOOD	PORTION	CALS	FAT	CARB	CHOL	SOD
Bartles & Jaymes						
Berry	12 fl oz	210	0	32	0	0
Margarita	12 fl oz	260	0	46	0	40
Original	12 fl oz	190	0	28	0	10
Peach	12 fl oz	210	0	33	0	5
Pina Colada	12 fl oz	280	0	49	0	0
Planter's Punch	12 fl oz	230	0	36	0	0
Strawberry	12 fl oz	210	0	32	0	0
Strawberry Daiquiri	12 fl oz	230	0	37	0	5
Tropical	12 fl oz	230	0	38	0	0

YOGURT

FOOD	PORTION	CALS	FAT	CARB	CHOL	SOD
coffee lowfat	8 oz	194	3	31	11	149
fruit lowfat	4 oz	113	1	21	5	60
fruit lowfat	8 oz	225	3	42	10	121
plain	8 oz	139	7	11	29	105
plain lowfat	8 oz	144	4	16	14	159

FOOD	PORTION	CALS	FAT	CARB	CHOL	SOD
plain no fat	8 oz	127	tr	17	4	174
vanilla lowfat	8 oz	194	3	31	11	149
Breyers						
1% Fat Black Cherry	8 oz	260	3	50	15	110
1% Fat Blueberry	8 oz	250	3	48	15	110
1% Fat Mixed Berry	8 oz	250	3	48	15	110
1% Fat Peach	8 oz	250	3	48	15	110
1% Fat Pineapple	8 oz	250	3	49	15	110
1% Fat Red Raspberry	8 oz	250	3	48	15	110
1% Fat Strawberry	8 oz	250	3	47	15	110
1% Fat Strawberry Banana	8 oz	250	3	50	15	115
1.5% Fat Coffee	8 oz	220	3	38	20	135
1.5% Fat Plain	8 oz	130	3	15	20	150
1.5% Fat Vanilla	8 oz	220	3	38	20	135
Cabot						
All Flavors	8 oz	220	3	42	10	120
Plain	8 oz	140	4	16	14	160
Colombo						
Banana Strawberry	8 oz	210	4	39	15	110
Black Cherry	8 oz	200	4	36	15	115
Blueberry	8 oz	200	4	36	15	110
Fat Free Apples 'n Spice	8 oz	190	0	39	5	130
Fat Free Apricot	8 oz	190	0	39	5	130
Fat Free Banana Strawberry	8 oz	200	0	42	5	130
Fat Free Blueberry	8 oz	190	0	39	5	130
Fat Free Cappuccino	8 oz	180	0	35	<5	140
Fat Free Cherry	8 oz	190	0	39	5	135
Fat Free Cranberry Strawberry	8 oz	200	0	43	5	120
Fat Free French Roast	8 oz	180	0	35	<5	140
Fat Free Fruit Cocktail	8 oz	190	0	39	5	130
Fat Free Lemon	8 oz	170	0	33	<5	150
Fat Free Peach	8 oz	190	0	33	5	130
Fat Free Plain	8 oz	110	0	16	5	170
Fat Free Raspberry	8 oz	190	0	39	5	130
Fat Free Strawberry	8 oz	190	0	39	5	130
Fat Free Strawberry Pineapple Orange	8 oz	190	0	38	5	125
Fat Free Vanilla	8 oz	170	0	32	5	150
French Vanilla	8 oz	180	4	29	20	130
Light 100 Blueberry	8 oz	100	0	16	<5	140

FOOD	PORTION	CALS	FAT	CARB	CHOL	SOD
Colombo (CONT.)						
Light 100 Cherry Vanilla	8 oz	100	0	16	<5	120
Light 100 Coffee & Cream	8 oz	100	0	16	<5	120
Light 100 Creamy Vanilla	8 oz	100	0	16	<5	130
Light 100 Fruit Medley	8 oz	100	0	16	<5	120
Light 100 Juicy Peach	8 oz	100	0	16	<5	140
Light 100 Lemon Creme	8 oz	100	0	16	<5	160
Light 100 Mandarin Orange	8 oz	100	0	16	<5	120
Light 100 Mixed Berries	8 oz	100	0	16	<5	110
Light 100 Raspberry	8 oz	100	0	16	<5	140
Light 100 Strawberry	8 oz	100	0	16	<5	140
Peach Melba	8 oz	200	4	36	15	115
Plain	8 oz	120	5	12	20	150
Raspberry	8 oz	200	4	36	15	115
Strawberry	8 oz	200	4	36	15	110
Dannon						
Blended Nonfat Blueberry	6 oz	160	0	33	<5	105
Blended Nonfat French Vanilla	6 oz	160	0	31	<5	100
Blended Nonfat Lemon Chiffon	6 oz	150	0	31	<5	110
Blended Nonfat Peach	6 oz	150	0	31	<5	100
Blended Nonfat Raspberry	6 oz	160	0	32	<5	100
Blended Nonfat Strawberry	6 oz	150	0	31	<5	105
Blended Nonfat Strawberry Banana	6 oz	150	0	31	<5	105
Danimals Lowfat Blueberry	4.4 oz	140	2	25	10	90
Danimals Lowfat Grape Lemonade	4.4 oz	130	2	23	10	80
Danimals Lowfat Lemon Ice	4.4 oz	130	2	22	10	90
Danimals Lowfat Orange Banana	4.4 oz	140	2	24	10	80
Danimals Lowfat Strawberry	4.4 oz	140	2	24	10	85

FOOD	PORTION	CALS	FAT	CARB	CHOL	SOD
Dannon (CONT.)						
Danimals Lowfat Tropical Punch	4.4 oz	140	2	25	10	85
Danimals Lowfat Vanilla	4.4 oz	140	2	24	10	80
Danimals Lowfat Wild Raspberry	4.4 oz	130	2	22	10	80
Fruit On The Bottom Lowfat Apple Cinnamon	8 oz	240	3	46	15	140
Fruit On The Bottom Lowfat Blueberry	8 oz	240	3	46	15	140
Fruit On The Bottom Lowfat Boysenberry	8 oz	240	3	45	15	150
Fruit On The Bottom Lowfat Cherry	8 oz	240	3	46	15	135
Fruit On The Bottom Lowfat Mixed Berries	8 oz	240	3	45	15	150
Fruit On The Bottom Lowfat Orange	8 oz	240	3	45	15	135
Fruit On The Bottom Lowfat Peach	8 oz	240	3	45	15	140
Fruit On The Bottom Lowfat Pear	8 oz	240	3	45	15	135
Fruit On The Bottom Lowfat Raspberry	8 oz	240	3	45	15	150
Fruit On The Bottom Lowfat Strawberry	8 oz	240	3	46	15	135
Fruit On The Bottom Lowfat Strawberry Banana	8 oz	240	3	43	15	140
Light Nonfat Banana Cream Pie	4.4 oz	60	0	9	0	80
Light Nonfat Cherry Vanilla	1 cup (3.5 oz)	110	0	19	<5	160
Light Nonfat Lemon Chiffon	4.4 oz	60	0	9	0	75
Light Nonfat Peach	4.4 oz	50	0	8	0	70
Light Nonfat Strawberry	1 cup (3.5 oz)	110	0	19	<5	160
Light Nonfat Strawberry	4.4 oz	50	0	8	0	70

FOOD	PORTION	CALS	FAT	CARB	CHOL	SOD
Dannon (CONT.)						
Light Nonfat Vanilla	1 cup (3.5 oz)	110	0	18	<5	160
Light 'N Crunchy Nonfat Cappuccino w/ Chocolate	1 pkg	150	0	27	<5	170
Light 'N Crunchy Nonfat Caramel Apple Crunch	1 pkg	150	0	28	<5	180
Light 'N Crunchy Nonfat Lemon Chiffon w/ Blueberry	1 pkg	140	0	26	<5	150
Light 'N Crunchy Nonfat Raspberry w/ Granola	1 pkg	150	0	17	<5	135
Light 'N Crunchy Nonfat Vanilla w/ Chocolate	1 pkg	150	0	26	<5	170
Light Nonfat Banana Cream Pie	8 oz	100	0	17	<5	150
Light Nonfat Blueberry	8 oz	100	0	20	<5	140
Light Nonfat Creme Caramel	8 oz	100	0	15	<5	125
Light Nonfat Lemon	8 oz	100	0	17	<5	140
Light Nonfat Peach	8 oz	100	0	18	<5	140
Light Nonfat Raspberry	8 oz	100	0	18	<5	150
Light Nonfat Strawberry	8 oz	100	0	18	<5	140
Light Nonfat Strawberry Banana	8 oz	100	0	18	<5	140
Light Nonfat Tropical Fruit	8 oz	100	0	19	<5	140
Light Nonfat Vanilla	8 oz	100	0	17	<5	140
Lowfat Coffee	1 cup (8.7 oz)	230	4	39	20	170
Lowfat Coffee	8 oz	210	3	36	15	160
Lowfat Cranberry Raspberry	8 oz	210	3	36	15	160
Lowfat Lemon	1 cup (8.7 oz)	230	4	39	20	170
Lowfat Lemon	8 oz	210	3	36	15	160
Lowfat Plain	1 cup (8.7 oz)	150	4	17	20	170
Lowfat Plain	8 oz	140	4	16	20	150
Lowfat Vanilla	1 cup (8.7 oz)	230	4	39	20	170
Lowfat Vanilla	8 oz	210	3	36	15	160

FOOD	PORTION	CALS	FAT	CARB	CHOL	SOD
Dannon (CONT.)						
Minipack Blended Nonfat Blueberry	4.4 oz	120	0	23	<5	105
Minipack Blended Nonfat Cherry	4.4 oz	110	0	23	<5	75
Minipack Blended Nonfat Peach	4.4 oz	110	0	23	<5	75
Minipack Blended Nonfat Raspberry	4.4 oz	120	0	23	<5	75
Minipack Blended Nonfat Strawberry	4.4 oz	110	0	23	<5	105
Minipack Blended Nonfat Strawberry Banana	4.4 oz	110	2	23	<5	105
Nonfat Light Cherry Vanilla	8 oz	100	0	17	<5	140
Nonfat Light Strawberry Fruit Cup	8 oz	100	0	18	<5	140
Nonfat Plain	1 cup (8.7 oz)	120	0	17	0	170
Nonfat Plain	8 oz	110	0	16	5	150
Sprinkl'ins Banana	4.1 oz	140	3	24	10	85
Sprinkl'ins Cherry Vanilla	4.1 oz	140	3	24	10	95
Sprinkl'ins Crazy Crunch Cherry w/ Honey Grahams	4.4 oz	170	3	30	10	150
Sprinkl'ins Crazy Crunch Grape w/ Chocolate Grahams	4.4 oz	160	3	29	10	170
Sprinkl'ins Crazy Crunch Vanilla w/ Chocolate Grahams	4.4 oz	160	3	29	10	140
Sprinkl'ins Crazy Crunch Vanilla w/ Honey Grahams	4.4 oz	170	3	30	10	135
Sprinkl'ins Strawberry	4.1 oz	140	3	24	10	95
Sprinkl'ins Strawberry Banana	4.1 oz	140	3	24	10	95
Tropifruta Nonfat Banana	6 oz	150	0	31	5	105
Tropifruta Nonfat Guava	6 oz	150	0	29	5	105

FOOD	PORTION	CALS	FAT	CARB	CHOL	SOD
Dannon (CONT.)						
Tropifruta Nonfat Mango	6 oz	150	0	31	5	105
Tropifruta Nonfat Papaya Pineapple	6 oz	150	0	30	5	105
Tropifruta Nonfat Pina Colada	6 oz	150	0	30	5	105
Tropifruta Nonfat Strawberry	6 oz	150	0	31	5	105
Tropifruta Nonfat Strawberry Banana	6 oz	150	0	31	5	105
Tropifruta Nonfat Strawberry Kiwi	6 oz	150	0	30	5	105
With Fruit Toppings Banana Creme Strawberry	6 oz	170	3	30	10	90
With Fruit Toppings Bavarian Creme Raspberry	6 oz	170	3	31	10	115
With Fruit Toppings Cheesecake Cherry	6 oz	170	3	31	10	90
With Fruit Toppings Cheesecake Strawberry	6 oz	170	3	30	10	90
With Fruit Toppings Vanilla Peach & Apricot	6 oz	170	3	30	10	90
With Fruit Toppings Vanilla Strawberry	6 oz	170	3	30	10	90
Friendship						
Coffee	8 oz	210	3	30	20	170
Fruit Crunch Blueberry	6 oz	190	4	32	10	125
Fruit Crunch Peach	6 oz	190	5	31	10	125
Fruit Crunch Strawberry	6 oz	190	5	31	10	125
Fruit Crunch Strawberry Banana	6 oz	190	4	32	10	125
Plain	8 oz	150	3	13	20	190
Hood						
Fat Free Blueberry	1 (8 oz)	190	0	40	5	120
Fat Free Cherry	1 (8 oz)	190	0	40	5	120
Fat Free Peach	1 (8 oz)	190	0	40	5	120
Fat Free Plain	1 (8 oz)	130	0	18	5	190
Fat Free Raspberry	1 (8 oz)	190	0	40	5	120

FOOD	PORTION	CALS	FAT	CARB	CHOL	SOD
Hood (CONT.)						
Fat Free Strawberry	1 (8 oz)	190	0	39	5	120
Fat Free Strawberry Banana	1 (8 oz)	190	0	40	5	120
Fat Free Swiss Blueberry	1 (8 oz)	210	0	45	5	110
Fat Free Swiss Lemon	1 (8 oz)	210	0	45	5	110
Fat Free Swiss Raspberry	1 (8 oz)	210	0	45	5	110
Fat Free Swiss Strawberry	1 (8 oz)	210	0	45	5	105
Fat Free Swiss Strawberry Banana	1 (8 oz)	210	0	45	5	110
Fat Free Swiss Vanilla	1 (8 oz)	210	0	45	5	105
Fat Free Vanilla	1 (8 oz)	190	0	34	5	170
Knudsen						
1.5% Fat Creamy Lemon	8 oz	220	3	38	20	140
70 Calories Black Cherry	6 oz	70	0	12	<5	85
70 Calories Blueberry	6 oz	70	0	12	5	80
70 Calories Lemon	6 oz	70	0	11	5	100
70 Calories Peach	6 oz	70	0	11	5	80
70 Calories Pineapple	6 oz	70	0	11	5	80
70 Calories Red Raspberry	6 oz	70	0	11	5	75
70 Calories Strawberry	6 oz	70	0	11	5	85
70 Calories Strawberry Banana	6 oz	70	0	11	5	85
70 Calories Strawberry Fruit Basket	6 oz	70	0	11	5	90
70 Calories Vanilla	6 oz	70	0	11	5	80
Free Lemon	6 oz	160	0	33	5	105
Free Mixed Berry	6 oz	170	0	33	5	105
Free Peach	6 oz	170	0	33	5	105
Free Red Raspberry	6 oz	170	0	31	5	105
Free Strawberry	6 oz	170	0	32	5	105
Free Vanilla	6 oz	170	0	32	5	100
La Yogurt						
French Style Banana	6 oz	180	3	32	10	100
French Style Blueberry	6 oz	180	3	32	10	100
French Style Cherry	6 oz	180	3	32	10	100

FOOD	PORTION	CALS	FAT	CARB	CHOL	SOD
La Yogurt (CONT.)						
French Style Cherry Vanilla	6 oz	190	3	35	10	95
French Style Guava	6 oz	180	3	32	10	100
French Style Key Lime	6 oz	180	3	32	10	100
French Style Mango	6 oz	180	3	32	10	100
French Style Mixed Berry	6 oz	180	3	32	10	100
French Style Nonfat Blueberry	6 oz	70	0	12	5	90
French Style Nonfat Cherry	6 oz	75	0	13	5	90
French Style Nonfat Raspberry	6 oz	70	0	12	5	90
French Style Nonfat Strawberry	6 oz	70	0	12	5	90
French Style Nonfat Strawberry Banana	6 oz	70	0	12	5	90
French Style Peach	6 oz	180	3	32	10	100
French Style Pina Colada	6 oz	180	3	32	10	100
French Style Raspberry	6 oz	180	3	32	10	100
French Style Strawberry	6 oz	180	3	32	10	100
French Style Strawberry Banana	6 oz	180	3	32	10	100
French Style Strawberry Fruit Cup	6 oz	180	3	32	10	100
French Style Tropical Orange	6 oz	180	4	32	10	100
French Style Vanilla	6 oz	170	3	28	15	110
Latin Style Banana	6 oz	190	3	34	10	105
Latin Style Guava	6 oz	190	3	34	10	105
Latin Style Mango	6 oz	190	3	34	10	105
Latin Style Papaya	6 oz	190	3	34	10	105
Latin Style Passion Fruit	6 oz	190	3	34	10	105
Latin Style Strawberry Kiwi	6 oz	180	3	32	10	100
Light N'Lively						
Free Blueberry	6 oz	190	0	38	5	105
Free Lemon	6 oz	170	0	35	5	105

FOOD	PORTION	CALS	FAT	CARB	CHOL	SOD
Light N'Lively (CONT.)						
Free Mixed Berry	6 oz	170	0	34	5	105
Free Peach	6 oz	170	0	35	5	105
Free Red Raspberry	6 oz	180	0	36	5	105
Free Strawberry	6 oz	180	0	36	5	105
Free Strawberry Fruit Cup	6 oz	170	0	35	5	105
Free Vanilla	6 oz	160	0	32	5	105
Free 50 Calories Blueberry	4.4 oz	50	0	8	<5	60
Free 50 Calories Peach	4.4 oz	50	0	9	<5	60
Free 50 Calories Red Raspberry	4.4 oz	50	0	8	<5	60
Free 50 Calories Strawberry	4.4 oz	50	0	8	<5	60
Free 50 Calories Strawberry Banana	4.4 oz	50	0	8	<5	60
Free 50 Calories Strawberry Fruit Cup	4.4 oz	50	0	8	<5	60
Free 70 Calories Black Cherry	6 oz	70	0	11	<5	85
Free 70 Calories Blueberry	6 oz	70	0	11	<5	80
Free 70 Calories Lemon	6 oz	70	0	12	<5	120
Free 70 Calories Peach	6 oz	70	0	12	<5	80
Free 70 Calories Red Raspberry	6 oz	70	0	11	<5	80
Free 70 Calories Strawberry	6 oz	70	0	11	<5	85
Free 70 Calories Strawberry Banana	6 oz	70	0	11	<5	85
Free 70 Calories Strawberry Fruit Cup	6 oz	70	0	11	<5	80
Kidpack Banana Berry	4.4 oz	130	1	24	10	65
Kidpack Berry Blue	4.4 oz	150	1	30	10	65
Kidpack Cherry	4.4 oz	140	1	27	10	65
Kidpack Grape	4.4 oz	130	1	24	10	65
Kidpack Outrageous Orange	4.4 oz	150	1	29	10	65

FOOD	PORTION	CALS	FAT	CARB	CHOL	SOD
Light N'Lively (CONT.)						
Kidpack Tropical Punch	4.4 oz	140	1	28	10	65
Kidpack Wild Berry	4.4 oz	140	1	27	10	65
Kidpack Wild Strawberry	4.4 oz	140	1	28	10	65
Multipack Blueberry	4.4 oz	140	1	27	10	65
Multipack Peach	4.4 oz	140	1	27	10	65
Multipack Pineapple	4.4 oz	140	1	27	5	60
Multipack Red Raspberry	4.4 oz	130	1	24	10	65
Multipack Strawberry	4.4 oz	140	1	26	10	65
Multipack Strawberry Banana	4.4 oz	140	1	28	10	60
Multipack Strawberry Fruit Cup	4.4 oz	140	1	27	10	60
Lite Line						
Swiss Style Cherry Vanilla	1 cup	240	2	45	—	150
Swiss Style Peach	1 cup	230	2	42	—	150
Swiss Style Plain	1 cup	140	2	16	—	150
Swiss Style Strawberry	1 cup	240	2	46	—	150
Meadow Gold						
Plain	1 cup	160	5	16	—	160
Sundae Style Raspberry	1 cup	250	4	42	—	160
Mountain High						
Blueberry	1 cup	220	6	31	—	140
Plain	1 cup	200	9	16	—	140
Weight Watchers						
Ultimate 90 Blueberries 'n Creme	1 cup	90	0	14	5	140
Ultimate 90 Cappuccino	1 cup	90	0	14	5	140
Ultimate 90 Cherries Jubilee	1 cup	90	0	14	5	140
Ultimate 90 Cranberry Raspberry	1 cup	90	0	14	5	140
Ultimate 90 Lemon Chiffon	1 cup	90	0	14	5	140
Ultimate 90 Peach	1 cup	90	0	14	5	140
Ultimate 90 Plain	1 cup	90	0	14	5	150

FOOD	PORTION	CALS	FAT	CARB	CHOL	SOD
Weight Watchers (CONT.)						
Ultimate 90 Raspberries 'n Creme	1 cup	90	0	14	5	140
Ultimate 90 Strawberry	1 cup	90	0	14	5	140
Ultimate 90 Strawberry Banana	1 cup	90	0	14	5	140
Ultimate 90 Vanilla	1 cup	90	0	14	5	140
Yoplait						
Custard Style Banana	6 oz	190	4	32	20	95
Custard Style Blueberry	6 oz	190	4	32	20	95
Custard Style Cherry	6 oz	180	4	30	20	95
Custard Style Lemon	6 oz	190	4	32	20	95
Custard Style Mixed Berry	6 oz	180	4	30	20	95
Custard Style Raspberry	6 oz	190	4	32	20	95
Custard Style Strawberry	4 oz	130	3	21	15	60
Custard Style Strawberry	6 oz	190	4	32	20	95
Custard Style Strawberry Banana	6 oz	190	4	32	20	95
Custard Style Strawvberry Banana	4 oz	130	3	21	15	60
Custard Style Vanilla	4 oz	130	3	20	15	70
Custard Style Vanilla	6 oz	180	4	30	20	110
Fat Free Blueberry	6 oz	150	0	31	5	95
Fat Free Cherry	6 oz	150	0	31	5	95
Fat Free Mixed Berry	6 oz	150	0	31	5	95
Fat Free Peach	6 oz	150	0	31	5	95
Fat Free Raspberry	6 oz	150	0	31	5	95
Fat Free Strawberry	6 oz	150	0	31	5	95
Fat Free Strawberry Banana	6 oz	150	0	31	5	95
Light Blueberry	4 oz	60	0	9	<5	75
Light Blueberry	6 oz	80	0	13	<5	80
Light Cherry	4 oz	60	0	9	<5	75
Light Cherry	6 oz	80	0	13	<5	80
Light Peach	4 oz	60	0	9	<5	75
Light Peach	6 oz	80	0	13	<5	80

FOOD	PORTION	CALS	FAT	CARB	CHOL	SOD
Yoplait (CONT.)						
Light Raspberry	4 oz	60	0	9	<5	75
Light Raspberry	6 oz	80	0	13	<5	80
Light Strawberry	4 oz	60	0	9	<5	75
Light Strawberry	6 oz	80	0	13	<5	110
Light Strawberry Banana	4 oz	60	0	9	<5	75
Light Strawberry Banana	6 oz	80	0	13	<5	80
Nonfat Plain	8 oz	120	0	18	5	160
Nonfat Vanilla	8 oz	180	0	35	5	140
Original Apple	6 oz	190	3	32	10	110
Original Blueberry	4 oz	120	2	21	5	75
Original Blueberry	6 oz	190	3	32	10	110
Original Boysenberry	6 oz	190	3	32	10	110
Original Cherry	6 oz	190	3	32	10	110
Original Lemon	6 oz	190	3	32	10	110
Original Mixed Berry	6 oz	190	3	32	10	110
Original Orange	6 oz	190	3	32	10	110
Original Peach	4 oz	120	2	21	5	75
Original Peach	6 oz	190	3	32	10	110
Original Pina Colada	6 oz	190	3	32	10	110
Original Pineapple	6 oz	190	3	32	10	110
Original Plain	6 oz	130	3	15	15	140
Original Raspberry	4 oz	120	2	21	5	75
Original Raspberry	6 oz	190	3	32	10	110
Original Strawberry	4 oz	120	2	21	5	75
Original Strawberry	6 oz	190	3	32	10	110
Original Strawberry Banana	6 oz	190	3	32	10	110
Original Strawberry Rhubarb	6 oz	190	3	32	10	110
Original Vanilla	6 oz	180	3	29	10	120

YOGURT FROZEN

FOOD	PORTION	CALS	FAT	CARB	CHOL	SOD
chocolate soft serve	½ cup (4 fl oz)	115	4	18	3	71
vanilla soft serve	½ cup (4 fl oz)	114	4	17	2	63
Bee-Lite						
Chocolate	4 oz	100	tr	23	0	55
Vanilla	4 oz	110	tr	23	0	55
Ben & Jerry's						
Cherry Garcia	½ cup (3.7 oz)	170	3	31	10	70
Chocolate Fudge Brownie	½ cup (3.7 oz)	190	4	35	10	130

FOOD	PORTION	CALS	FAT	CARB	CHOL	SOD
Ben & Jerry's (CONT.)						
Coffee Almond Fudge	½ cup (3.7 oz)	200	7	30	15	85
English Toffee Crunch	½ cup (3.7 oz)	190	6	32	10	110
No Fat Cappuccino	½ cup (3.3 oz)	140	0	32	0	85
Pop Cherry Garcia	1 (3.8 oz)	290	16	34	20	60
Borden						
Strawberry	½ cup	100	2	19	—	50
Bresler's						
All Flavors	5 oz	145	2	28	9	—
All Flavors Lite	5 oz	135	0	30	0	—
Breyers						
Chocolate	½ cup (2.7 oz)	150	4	25	15	45
Light Fat Free Apple Pie A La Mode	1 cup (8 oz)	130	0	23	5	110
Light Fat Free Black Cherry Jubilee	1 cup (8 oz)	130	0	23	5	110
Light Fat Free Blueberries n' Cream	1 cup (8 oz)	130	0	23	5	110
Light Fat Free Cherry Chocolate	1 cup (8 oz)	130	0	23	5	110
Light Fat Free Classic Strawberry	1 cup (8 oz)	130	0	23	5	110
Light Fat Free Key Lime Pie	1 cup (8 oz)	130	0	23	5	110
Light Fat Free Lemon Chiffon	1 cup (8 oz)	130	0	23	5	110
Light Fat Free Peaches n'Cream	1 cup (8 oz)	130	0	23	5	110
Light Fat Free Strawberry Cheesecake	1 cup (8 oz)	130	0	23	5	110
Red Raspberry	½ cup (2.7 oz)	140	4	24	15	40
Strawberry Banana	½ cup (2.7 oz)	140	3	24	15	40
Vanilla	½ cup (2.7 oz)	140	4	24	15	45
Dannon						
Coco-Nut Fudge	½ cup (3 oz)	160	3	28	15	70
Light Cappuccino	½ cup (2.8 oz)	80	0	19	0	70
Light Cherry Vanilla Swirl	½ cup (2.8 oz)	90	0	21	0	65
Light Chocolate	½ cup (2.7 oz)	80	0	21	0	60
Light Lemon Chiffon	½ cup (2.8 oz)	90	0	22	0	65
Light Nonfat Cappuccino	8 oz	100	0	17	<5	140

FOOD	PORTION	CALS	FAT	CARB	CHOL	SOD
Dannon (CONT.)						
Light Peach Raspberry Melba	½ cup (2.8 oz)	90	0	21	0	65
Light Strawberry Cheesecake	½ cup (2.8 oz)	90	0	22	0	60
Light Vanilla	½ cup (2.8 oz)	80	0	21	0	65
Light'N Crunchy Banana Cream Pie	½ cup (2.8 oz)	110	1	24	0	65
Light'N Crunchy Mocha Chocolate Chunk	½ cup (2.8 oz)	110	1	26	0	60
Light'N Crunchy Peanut Chocolate Crunch	½ cup (2.8 oz)	110	0	29	0	65
Light'N Crunchy Triple Chocolate	½ cup (2.8 oz)	110	0	28	0	60
Light'N Crunchy Vanilla Blueberry Swirl	½ cup (2.8 oz)	110	1	26	0	65
Pure Indulgence Cherry Chocolate Cherry	½ cup (3 oz)	150	3	26	15	85
Pure Indulgence Chunky Chocolate Nut	½ cup (3 oz)	150	3	25	0	65
Pure Indulgence Cookies'n Cream	½ cup (3 oz)	150	3	24	0	105
Pure Indulgence Crunchy Espresso	½ cup (3 oz)	150	3	26	15	85
Pure Indulgence Heath Toffee Crunch	½ cup (3 oz)	150	3	25	5	105
Pure Indulgence Vanilla Raspberry Truffle	½ cup (3 oz)	150	3	25	15	70
Desserve						
All Flavors	4 oz	70	0	16	0	57
Dutch Chocolate	4 oz	80	0	18	0	62
Edy's						
Banana Strawberry	3 oz	80	1	15	5	40
Blueberry	3 oz	80	1	15	5	40
Cherry	3 oz	80	1	15	5	40
Chocolate	3 oz	80	1	15	5	40
Chocolate Chip	3 oz	100	1	20	5	55

FOOD	PORTION	CALS	FAT	CARB	CHOL	SOD
Edy's (CONT.)						
Citrus Heights	3 oz	80	1	15	5	40
Cookies'N'Cream	3 oz	100	1	20	5	55
Marble Fudge	3 oz	100	1	20	5	55
Perfectly Peach	3 oz	80	1	15	5	40
Raspberry	3 oz	80	1	15	5	40
Raspberry Vanilla Swirl	3 oz	80	1	15	5	45
Strawberry	3 oz	80	1	15	5	40
Vanilla	3 oz	80	1	15	5	50
Elan						
Blueberry	4 oz	130	3	23	11	50
Caramel Almond Praline	4 oz	150	4	26	10	90
Chocolate	4 oz	130	3	24	10	50
Chocolate Almond	4 oz	160	6	22	10	50
Coffee	4 oz	130	3	22	11	60
Coffee Decaffeinated	4 oz	130	3	22	11	60
Peach	4 oz	130	3	23	10	50
Rum Raisin	4 oz	135	3	25	12	55
Strawberry	4 oz	125	3	22	10	50
Vanilla	4 oz	130	3	22	11	60
Fi-Bar						
Chocolate	1	190	7	26	0	160
Strawberry	1	190	7	26	0	150
Vanilla	1	190	7	26	0	150
Friendly's						
Apple Bettie	½ cup (2.6 oz)	140	3	25	10	75
Fabulous Fudge Swirl	½ cup (2.6 oz)	140	3	23	10	80
Fudge Berry Swirl	½ cup (2.6 oz)	150	4	25	10	75
Lowfat Perfectly Peach	½ cup (2.6 oz)	110	2	21	10	55
Lowfat Purely Chocolate	½ cup (2.6 oz)	120	3	20	10	65
Lowfat Raspberry Delight	½ cup (2.6 oz)	120	3	21	10	60
Lowfat Simply Vanilla	½ cup (2.6 oz)	120	3	19	10	70
Lowfat Strawberry Patch	½ cup (2.6 oz)	110	2	20	10	55
Mint Chocolate Chip	½ cup (2.6 oz)	130	4	21	10	65
Strawberry Cheesecake Blast	½ cup (2.6 oz)	140	4	22	15	75
Toffee Almond Crunch	½ cup (2.6 oz)	160	5	24	15	85

FOOD	PORTION	CALS	FAT	CARB	CHOL	SOD
Good Humor						
Creamsicle Raspberry	1 (2.8 oz)	100	1	23	<5	20
Frista Cup	1 (6.2 oz)	220	5	38	15	125
Haagen-Dazs						
Banana Nut Blast	½ cup (3.5 oz)	220	8	29	40	65
Bars Cherry Chocolate Fudge	1 (2.6 oz)	240	13	26	35	45
Bars Peach	1 (2.5 oz)	90	1	19	15	20
Bars Pina Colada	1 (2.5 oz)	100	1	19	15	45
Bars Raspberry & Vanilla	1 (2.5 oz)	90	1	19	15	25
Bars Strawberry Daiquiri	1 (2.5 oz)	90	1	18	15	20
Chocolate	½ cup (3.4 oz)	160	3	26	30	60
Coffee	½ cup (3.4 oz)	160	3	26	45	55
Fat Free Bar Raspberry & Vanilla	1 (2.5 oz)	90	0	20	0	15
Fat Free Cherry Vanilla	½ cup (3.3 oz)	140	0	30	<5	40
Fat Free Chocolate	½ cup (3.3 oz)	140	0	28	<5	45
Fat Free Coffee	½ cup (3.3 oz)	140	0	29	<5	45
Fat Free Vanilla	½ cup (3.3 oz)	140	0	29	<5	45
Fat Free Vanilla Fudge	½ cup (3.3 oz)	160	0	34	<5	100
Orange Tango	½ cup (3.5 oz)	130	1	26	20	25
Pina Colada	½ cup (3.4 oz)	130	2	26	25	25
Raspberry Rendezvous	½ cup (3.5 oz)	130	2	26	20	25
Strawberry Cheesecake Craze	½ cup (3.6 oz)	220	8	31	65	140
Strawberry Duet	½ cup (3.4 oz)	130	2	26	25	25
Vanilla	½ cup (3.4 oz)	160	3	26	45	55
Hood						
Bavarian Truffle & Twist	½ cup (2.6 oz)	150	4	26	10	60
Coffee Toffee Chunk Sundae	½ cup (2.6 oz)	150	4	27	10	75
Combo Bars	1 (2.2 oz)	90	2	17	5	40
Cookies & Cream	½ cup (2.6 oz)	140	4	25	10	75
Grandma's Raisin Oatmeal Cookie Dough	½ cup (2.6 oz)	140	3	25	10	75
Mixed Berry Swirl	½ cup (2.6 oz)	120	2	24	10	45
Natural Strawberry	½ cup (2.6 oz)	110	3	21	10	50
Natural Strawberry Banana	½ cup (2.6 oz)	110	3	21	10	50

FOOD	PORTION	CALS	FAT	CARB	CHOL	SOD
Hood (CONT.)						
Natural Vanilla	½ cup (2.6 oz)	120	3	22	10	55
Nonfat Caramel & Brownie Sundae	½ cup (2.6 oz)	120	0	28	0	60
Nonfat Chocolate Marshmallow	½ cup (2.6 oz)	110	0	26	0	60
Nonfat Double Raspberry	½ cup (2.6 oz)	120	0	26	0	55
Nonfat Mocha Fudge	½ cup (2.6 oz)	120	0	27	0	55
Nonfat Olde Fashioned Vanilla	½ cup (2.6 oz)	110	0	24	0	55
Nonfat Peach Cobbler A La Mode	½ cup (2.6 oz)	110	0	25	0	50
Nonfat Strawberry	½ cup (2.6 oz)	100	0	23	0	50
Nonfat Vanilla Fudge	½ cup (2.6 oz)	120	0	27	0	55
Raspberry Swirl	½ cup (2.6 oz)	130	2	25	10	55
Sundae Cups Chocolate & Strawberry	1 (2.2 oz)	110	2	24	5	55
Vanilla Chocolate Strawberry	½ cup (2.6 oz)	120	3	22	10	50
Vanilla Swiss Almond Sundae	½ cup (2.6 oz)	150	4	25	10	60
Just 10						
All Flavors	1 oz	10	0	3	0	14
Kissed With Honey						
Chocolate	3.5 oz	100	3	18	9	50
Nonfat Chocolate	3.5 oz	85	tr	19	0	60
Nonfat Vanilla	3.5 oz	85	tr	18	0	50
Vanilla	3.5 oz	100	3	17	9	75
Meadow Gold						
Strawberry	½ cup	100	2	19	—	50
Sealtest						
Chocolate	½ cup (2.7 oz)	120	2	24	5	45
Mocha Fudge	½ cup (2.6 oz)	130	2	25	10	45
Vanilla	½ cup (2.6 oz)	120	2	24	10	45
Tofutti						
Better Than Yogurt Chocolate Fudge	4 fl oz	120	2	25	0	98
Better Than Yogurt Coffee Mashmallow Swirl	4 fl oz	100	1	24	0	77
Better Than Yogurt Passion Island Fruit	4 fl oz	100	1	21	0	100

FOOD	PORTION	CALS	FAT	CARB	CHOL	SOD
Tofutti (CONT.)						
Better Than Yogurt Peach Mango	4 fl oz	100	1	23	0	102
Better Than Yogurt Strawberry Banana	4 fl oz	100	1	23	0	92
Better Than Yogurt Vanilla Fudge	4 fl oz	120	2	24	0	90
Turkey Hill						
Chocolate Cherry Cordial	½ cup (2.6 oz)	130	3	22	10	60
Chocolate Chip Cookie Dough	½ cup (2.6 oz)	140	5	23	10	120
Death By Chocolate	½ cup (2.6 oz)	150	4	25	10	90
Nonfat Chocolate Cherry Cordial	½ cup (2.4 oz)	100	0	24	0	70
Nonfat Chocolate Marshmallow	½ cup (2.4 oz)	130	0	30	0	40
Nonfat Coffee Cappuccino	½ cup (2.4 oz)	110	0	23	0	60
Nonfat Mint Cookie 'N Cream	½ cup (2.4 oz)	110	0	24	0	80
Nonfat Neapolitan	½ cup (2.4 oz)	100	0	22	0	50
Nonfat Raspberry Chocolate Bliss	½ cup (2.4 oz)	110	0	25	0	100
Nonfat Southern Lemon Pie	½ cup (2.4 oz)	110	0	25	0	90
Nonfat Vanilla Fudge	½ cup (2.4 oz)	110	0	24	0	80
Peach Raspberry	½ cup (2.6 oz)	110	2	20	10	60
Strawberry	½ cup (2.6 oz)	110	2	20	10	60
Tin Roof Sundae	½ cup (2.6 oz)	140	5	21	10	100
Vanilla & Chocolate	½ cup (2.6 oz)	110	3	19	10	70
Vanilla Bean	½ cup (2.6 oz)	110	3	17	10	70